TOXICOLOGY IN RISK ASSESSMENT

TOXICOLOGY IN RISK ASSESSMENT

Edited by

Harry Salem and Eugene J. Olajos
U.S. Army Edgewood Chemical and Biological Center
Aberdeen Proving Ground, Maryland, USA

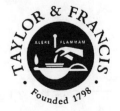

USA	Publishing Office:	Taylor & Francis 325 Chestnut Street Philadelphia, PA 19106 Tel: (215) 625–8900 Fax: (215) 625–2940
	Distribution Center:	Taylor & Francis 47 Runway Road, Suite G Levittown, PA 19057-4700 Tel: (215) 269-0400 Fax: (215) 269-0363
UK		Taylor & Francis Ltd. 11 New Fetter Lane London EC4P 4EE Tel: 44-171-583-9855 Fax: 44-171-842-2298

TOXICOLGY IN RISK ASSESSMENT

Copyright © 2000 Taylor & Francis. All rights reserved. Printed in the United States of America. Except as permitted under the United States Copyright Act of 1976, no part of this publication may be reproduced or distributed in any form or by any means, or stored in a database or retrieval system, without prior written permission of the publisher.

1 2 3 4 5 6 7 8 9 0

Printed by Sheridan Books, Ann Arbor, Michigan, 1999.
Cover Design by Claire O'Neill.

A CIP catalog record for this book is available from the British Library.
   The paper in this publication meets the requirements of the ANSI Standard Z39.48–1984 (Permanence of Paper). Library of Congress Cataloging-in-Publication data available from the publisher.

ISBN 1-56032-837-1 (case)

DEDICATION

This book is also dedicated to the memory of two cherished friends and colleagues: Leo G. Abood and George B. Koelle. Their contributions as consultants to the Department of Defense and to us personally over the years have been both inspiring and invaluable.

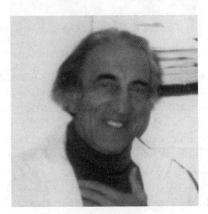

Leo G. Abood (1922–1998)

Leo G. Abood, renowned Professor of Pharmacology and Biochemistry at the School of Medicine and Dentistry at the University of Rochester, was a native of Erie, Pennsylvania, and a graduate of Ohio State University. He earned a doctorate in pharmacology at the University of Chicago. Prior to his appointment at the University of Rochester, Dr. Abood served as Professor of Neurophysiology and Biochemistry at the College of Medicine, University of Illinois, and Director of Research Labs at the Neuropsychiatric Institute at the University of Rochester. He became Professor of Biochemistry in 1965, Professor of Pharmacology in 1987, and Distinguished Professor of Neurosciences in 1987 at the University of Toledo. He retained all three of these positions until his death. At the University of Rochester he was one of the first faculty members involved in creating the Center for Brain Research. Through the center's work, Rochester became the second university in the country to grant a doctoral degree in neurosciences. Dr. Abood was the author of more than 200 research papers and served on many scientific committees and editorial boards. He served on the National Research Council and as a trustee on the Brain Research Foundation at the University of Chicago. Among the many national and international committees on which he served was the Life Sciences Advisory Committee at the U.S. Army Chemical Research and Development Center.

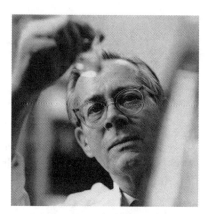

George B. Koelle (1919–1997)

George B. Koelle, distinguished professor of pharmacology at the University of Pennsylvania School of Medicine, lived in Swarthmore, Pennsylvania, for over 40 years. He was recognized as an international expert in neurophysiology and pharmacology. A native of Philadelphia, Dr. Koelle was a graduate of the Philadelphia College of Pharmacy and Science. He earned a doctorate degree in pharmacology at the University of Pennsylvania and a medical degree at Johns Hopkins University. During World War II, he served as an Army Lieutenant assigned to the Chemical Warfare Service at Edgewood Arsenal in Maryland. Dr. Koelle was named Distinguished Professor at the University of Pennsylvania School of Medicine, where he taught from 1952 through 1989. Throughout his career, he served as visiting professor and lecturer to many universities worldwide. Dr. Koelle was the author of more than 200 publications in journals and books. He was elected to the National Academy of Sciences in 1972. Among the many distinguished honors and awards he received were the John Jacob Able and the Torald Sollmann awards. He served on many editorial boards and was a member of many scientific societies. Among the many national and international committees on which he served was the Life Sciences Advisory Committee at the U.S. Army Chemical Research and Development Center.

DEDICATION

THE ZERO-TOLERANCE CONCEPT

George B. Koelle

Department of Pharmacology, Medical School, University of Pennsylvania, Philadelphia, Pennsylvania.

In a memorable scene from Samuel Butler's *The Way of All Flesh*, old George Pontifex drops and breaks a pint bottle of Jordan water that he has been saving for many years for his first grandson's christening. The quick-thinking butler averts an impending crisis (he has been blamed for having misplaced the hamper that Pontifex has tripped over) by snatching up a sponge, recovering half the treasured liquid from the floor, and filtering it through a bit of blotting paper. On reflection, the same purpose would have been served by the simpler expedient of turning an adjacent tap and drawing a fresh pint from the local English water supply. It has been calculated that the Jordan daily pours 6.5×10^6 tons of water into the Dead Sea [1]. Thus, when a single day's effluent has equilibrated with the remaining water of the world (which over the course of a few million years it undoubtedly would), estimated as 3.3×10^8 cu mi [2] or 1.5×10^{18} tons, a pint of water sampled from any source will contain 3.7×10^{12} molecules of Jordan water. To extend this concept still further, if a pint of water is poured into the sea and allowed to mix completely with all the water on the surface of the earth, over 5,000 molecules of the original sample will be present in any pint taken subsequently.

The general conclusion to be drawn from these calculations is that nothing is completely uncontaminated by anything else. Yet this conclusion is in conflict

Presented as a tribute to the late Dr. Koelle.
Reprinted from *Perspectives in Biology and Medicine*, Vol. 20, No. 4, Summer 1977, with permission. © 1977 by the University of Chicago. All rights reserved.

with both the implications and applications of certain items of federal legislation that have led to serious limitations in the production of foods and drugs. The best known and most controversial of these is the Delaney Amendment to the Food Additives Amendment of 1958, sec. 409 (c) (3) (A) of the Federal Food, Drug, and Cosmetic Act. Paraphrased, the amendment states simply that no additive found to induce cancer in any animal species following oral ingestion shall be deemed safe. On first consideration, this seems quite reasonable. However, as was brought out in extensive hearings before a subcommittee of the Committee on Appropriations of the House of Representatives in May 1974 [3], its interpretation and enforcement have followed lines that seem to have ignored both the well-established pharmacological principle of "threshold dose" (that below which no effect is detectable) and the remarkable degrees of improvement in the sensitivity and specificity of analytical methods that have now been developed. Thus, the enforcement agency has labeled as unsafe any compound that can be demonstrated to cause a higher incidence than in controls of any type of cancer in any species when added to the diet in any concentration for any period of time. By extrapolation from the test animals to human subjects, it has been estimated that the latter would have to consume up to 500 12-oz bottles of soft drink daily to achieve a carcinogenic dose of cyclamate. For oil of calamus, which has been used as a constituent of vermouth, the extrapolation is truly staggering; attainment of a carcinogenic level would require the daily consumption of 250 qt of vermouth, which in a standard ratio of 1 part to 9 parts of gin represents over 50,000 1.5-oz martinis. Yet despite such figures, these compounds and others have been proscribed as additives. In the former case, the consumer has the choice to weigh the great or small hazard of consuming an equivalent amount of sugar or of some other synthetic substitute of yet unproven carcinogenic potential against his desire for soft drinks; in both cases, the manufacturer may no longer include the condemned compound in his product.

No such simple solutions are afforded by a more recent proposal issued by the Food and Drug Administration in April 1976 [4]. This relates to the finding that when male rats were given chloroform in a dose of 90 or 180 mg per kilogram orally five times weekly for 78 weeks, significant numbers (8 and 24 percent, respectively) developed kidney epithelial tumors; at higher dose levels, mice developed hepatocellular carcinoma. Accordingly, it was recommended that chloroform be banned as an unsafe ingredient and any drug containing it be deemed misbranded and subject to withdrawal. As with other additives, producers of cough syrups and other products to which chloroform has been added as a flavoring agent will now have to find substitutes for this purpose. Much more serious is the problem this presents for the preparation of tablets of some digitalis glycosides. One of the major advances in the treatment of chronic congestive heart failure over the past few decades has been the replacement of crude extracts of digitalis leaf of variable potency by pure, consistent preparations of digitoxin, digoxin, and other glycosides. A critical step in the production of digitoxin and perhaps other glycosides involves the use of chloroform as a solvent. The final product may contain a nearly infinitesimal quantity of chloroform, which by the analytical techniques available a few years ago would have been undetectable. However, refinements in gas chromatography, mass spectrometry, and other methods have now reduced by several magnitudes the levels at which such substances can be identified and hence at which tablets or other dosage forms containing chloroform would be considered carcinogenic. Enforcement of this proposal, as in many other cases of "zero tolerance," will thus involve an extremely prolonged and costly program for the development of alternate means of extracting and purifying the glycosides and might entail for an unpredictable period the same uncertainty of the uniformity of the tablets as prevailed in the days of galenical preparations. Meanwhile, cardiac patients and everyone else will continue to consume every day similarly detectable amounts of chloroform, along with undetectable amounts of Jordan water, in their drinking water.

The solution to this dilemma is obvious. There should be no such thing as "zero tolerance" any more than there is "zero concentration" of a potentially toxic synthetic chemical or naturally occurring heavy metal in the environment. It is the task of the toxicologist to establish the minimal safe levels of such components and that of enforcement agencies to assure that scientifically determined, reasonable requirements are met.

REFERENCES

1. Encyclopaedia Britannica, 1966 ed., s.v. "Dead Sea."
2. Encyclopaedia Britannica, 1966 ed., s.v. "Ocean and Oceanography."
3. U.S. Congress, House, Agriculture-environmental, and consumer protection appropriations for 1975: hearings before a subcommittee of the committee on appropriations. 93d Cong., 2d sess., pt. 8, 1974.
4. Federal Register, 41:15026, 1976.

CONTENTS

Preface	xv
List of Contributors	xvii

1 A WINDOW OF OPPORTUNITY FOR TOXICOLOGY 1
John Doull

2 THE EVOLVING PRINCIPLES OF RISK ANALYSIS 7
Margaret M. MacDonell, Kirpal S. Sidhu, and Jasvinder S. Sidhu

**3 HOW TO COMMUNICATE RISK IN A LOW TRUST / HIGH
    CONCERN ENVIRONMENT** 33
Keith A. Fulton

**4 VALUES AND ETHICAL CHOICES THAT UNDERLIE
    TOXICOLOGIC AND RISK-ANALYSIS DECISIONS** 39
C. Richard Cothern

5 IMPROVING THE RISK-ASSESSMENT PROCESS 47
Leo G. Abood

**6 IMPROVING RISK CHARACTERIZATION AT THE
    U.S. ENVIRONMENTAL PROTECTION AGENCY** 51
Edward V. Ohanian

7 MULTIPLE FACTORS IN RISK ASSESSMENT 57
Leo G. Abood

**8 ENVIRONMENTAL FACTORS MODIFYING SENSITIVITY
    TO CHEMICALS** 65
Bernard Weiss

9 ANIMAL MODEL OF CHEMICAL SENSITIVITY
    INVOLVING CHOLINERGIC AGENTS   75
    *David H. Overstreet, Amir H. Rezvani, Ying Yang, Mani Hamedi,
    and David S. Janowsky*

10 APPLICATION OF CHEMICAL HORMESIS CONCEPT
   TO RISK ASSESSMENT: REPRODUCTIVE TOXICITY
   AS AN EXAMPLE   95
   Edward J. Calabrese and Linda A. Baldwin

11 TRENDS IN TOXICOLOGY MODELING FOR
   RISK ASSESSMENT   107
   Shayne C. Gad

12 OVERVIEW OF ENVIRONMENTAL DECISION-SUPPORT
   SOFTWARE   147
   T. M. Sullivan, P. D. Moskowitz, and M. Gitten

13 APPLICATION OF RISK-ASSESSMENT TECHNIQUES TO
   MILITARY DEPLOYMENTS: OPERATION DESERT STORM,
   OPERATION JOINT ENDEAVOR, OPERATION
   DESERT FOCUS   163
   Jack M. Heller

14 APPLICATION OF RISK-ASSESSMENT TECHNIQUES
   TO MILITARY SCENARIOS: MULTIPATHWAY EXPOSURE
   ASSESSMENT FOR CHEMICAL AGENT INCINERATORS   183
   Hsieng-Ye Chang

15 A DRINKING WATER ADVISORY: CONSUMER
   ACCEPTABILITY ADVICE AND HEALTH EFFECTS
   ANALYSIS ON METHYL TERTIARY-BUTYL ETHER   191
   *Charles O. Abernathy, Julie T. Du, Amal Mahfouz,
   Maria M. Gomez-Taylor, and Joyce M. Donohue*

16 ARSENIC: MOVING TOWARD A REGULATION   211
   *Charles O. Abernathy, Irene S. Dooley, James Taft,
   and Jennifer Orme-Zavaleta*

17 THE EVOLUTION OF HEALTH-RISK ASSESSMENT:
   TRICHLOROETHYLENE AS A CASE STUDY   223
   Elizabeth A. Maull and Harvey J. Clewell

18 HISTORY OF METHYLENE CHLORIDE IN CONSUMER
   PRODUCTS: TRACING SCIENTIFIC KNOWLEDGE,
   REGULATIONS, AND PERCEPTIONS   235
   Donna M. Riley and Paul S. Fischbeck

19 RISK ASSESSMENT AND RISK MANAGEMENT IN
REGULATORY DECISION MAKING: RECOMMENDATIONS
OF THE COMMISSION ON RISK ASSESSMENT AND
RISK MANAGEMENT 261
*Gail Charnley and the Members of the Commission
on Risk Assessment and Risk Management*

20 RISK ASSESSMENT AND RISK MANAGEMENT:
PATHWAYS TOWARD PROCESS ENHANCEMENT 269
Eugene J. Olajos and Harry Salem

Index 311

PREFACE

Toxicology is an integral part of the risk-assessment process. In this book, investigators from the scientific and regulatory communities describe recent technical developments in risk assessment embracing toxicology and its allied sciences, risk quantification and characterization, risk management, and risk communication. Case studies pertaining to current issues involving chemical and environmental risks include military and industrial scenarios. Chapters describing values and ethical choices underlying toxicologic decisions, economic and legal implications of regulations, understanding the risk, and recommendations of the Commission on Risk Assessment and Risk Management also are included.

This book evolved from a symposium sponsored by the editors entitled *Toxicology in Risk Assessment*. Because of the success of the symposium, and the interest generated, invitations were extended to the participants who made a significant contribution and impact at the symposium to contribute chapters tailored to meet the framework and objectives of this book. Additionally, we solicited a mix of "heavy hitters" in the fields of toxicology and risk assessment, as well as "up-and-coming stars" recommended from prestigious academic institutions and organizations that have been prominent in these politically charged and socially relevant fields.

We thank all of those who helped to make this publication possible and hope that this will enhance the careers of the up-and-coming contributors and help them gain prominence in the field.

We also want to thank our families and hope that this will inspire them to seek knowledge and apply it to help make this a better and safer world to live in. We dedicate this book to you, Flo, Jerry, Amy, Joel, Marshall, and Abby-Rose, and Elizabeth, Stephanie, Andrew, and Allison.

Harry Salem
Eugene J. Olajos

LIST OF CONTRIBUTORS

CHARLES O. ABERNATHY
U.S. Environmental Protection Agency
Washington, DC

LEO G. ABOOD*
Department of Pharmacology and Physiology
University of Rochester Medical Center
Rochester, New York

LINDA A. BALDWIN
Environmental Health Sciences Department
School of Public Health
University of Massachusetts
Amherst, Massachusetts

EDWARD J. CALABRESE
Environmental Health Sciences Department
School of Public Health
University of Massachusetts
Amherst, Massachusetts

*Deceased.

HSIENG-YE CHANG
U.S. Army Center for Health Promotion and Preventive Medicine
Aberdeen Proving Ground, Maryland

GAIL CHARNLEY
HealthRisk Strategies
Washington, DC

HARVEY J. CLEWELL
KS Crump Group, Inc.
ICF Consulting
Ruston, Louisiana

C. RICHARD COTHERN
University of Maryland (University College)
College Park, Maryland; and
The George Washington University
Washington, DC

JOYCE M. DONOHUE
U.S. Environmental Protection Agency
Washington, DC

IRENE S. DOOLEY
U.S. Environmental Protection Agency
Washington, DC

JOHN DOULL
University of Kansas Medical Center
Kansas City, Kansas

JULIE T. DU
U.S. Environmental Protection Agency
Washington, DC

PAUL S. FISCHBECK
Department of Engineering and
  Public Policy and Department of
  Social and Decision Sciences
Carnegie Mellon University
Pittsburgh, Pennsylvania

KEITH A. FULTON
Fulton Communication
Houston, Texas

SHAYNE C. GAD
Gad Consulting Services
Raleigh, North Carolina

M. GITTEN
Environmental Project Control
Maynard, Massachusetts

MARIA M. GOMEZ-TAYLOR
U.S. Environmental Protection Agency
Washington, DC

MANI HAMEDI
Skipper Bowles Center for Alcohol
  Studies and Department of
  Psychiatry
University of North Carolina School
  of Medicine
Chapel Hill, North Carolina

JACK M. HELLER
U.S. Army Center for Health
  Promotion and Preventive Medicine
Aberdeen Proving Ground, Maryland

DAVID S. JANOWSKY
Skipper Bowles Center for Alcohol
  Studies and Department of
  Psychiatry
University of North Carolina School
  of Medicine
Chapel Hill, North Carolina

MARGARET M. MACDONELL
Environmental Assessment Division
Argonne National Laboratory
Argonne, Illinois

AMAL MAHFOUZ
U.S. Environmental Protection Agency
Washington, DC

ELIZABETH A. MAULL
Institute for Environment, Safety and
  Occupational Health Risk Analysis
Brooks Air Force Base, Texas

P. D. MOSKOWITZ
Brookhaven National Laboratory
Upton, New York

EDWARD V. OHANIAN
Office of Water
U.S. Environmental Protection Agency
Washington, DC

EUGENE J. OLAJOS
U.S. Army Chemical and Biological
  Center
Aberdeen Proving Ground, Maryland

JENNIFER ORME-ZAVALETA
U.S. Environmental Protection Agency
Research Triangle Park,
North Carolina

DAVID H. OVERSTREET
Skipper Bowles Center for Alcohol
  Studies and Department of
  Psychiatry
University of North Carolina School
  of Medicine
Chapel Hill, North Carolina

AMIR H. REZVANI
Skipper Bowles Center for Alcohol
  Studies and Department of
  Psychiatry
University of North Carolina School
  of Medicine
Chapel Hill, North Carolina

DONNA M. RILEY
Department of Engineering and
  Public Policy
Carnegie Mellon University
Pittsburgh, Pennsylvania

HARRY SALEM
U.S. Army Chemical and Biological
  Center
Aberdeen Proving Ground, Maryland

JASVINDER S. SIDHU
Internal Medicine Residency Program
University Hospitals of Cleveland
Case Western Reserve University
Cleveland, Ohio

KIRPAL S. SIDHU
Division of Environmental
  Epidemiology
Michigan Department of Community
  Health
Lansing, Michigan

T. M. SULLIVAN
Brookhaven National Laboratory
Upton, New York

JAMES TAFT
U.S. Environmental Protection Agency
Washington, DC

BERNARD WEISS
Department of Environmental
  Medicine
University of Rochester School of
  Medicine and Dentistry
Rochester, New York

YING YANG
Skipper Bowles Center for Alcohol
  Studies and Department of
  Psychiatry
University of North Carolina School
  of Medicine
Chapel Hill, North Carolina

CHAPTER
ONE

A WINDOW OF OPPORTUNITY FOR TOXICOLOGY

John Doull

University of Kansas Medical Center, Kansas City, Kansas

When Congress passed the Clean Air Act Amendments of 1990, they included two provisions that were intended to improve our ability to assess and manage risks to human health resulting from exposure to chemicals. The first of these was to request that the National Academy of Sciences "review the methods used to assess the carcinogenic risk associated with exposure to hazardous air pollutants and to recommend improvements." Congress also requested that the Academy "look at other chronic effects and non-cancer effects for which safe thresholds might not exist." When the National Research Council (NRC) accepted this charge they narrowed the mandate to include only toxicologic risk, and the resulting report, which was called *Science and Judgment in Risk Assessment* (NRC, 1994), was focused on topics such as uncertainty and variation, the use of defaults and iteration, exposure and mixtures, sensitive populations and comparative risk, bright lines, peer review, and other toxicologic issues. The committee concluded that the current Environmental Protection Agency (EPA) health risk assessment methodology needs to establish more clearly both its scientific and policy bases but was unable to reach a consensus on whether "plausible conservatism" or "best science" should be the primary basis for risk assessment. Position statements were developed for both arguments, and these can be found in Appendices N1 and N2 of the report. This report is available in both hard copy and paper back editions from the National Academy Press in Washington, DC.

The second provision of the 1990 Clean Air Act was to create a risk assessment and management commission to "investigate the policy implications and appropriate use of risk assessment and risk management in regulatory programs to prevent cancer and other chronic human health effects from exposure to hazardous substances." The commission has 10 members, three members appointed by the president, six by congressional leaders, and one by the president of the National Academy of Sciences (NAS). Dean Gil Omen was the chair and Dr. Gail Charnley was the executive director. The first meeting was held in May 1994 and for the subsequent 2 years, public hearings were held both in Washington and across the country to obtain local input from the various stakeholders. A draft report was issued in June of 1996 and a final report was released in 1997 (Presidential Commission, 1996, 1997).

The major focus of the final report is on risk management, but there are three recommendations in the risk-assessment or toxicity area that are discussed in this chapter. First and most important, the use of a common metric is recommended for extrapolating both cancer and noncancer effects, and it is suggested that the margin-of-exposure approach, as defined by EPA (1996) in the new cancer guidelines, be considered as one option. Second, although Congress was urged to repeal the Delaney Amendment, regulators also were urged to recognize that agents that cause cancer in rodents by mechanisms or doses that are not relevant to humans should not be regulated as carcinogens. Third, it was recommended that the risks of chemicals in mixtures should be added if their mechanisms are similar or unknown but that for chemicals having different mechanisms, the risks should not be added but considered to be independent. The report is available on the Internet at www.riskworld.com.

Several major developments in risk assessment have occurred since the release of the draft report. Congress has partially repealed Delaney, and the EPA has released new cancer guidelines that no longer mandate the linear multistage extrapolation for carcinogens but encourage other options based on mode of action or mechanistic data (U.S. EPA, 1996). There is growing acceptance and enthusiasm for the common metric recommendation and a willingness on the part of risk managers to consider thresholds as the primary approach for regulating mixtures. These are exciting changes and they provide a window of opportunity for toxicologists to reestablish their role in risk assessment, which they have pretty well lost by default to the modelers. It seems that the best way for toxicologists to get back in the risk-assessment ball game is to go back to the basic principles of their discipline and to reaffirm the importance of the basic principles of toxicology in every aspect of risk assessment.

The first and most important principle of toxicology is that of dose response, which says that there is a toxic dose and a safe dose for every chemical. Just as there are no inherently "safe" chemicals (safe under all conditions of exposure), there are also no chemicals that cannot be used safely simply by reducing the exposure. Toxicologists recognize that thresholds would not exist for any toxic effect if they were dealing with a population of infinite size and eternal life. However, in the real world, in which the total population is less than 6 billion and the average life span is less than 100 years, practical or pragmatic thresholds exist for all chemicals including mutagens and carcinogens. The recognition that all toxic effects are dose-related also means that the use of labels such as *toxic chemical, liver poison, irritant, carcinogen,* and *teratogen* has little descriptive or regulatory value unless information is included about the exposure and species. As toxicologists, our message should be that labels are not bright lines providing yes or no answers to safety questions, but it is necessary to emphasize that exposure includes both dose and time. When Paracelsus made his dose–response observations over 500 years ago, it is interesting that he did not specifically include time as a variable. Time was formally included in the dose–response equation in 1921 by Flury (Deichman et al., 1986) and of course by Haber in 1924. Druckrey and Kupfmuller (1948) subsequently proved that time is a response variable, and Rozman et al. (1996) showed that it is necessary to include both calendar and kinetic time scales in the toxicity equation. Recognizing that toxicity is determined by both dose and time, we can define thresholds in terms of reversibility of effect or the ability of the organisms to repair to adapt to the toxic insult.

The second major principle of toxicology is that the results of studies in a test species, if properly interpreted, can be used to make predictions in a target species. Although this is the basis for using animal tests to predict effects in man, it is recognized that because animal studies do not always give the right answers, the only absolutely reliable basis for predicting adverse effects in man is to base the prediction on human studies. Most toxicologists recognize that good epidemiology takes precedence over toxicologic data as a basis for making predictions for humans and attempt to utilize fully all of the available epidemiologic and toxicologic evidence in a weight-of-evidence risk assessment.

Predictions in toxicology traditionally are based on three kinds of information: first something about the chemical and its adverse effects needs to be known; second the dose and exposure conditions must be known; and third information on the test species is necessary. These same criteria—adverse effect, exposure scenario, and susceptibility of the exposed population—are also the criteria for setting exposure standards in humans, and the ideal situation for establishing the correct exposure standard is to have data with the right chemical, the right dose range and exposure situation, and the right population. Anything less than this requires extrapolation. In principle it is only if we do not have adequate human data on the test chemical or on a surrogate with similar chemical and biological properties that we use studies in a surrogate species, but in practice, animal studies almost always are used to validate the human studies or as a part of the predictive process.

The first step in what used to be called *hazard evaluation* in toxicology is to identify all of the adverse effects that can be produced by either acute or chronic exposure to the chemical, and the second step is to establish dose–response relationships for each of these adverse effects. Studies that do not provide this dose–response information, such as single dose or maximum tolerated dose studies, are safety studies rather than true toxicologic studies. Ideally, these studies also would provide information on the effects of administration by different routes and with different rates and durations of exposure, and information on other species. This information, together with data on the chemical and physical properties of the agent, kinetic data in various species, gene-tox studies, teratology, reproduction, and other types of end-organ damage plus whatever mechanistic information is available, constitutes the toxicology data base for the test chemical. The next step is to determine whether this information is relevant for the target species and the exposure scenario and of sufficient quality to support a risk assessment or regulation. If the information is reliable and relevant and there is a threshold or no-effect level, the final step is to simply divide the no-observed-adverse-effect level by an appropriate safety factor to establish the exposure limit. The advantage of the threshold approach is that it is easy to understand and that it has been used effectively for over 50 years by the Food and Drug Administration, the NAS/NRC Committee on Toxicology, the American Conference of Governmental Industrial Hygienists Threshold Limit Values committee, and many other groups both in this country and in Europe to establish exposure limits for chemicals in our environment. One problem with this approach is that it can be used only with threshold effects. Perhaps the greatest problem with this approach is that we have not incorporated the newer science and methods into the process. The traditional acute, subchronic, and two-species chronic and some special studies still are being used as the basis for predictions, and it is time to utilize the exciting new developments in kinetics, receptor theory, and other mechanistic areas that are part of today's toxicology. It is also necessary to explore new approaches like the benchmark dose, which does not require a threshold to evaluate dose–response data. Most important, we need one approach that works for both carcinogens and noncarcinogens. The dichotomy that exists between the ways we handle noncancer and cancer risks makes it almost impossible to achieve rational and effective regulation of these risks, and the recommendation of the Presidential Risk Assessment and Management Commission is an effort to provide a level playing field for extrapolating the results of animal studies for cancer and noncancer effects. It should be pointed out that this is not an original recommendation. In 1995 Purchase and Auton made a similar suggestion in a paper on thresholds in chemical carcinogenesis, and many other toxicologists have been saying this for years. The future of toxicology may well be determined in large part by how the issues of extrapolating cancer and noncancer effects and the use of thresholds versus models are resolved.

Another recommendation from the commission report deals with the risk assessment of mixtures, which is a very old problem in toxicology but one that needs new answers. Part of the problem here is that when the number of possible combinations with even a small number of mixture components is calculated, the testing requirements scare us away, and thus we do not have many actual data. Recently, however, several groups have shown that exposure to combinations of pollutants at doses less than the no-observed-adverse-effect levels does not produce additive toxicity and in fact is often antagonistic. Previous recommendations of NRC/NAS committee reports, as in *Complex Mixtures* (1995) and in *Science and Judgment* (1994), as well as those of the EPA and other groups have been to add risks in all cases unless there is evidence of synergism or antagonism. The Presidential Commission on Risk Assessment and Risk Management is recommending that risks should not be added for chemicals acting through different mechanisms; they should be added only if the mechanisms are identical or unknown. This recommendation would permit regulators to use a threshold of regulation approach similar to that proposed by the FDA for trivial risks and would markedly improve our ability to clean up waste dump sites. Scientifically this is a good recommendation, and hopefully it eventually will become another principle of toxicology.

In conclusion, a short sermon accountability: Some time ago, Neal and I (1995) published a commentary in which we argue that toxicologists need to accept more responsibility for their part in the risk-assessment process. One way that we could do this would be to indicate how the toxicologic risks that we are predicting fit into the broader public-health picture. For example, when we pointed out the risk of cancer resulting from the chlorination of our drinking water, we should also have pointed out the microbial risk of nonchlorination. This might have avoided a cholera epidemic in Peru that occurred in part because they stopped chlorinating the water to prevent cancer. Similarly, at a recent NAS conference on the use of alternatives for halon and other chlorofluorocarbons, there was concern about increased fire deaths resulting from our concerns about the possible adverse effects of halon in fire extinguishers on the ozone layer. As toxicologists, we tend to focus our attention on the trees of individual adverse effects rather than on the forest of public health. In the final analysis, our mandate is not to use what-if toxicology to produce media headlines and stimulate funding for the investigation of phantom risks but to improve public health, and that is or should be the most basic principle of toxicology and all science.

REFERENCES

Deichman, W. B., Henschler, D., Holmstadt, B., and Keil, G. 1986. What is there that is not a poison: A study of the Third Defense by Paracelsus, *Toxicology* 58:207–213.
Druckrey, V. H., and Kupfmuller, K. 1948. Quantative Analyse der Krebsentstehung. *Z. Naturforschg.* 36:254–266.
Haber, F. 1924. Zur Geschichte des Gakrieges. In *Fuenf Vortraege aus den Jahren 1920–1923*, pp. 74–94. Berlin: Julius Springer.
National Research Council. 1995. *Complex mixtures: Methods for in-vivo toxicity testing.* Washington, DC: National Academy Press.
National Research Council. 1994. *Science and judgment in risk assessment.* Washington, DC: National Academy Press.
Neal, R. R., and Doull, J. 1995. Commentary: The discipline of toxicology, *Fundam. Appl. Toxicol.* 24:151–153.
Presidential Commission on Risk Assessment and Risk Management. 1997. *Final report*, Washington, DC: Author.
Presidential Commission on Risk Assessment and Risk Management. 1996. *Risk assessment and risk management in regulatory decision-making.* Draft Report for Public Review and Comment. Washington, DC: Author.

Purchase, I. F. H., and Auton, T. R. 1995. Thresholds in chemical carcinogenesis. *R. Toxicol. Pharmacol.* 22:199–205.

Rozman, K. K., Kerecsen, L., Viluksela, M. K., Osterle, D., Deml, E., Viluksela, M., Stahl, B. B., Greim, H., and Doull, J. 1996. A toxicologists view of cancer risk assessment. *Drug Metab Rev* 28:29–52.

U.S. Environmental Protection Agency. 1996. *Proposed guidelines for carcinogen risk assessment.* EPA/600P-92/003C. Washington, DC: Office of Research and Development.

CHAPTER
TWO

THE EVOLVING PRINCIPLES OF RISK ANALYSIS

Margaret M. MacDonell

Environmental Assessment Division, Argonne National Laboratory, Argonne, Illinois

Kirpal S. Sidhu

Division of Environmental Epidemiology, Michigan Department of Community Health, Lansing, Michigan

Jasvinder S. Sidhu

Internal Medicine Residency Program, University Hospitals of Cleveland, Case Western Reserve University, Cleveland, Ohio

BACKGROUND ON RISK PRINCIPLES

Four-step Assessment Process

Nearly 15 years have elapsed since the father of risk-assessment reports—*Risk Assessment in the Federal Government: Managing the Process*, commonly referred to as the "Red Book"—was issued by the National Academy of Sciences (1986). In this book, the National Research Council laid out four basic steps for risk assessment, as shown in Figure 2.1. This model served as the framework that was swept forward into nationwide implementation through the U.S. Environmental Protection Agency's (EPA's) Superfund Program (U.S. EPA, 1989b,c) and other risk-based initiatives.

In the context of chemical risks, the four steps perform the following functions: (1) The hazard identification addresses whether a chemical that could be linked to a particular health effect is present; (2) the exposure assessment evaluates whether a receptor might come into contact with the chemical; (3) the toxicity or dose–response assessment presents information from the scientific literature on the potential harm that could be incurred following an exposure, considering its magnitude as well as the probability that the indicated health effect will occur; and (4) risk characterization provides the integrated endpoint

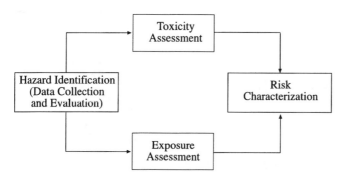

Figure 2.1 Four-step assessment process. Adapted from National Academy of Sciences (1986).

of this stepwise analysis, answering the question of what is the nature and magnitude of a potential receptor's risk.

The National Research Council framework has proved both general and flexible enough to accommodate a variety of applications. Over the years it has served as the foundation for assessing risks ranging from the health effects of chemical, radiological, and microbial exposures to ecological impacts. Just as life forms have evolved from simple to complex systems still anchored by four basic building blocks, the current paradigm for risk analysis is a model of interconnected processes that still can be distilled into the four basic steps.

Estimating Risk from Exposure and Toxicity Data

The EPA (1989b) incorporated the four-step model into its current guidelines for assessing health risks at contaminated sites. Under this process, contaminant hazards at a site are identified and various exposures are assumed so risks can be estimated to guide cleanup plans. For these estimates, intakes are calculated for generally hypothetical receptors by multiplying an environmental concentration (e.g., in soil, surface water, groundwater, or air) by an intake rate and amount of exposure (considering time, frequency, and duration) that are appropriate for the exposure being evaluated. The product then is divided by a standard body weight and an averaging time that reflects the assumptions used to derive the carcinogenic or noncarcinogenic toxicity value, which is used to convert intake to risk.

Intakes from assumed exposures are calculated using the following basic equation:

$$I_i = \frac{C_i \times IR \times CF_1 \times ET \times EF \times ED}{BW \times AT}$$

where:

I_i = intake of contaminant i (mg/kg · day)
C_i = concentration of contaminant i (e.g., mg/m^3 in air, mg/kg in soil, or mg/L in water)

IR = intake rate (e.g., m³/h or day for inhalation, or L/day for water ingestion)
CF_1 = conversion factor, as needed (e.g., 10^{-6} kg/mg)
ET = exposure time (hours per exposure event, or exposure day)
EF = exposure frequency (exposure events or exposure days per year)
ED = exposure duration (years)
BW = average body weight over the exposure period (kg)
AT = averaging time, taken to be the exposure time (in days) for noncarcinogens and 70 years (in days) for carcinogens

The estimated intake then is multiplied by the toxicity value appropriate for a given exposure, if available. The EPA develops these contaminant- and route-specific toxicity values based on a review and interpretation of the scientific literature, and they are provided electronically through the Integrated Risk Information System (online at http://www.epa.gov/ngispgm3/iris).

The toxicity value for a carcinogen is termed the *slope factor*. It represents the upper 95% confidence limit of the slope of the dose–response curve, which conservatively assumes nonthreshold linearity. This conservative basis can result in considerable overprediction of likely risks, especially if dose–response data indicate that a threshold exists.

The toxicity value for a noncarcinogen is termed the *reference dose*. For chronic exposures, which commonly are assumed in developing clean-up levels for contaminated sites, this value represents the concentration determined to be safe for daily human exposure per the critical endpoint for a given contaminant. Individual uncertainty factors of 10 are applied to the derivation of a reference dose to account for (1) extrapolation from animals to humans, (2) variation in human sensitivity, (3) use of a lowest-observed-adverse-effect level versus a no-observed-adverse-effect level, and (4) use of a no-observed-adverse-effect level from a subchronic rather than chronic study, as indicated. Although this approach was developed to ensure health protectiveness in the face of uncertainty, the reference doses used to estimate noncarcinogenic effects are often a very small fraction (e.g., 0.1%) of the "safe" dose determined from scientific studies. Thus, decisions based on these estimates can be too conservative and inefficient.

At the last step, the cancer endpoint or risk is calculated by multiplying the estimated intake by the chemical- and route-specific slope factor. If more than one contaminant or pathway is present, individual risks are summed to a total risk estimate. The noncancer effect is calculated by dividing the intake by the chemical- and route-specific reference dose to arrive at a hazard quotient. Individual hazard quotients are summed to a collective hazard index.

General Risk Targets for Contaminated Sites

To limit the chance that someone could get cancer from contaminants at a clean-up site, the EPA (1990) has established a range of 1 in 1 million to 1 in 10,000 for the incremental lifetime risk of cancer associated with possible exposures. This target range represents the increased probability (above the background cancer rate) that someone could get cancer during his or her lifetime if repeatedly exposed to the contaminants from a given site.

For context, the American Cancer Society (1992) has estimated that about one in three Americans will develop cancer during his or her lifetime from all sources, including smoking, and about one in four will die of cancer. (However, with ongoing scientific developments in such fields as gene therapy, these estimates may drop substantially within several decades.) Further, the risk from exposure to radiation naturally present in the environment is estimated to be about 1 in 100 (U.S. EPA, 1989a,d). In other words, the EPA aims to manage risks associated with contaminated sites at a level that represents a small percentage of estimated "natural" risks and an extremely small fraction (0.003% or less) of the cancer risk currently expected in the general population from everyday exposures.

The EPA uses the hazard index to indicate the potential for noncarcinogenic health effects. An index greater than 1—as segregated by the target organ/mechanism of action—indicates that the exposure may result in an adverse effect. A similar index has been applied to estimate ecological risks, and benchmark ecotoxicity values that parallel human toxicity values continue to be developed (Opresko et al., 1995; U.S. EPA, 1996a).

The target endpoints for health effects are graphically shown in Figure 2.2. Again, the largest uncertainty in the four-step risk assessment process is in the toxicity step. Faced with a paucity of specific human data at environmental exposure levels, the EPA method built considerable safety margins into the slope factors and reference doses used to convert intakes to cancer risk and noncancer effects, to err on the side of protectiveness. Clearly, this can lead to very expensive clean-up actions with little risk-reduction benefit.

Three Elements of Risk Analysis

Although risk assessment was the original focus of risk analysis, by the early 1990s the other two legs of the stool—management and communication—also were enjoying considerable visibility. Of these three, the National Research Council (1994) was initially careful to present the assessment component as distinct from the management component.

In a subsequent critique of that delineation, the council clarified their intent. It was not that the two had no commonality (as indeed the interrelationships are strong) but that risk managers should not be allowed to "influence the science" of an inherently uncertain process. To direct the outcome would corrupt the assessment methodology and hence the integrity of the results. In other words, maintaining a distinction emphasized the importance of having information flow from the scientific assessor to the project manager rather than vice versa. The intent was to preclude the manager insisting that the assessment assume whatever was necessary to assure that the outcome would demonstrate no significant risk to any receptor (e.g., to assume only one

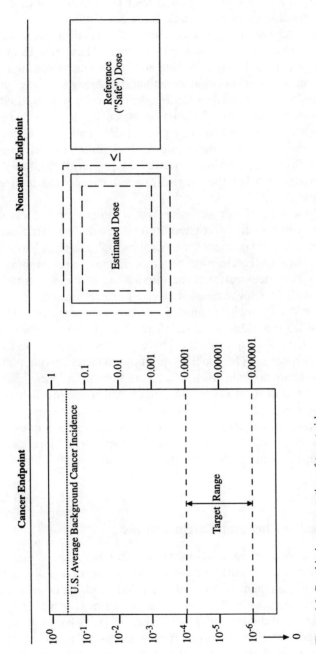

Figure 2.2 Graphical representation of target risks.

exposure event in 20 years, although a greater frequency such as one event per year might be considered more realistic for a given site).

That point having been made early on, the dichotomy between risk assessment and risk management began to blur. These two elements of risk analysis are now depicted as overlapping at the risk-characterization stage, with a dialectic process underlying that combination. Along the way, public policy and other decision factors were added explicitly to the mix. By 1995, the EPA was well into discussions on additional contributors to risk characterization, including technical, social, economic, legal, political, and other factors (Fig. 2.3). This acknowledgement of the major role "nonscientific" factors were playing in environmental decisions, previously viewed as primarily risk-based, dismayed technical assessors who felt that unencumbered science was getting the short end of the stick.

The third element of risk analysis—risk communication—was seen as the essential glue. The benefit of community and regulatory participation in risk assessment and risk management for environmental decisions had been obvious since the early days of the clean-up program. Extensive research and hundreds of case studies have demonstrated the importance of two-way interactions and meaningful stakeholder involvement to overall project success.

"Cancer" is itself a major communication issue. Compared with developing countries in which morbidity from such causes as infectious diseases and poor nutrition is a dominant concern, the United States can be characterized as a nation of cancerphobes. Our public's primary concerns about pollution have revolved around carcinogenic risks rather than noncarcinogenic health effects.

The EPA's recent draft cancer guidelines, which are highlighted elsewhere in this discussion, update the risk-assessment process per ongoing advances in our understanding of carcinogenesis. The following brief overview of chemical carcinogenesis is provided for background perspective. More detailed information can be found in reviews by Pitot and Dragan (1996) and Cotran et al. (1994).

Brief Overview of Chemical Carcinogenesis

A carcinogen is defined as a chemical or substance that causes or induces cancer. A tumor is an abnormal mass of new tissue or neoplasm and can be either benign or malignant (Cotran et al., 1994). Both types grow and expand, but a benign tumor does not invade or metastasize as a malignant neoplasm does (Cotran et al.; Williams and Wiseburger, 1991). Tissue growth exceeds and is uncoordinated with that of normal tissues, persisting in an excessive manner even after the stimulus that caused the growth stops (Pitot and Dragan, 1996). The current risk-assessment process does not distinguish between benign and malignant neoplasms (U.S. EPA, 1986), as both are included in tumor counts. However, the EPA's recent draft guidelines do consider this distinction.

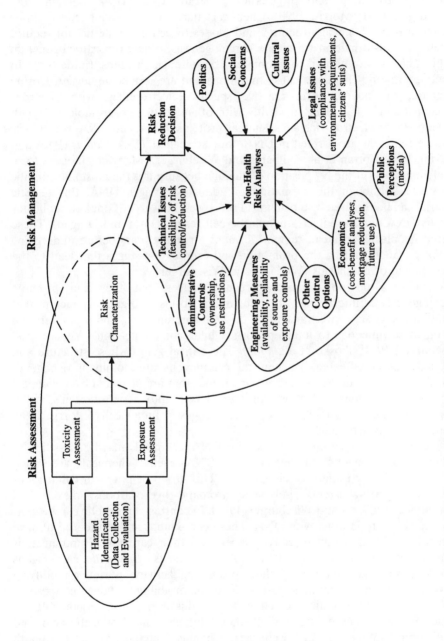

Figure 2.3 Relationship between risk assessment and risk management.

Chemical carcinogenesis is a complex, multistep process consisting of initiation, promotion, and progression (Cotran et al., 1994; Williams and Wiseburger, 1991; Morris, 1990). Chemicals that initiate carcinogenesis differ greatly in their chemical structures and modes of action. Some do not require metabolic transformation to initiate carcinogenesis; others (procarcinogens) do require biotransformation to ultimately become carcinogens (initiators). In general, initiating chemicals cause mutations and are termed *mutagens*. During initiation, carcinogens form reactive species (electrophiles, with electron-deficient atoms) that react covalently with other cellular macromolecules with nucleophilic or electron-rich sites, such as proteins, DNA, and RNA. If products of these reactions are formed in DNA, they are called *DNA adducts* (Pitot and Dragan, 1996; Cotran et al.; Williams and Wiseburger). Many carcinogens form covalent adducts at the N7 position of guanine because it is the most nucleophilic DNA site. Although the formation of adducts damages DNA, this genetic material can be repaired by biochemical processes. However, if one cell replicates with its DNA damage intact a neoplastic cell results (Pitot and Dragan). These altered neoplastic cells can remain dormant for many years before undergoing complex changes during the promotion and progression stages that lead to the development of neoplasms (Williams and Wiseburger).

Promoters do not themselves cause cancer, but they can promote carcinogenesis by interfering with cellular homeostasis. Regulatory factors that maintain homeostasis are transmitted through gap junctions, and promoters can act on these junctions to interrupt intracellular communication (Williams and Wiseburger, 1991; Trosko et al., 1983). The critical genes whose structure and function can be affected by chemical carcinogens are dominant oncogenes and recessive oncosuppressor genes. Oncogenes that are activated by a chemical (e.g., via a mutation) can transform normal cells into neoplastic cells; oncosuppressor genes can suppress neoplastic changes in tumor cells (Morris, 1990; Williams and Wiseburger).

Depending on how they interact with DNA, chemicals may be classified as genotoxic or epigenetic carcinogens. The DNA-reactive chemicals are called *genotoxic*, and they initiate carcinogenesis. This group of powerful carcinogens includes alkylating agents, polycyclic aromatic hydrocarbons, nickel, and nitrosamine (Williams and Wiseburger, 1991). In contrast, epigenetic carcinogens lack the ability to interact with DNA. These compounds are considered to have thresholds in their ability to cause cancer, and their carcinogenic potential is primarily attributed to their other biological effects. *Epigenetic* carcinogens include those characterized by their promoting activity, hormone-modifying activity, cytotoxicity, immune-suppression action, or ability to induce peroxisome proliferation. The chemical carcinogens in this group are organochlorine pesticides, saccharine, estrogen, diethylhexylphthalate, nitrilotriacetic acid, and cyclosporin A (Williams and Wiseburger). Chemical carcinogens that have both genotoxic and epigenetic characteristics are classified as genotoxics (Williams and Wiseburger). Although the standard risk-assessment process has not historically distinguished between these two classes of carcinogens (U.S. EPA, 1986; Morris, 1990), the EPA is moving the process in that direction by making the mode of action a cornerstone of their new cancer guidelines.

RISK AND ENVIRONMENTAL CLEANUP

Although intended as a tool to support environmental decision making, risk assessment often is waved as a compliance flag or enforcement threat. Emotional risk perceptions are commonly out of balance with existing scientific knowledge, and the public often has pushed for pristine "greenfields" as the endpoint of environmental clean-ups. A key challenge for risk analysts is to continue to strive for an improved sensibility, defensibility, and utility of risk assessments so sound science and good judgment will play stronger roles in environmental decisions.

Inefficiencies and Delays

A decade after Congress reauthorized the hazardous waste and Superfund regulations, the nation's clean-up programs still were slogging under the weight of management-heavy processes and confrontational interactions among the parties responsible for remediating contaminated sites, the regulatory community, and the public. There was a general feeling that waste had begotten waste, as billions of dollars had been spent on cleanup programs with very little to show for it. For example, few National Priorities List sites had qualified for delisting. Even straightforward clean-up activities at operating facilities (of which there are more than 5000—triple the number of National Priorities List sites) were being held up by extended administrative loops of oversight agency review and approval. Mounting criticism was directed not only at the responsible parties who were planning the work but also at the regulators administering these programs.

With the Federal deficit and cost accountability moving to the forefront of national concerns, the president signed Executive Order 12866 in October 1993. This order required that any significant regulatory action put before the American people be given a full review by the Office of Management and Budget—with "significant" defined as having an annual effect on the economy of $100 million or more, among other factors. This put a new spotlight on cost–benefit calculations and life-cycle assessments, which focused attention on more sensible and practicable risk analyses that addressed the "whole picture." This focus included considering more likely future land-use scenarios for contaminated sites, which directly affect residual contaminant levels and reasonable end states.

Stakeholder Involvement

A recent increase in coordinated risk-communication activities follows the pendulum swing toward more informed stakeholder involvement in environmental issues. Constructive engagement had been on the wane compared with the early years of involvement that began with the first Earth Day in 1970. Politics and drama often have held sway over science as the nation struggled with other problems such as the Federal budget, crime, and health care. However, pollution issues have remained in the public eye, and as technical advances in information access and the need for tax-dollar accountability gained strength, so did the emphasis on stakeholder participation in risk-based environmental decisions. Together with the broadened scope of risk management, this has lent further interesting complexity to the evolving paradigm for risk analysis.

Explicit requirements for public input and notification that were carried forward from the National Environmental Policy Act of 1970 into the Comprehensive Environmental Response, Compensation, and Liability Act of 1980 and the Superfund Amendments and Reauthorization Act of 1986 (including the latter's community right-to-know provisions) have also played a role in heightened public involvement. To encourage front-end participation, the EPA established such proactive mechanisms as technical-assistance grants under the Superfund program. These grants provided affected communities with the resources to support their involvement in local clean-ups, and citizens' advisory boards sprang up at sites across the country. Projects that meaningfully involve such groups and other stakeholders (including state and Federal regulators) in the assessment and decision-making processes have been successful in moving forward with remediation work; many others have remained mired in protracted battles arising from the old-guard mentality of forced community acceptance.

In 1996, the National Research Council's Committee on Risk Characterization identified increased stakeholder acceptance of risk assessments as the ultimate goal of risk characterization. Rather than simply viewing this process as the repackaging of technical risk information into lay terms, the committee described risk characterization as a more iterative, analytical-deliberative activity that is meant to involve stakeholders from the outset.

In fact, the committee interpreted this step as a prelude to decision making, rather than the endpoint itself. It further defined risk characterization as the processing of information that addresses the needs and interests of decision makers as well as other interested and affected parties. Interested parties are described as those who decide to become informed and involved in a given risk project, whereas affected parties are those who may incur harm or benefit from a given hazard, characterization process, or decision (National Research Council, 1996).

The recent report by the Presidential/Congressional Commission on Risk Assessment and Risk Management (1997) identifies stakeholders as parties who are concerned about or affected by a given risk-management problem. Consid-

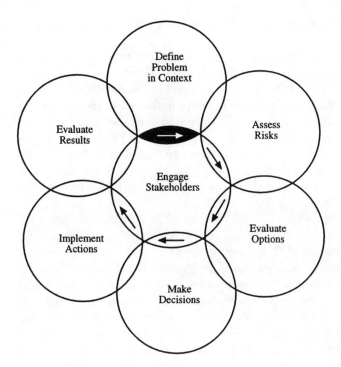

Figure 2.4 Iterative risk management framework. Modified from Presidential/Congressional Commission on Risk Assessment and Risk Management (1997).

ering the risk-assessment paradigm to be relatively well conceptualized, this group focused on the management component of risk analysis. The intent was to describe a process that would emphasize the importance of continuous communication and sensible implementation of risk principles. Toward this end, the commission developed a framework that captures the iterative nature of the process and identifies a central role for stakeholders (Fig. 2.4).

Recent Guidance Influencing Risk Analysis

Better incorporation of new scientific information and an expanded scope have led to a number of recent improvements in risk analysis. From 1989 through the mid-1990s, the EPA continued to refine its risk-assessment guidance for the Superfund program by building on the four fundamental steps (MacDonell et al., 1996; U.S. EPA, 1991a,b, 1992, 1995a).

Among these refinements was encouragement of more representative (versus simplistic and typically high-end default) values for the exposure parameters used to estimate contaminant intakes, especially if the outcome is sensitive to a given parameter. However, in many cases critical data are not readily available and cannot reasonably be obtained for the risk assessment—including toxicity data—so modeling is used to predict what has not yet been or cannot be practicably measured.

Advances in the hazard-identification step involve better approximations of the environmental behavior of site contaminants. Generic air and water dispersion and transport models have been enhanced to accommodate local and regional data. Clearly, the use of site-specific data in fate and exposure models can limit the overconservatism that leads to poor decisions such as unnecessary clean-ups. In fact, the use of representative site values for parameters ranging from environmental transport and fate indicators to exposure factors and risk estimators has resulted in risks within "acceptable" targets, where the use of default values resulted in estimates that exceeded those levels and implied that some action was warranted.

For certain sites, key local data are developed in conjunction with local researchers and students from universities, high schools, and grade schools, for example through "Partners in Education" programs and mentored science projects. Such cooperative studies have produced useful input data for parameters ranging from particle size distribution to organic content, soil/water distribution coefficients, hydraulic conductivity, and biouptake factors—in addition to valuable local buy-in of the risk-analysis process through personal involvement (MacDonell et al., 1996). These refined inputs have resulted in more realistic estimates, as borne out by monitoring results for air, soil, groundwater, and biota.

Exposure assumptions also have been refined to better reflect site conditions, considering land use and activity patterns per actual climatic conditions and related inhalation rates and ingestion rates, including for local food. For example, at a U.S. Department of Energy (DOE) National Priorities List site in Missouri that is surrounded by wildlife areas, data on recreational use, allowable hunting days, and fish-catch limits and consumption data provided by the state departments of conservation and natural resources were incorporated into a representative recreational scenario rather than using generic default values for a conservative residential scenario. This resulted in a more realistic depiction of likely future land use and related risks for the site (U.S. DOE, 1992a, b). The EPA subsequently relaxed its insistence on assumed residential use as essentially the sole driver for clean-up levels at such sites (U.S. EPA, 1995a).

Progress on the toxicity-assessment phase was not as striking during the late 1980s and early 1990s, except for the withdrawal of certain default assumptions that were inconsistent with empirical evidence (such as a nonspecific permeability coefficient of 0.01 for dermal exposures of metals). The more frequent use of surrogates to predict effects if no chemical-specific data were available held promise, as assessors initially were constrained by data developed through a much more formal, time-consuming process.

Additional interesting issues are associated with assessing risks at sites that are both radioactively and chemically contaminated. Many of these sites are Federal facilities, including more than 100 for the DOE alone (U.S. DOE, 1996).

Table 2.1 Comparison of toxicity assessments for chemicals and radionuclides

Component	Chemicals	Radionuclides
Primary data source	Little human data (primarily worker accidents), so toxicity values are generally derived from animal studies, with assumption of guilt unless proven innocent (using most sensitive species), exposures typically orders of magnitude higher than for environmental exposures, benign and malignant tumors often both included in the count, and durations often mismatched (e.g., short-term study used to predict chronic effects).	Human data exist for high doses (Chernobyl, Japanese bomb survivors, radium dial painters, patients), so toxicity values are primarily derived from human data
Effect of medium/absorption efficiency	Often not accounted for	Accounted for in the slope factor and dose-conversion factor
Distribution in the body	Can be preferential, not necessarily accounted for in the cancer assessment	Can also be preferential; accounted for in the slope factor and dose-conversion factor
Dose–response relationship	Poorly characterized, even at high doses	Relatively well characterized at high doses
Dose scaling	Different methods have been applied (with factors of 0.25 to 0.75)	Slope factors incorporate age-specific risk coefficients.
Carcinogenicity	Chemical- and route-specific; often dependent on biotransformation or bioactivation	Can cause cancer via multiple routes in nearly every tissue/organ (all are considered carcinogens)
Cancer slope factor	Upper 95% confidence level of the dose–response curve (no consideration of competing risks)	Best-estimate (50th percentile) from the dose–response curve; accounts for competing risks

A summary comparison that focuses on the toxicity-assessment step for chemicals and radionuclides based on the current framework is presented in Table 2.1.

As implementation of its clean-up program hit full stride, the EPA recognized the merit of screening-level assessments for identifying the key locations, contaminants, and pathways at a given site. Although this type of analysis is appropriately timely and more resource-efficient, it can generate overly conservative results, which if not qualified and understood can mislead decision makers and the public. More detailed assessments began to hone in on major problems and the parameters that dominated the results, which helped avoid wasting time and money on insignificant contributors to potential impacts. Uncertainty analysis was the tool applied to support this "focusing" effort, and its use became increasingly commonplace at the risk-characterization phase.

Probabilistic methods such as Monte Carlo simulations and Latin hypercube sampling often are applied to express the stochastic versus deterministic nature of environmental risks. Use of such analyses was formally encouraged in recent

Federal guidance (U.S. EPA, 1997) as a means of identifying sensitive parameters and focusing calculational refinements on those elements that significantly affect the final risk estimates. Although this approach can be applied across each of the elements of an ecological risk assessment, the EPA has not yet endorsed its use for all the human health assessment elements, notably the single largest contributor to uncertainty in risk estimates: the toxicity values.

Further Improvements

After the spate of focused EPA program documents in the early 1990s, new advancements in the underlying science have been reflected in an impressive round of supporting guidance with a strong emphasis on toxicity in risk assessment. These included recently proposed guidelines for assessing neurotoxicity (U.S. EPA, 1995b), reproductive toxicity (U.S. EPA, 1996e), carcinogenic risks (U.S. EPA, 1996c), and ecological risks (U.S. EPA, 1996d). Selected advances in the toxicity and risk areas are highlighted in the following discussion.

Toxicity and Risk Data. Flexibility to accommodate the wealth of new scientific information that will continue to be generated by toxicologists and other researchers is a major feature of the latest EPA guidelines. Considerable data are being generated by more efficient and effective testing programs that are frequently conducted as multiorganizational efforts.

Short-term animal studies and microbial tests have yielded extensive information that together with the results of other toxicity tests are providing insights into absorbed dose, metabolism and pharmacokinetics (distribution within the body), and pharmacodynamics (mechanism of action at the target tissue). New data are being incorporated into more sophisticated representations of what happens to a chemical following exposure, for example through molecular-level studies and time-dependent multivariate kinetic models (Sidhu and Sidhu, 1996; Moeller, 1997). If experimental data are limited or unavailable, quantitative structure–activity relationships (QSARs) have been developed from analogues to help predict chemical behaviors.

Bioavailability has long been an issue in transport and exposure modeling, especially for metals. Default assumptions can grossly overestimate chemical availability, and therefore the calculated health endpoint. In fact, the Presidential/Congressional Commission's report (1997) identifies bioavailability as among the primary areas warranting further study, along with mixtures and synergistic effects. Data from the current scientific literature have begun to be used in place of outdated and unrealistically conservative values.

Health-effect estimates can be significantly affected by speciation assumptions, for example for metals such as arsenic and lead. Although the EPA has not yet broken free of the traditional "100% available" conservative assumptions—as indicated by certain analyses supporting proposed hazardous-waste rulemakings—the Food and Drug Administration has considered bioavailability in recent decisions and relaxed the Delaney clause "zero cancer risk" approach for pesticide residues in food, per the 1996 Food Quality Protection Act. Thus, some progress is being made in incorporating new scientific information into Federal guidance and regulations.

Animal dose–response data also are being more closely scrutinized to refine interpretations vis-à-vis the potential for adverse health effects in humans. An "observed effect" now is evaluated carefully to determine whether that endpoint is indicative of a hazard, and further whether it necessarily represents a human hazard. One of the factors behind the improved toxicity data is the standardization of studies through the good laboratory practices program, which has allowed better cross-study interpretations and metaanalyses.

Harmonization has increased among agencies at the Federal and state levels and throughout the international community. For example, a multiagency radiation survey and site investigation effort is underway, with the U.S. Nuclear Regulatory Commission, Department of Defense, EPA, and DOE joining forces to develop a consistent approach for characterizing radioactively contaminated sites and verifying that health-protective clean-ups have been achieved. The U.S. Departments of Energy and Defense also have collaborated on ways to rank relative risks across multiple clean-up areas, to help prioritize remediation activities. Further collaboration also has occurred on the evaluation of common contamination problems and related risk issues (such as those associated with volatile organic compounds and metals in groundwater) to help guide technology development.

Similarly, U.S. EPA and California EPA scientists have worked together to harmonize approaches for evaluating specific chemical risks, and international collaboration is ongoing through the World Health Organization's Program on Chemical Safety. Extensive partnering also has occurred in the pharmaceutical industry with regard to protocols for genotoxicity and other tests. As a note, increased collaboration on broad-spectrum and focused, short-term studies combined with QSARs also has helped minimize the use of animal tests for new or uncharacterized chemicals, which has helped address concerns of animal-rights activists.

New Cancer Guidelines. In order to better reflect the wealth of toxicity information as it is generated, the EPA has proposed a new qualitative–descriptive classification system for carcinogens (U.S. EPA, 1996c). A brief summary of how the carcinogen classification system has evolved since the early 1980s is presented in Table 2.2. In previous guidelines, tumor findings in animals or humans constituted the main determinant of the classification decision, and other input served only as a modifier within the indicated category. Under the newly proposed system, other data on toxicological, metabolic, and other biological properties also are considered primary factors—including QSARs and results of mechanistic and precursor-effect tests. The combined evidence is now to be weighed together and narrative descriptors used in place of the letter categories.

Table 2.2 Evolution of cancer classification (1982–1996)

Indicated carcinogenicity	IARC (1982)	U.S. EPA (1986)	U.S. EPA (1996)
Human carcinogen	Group 1	Group A	Known/likely
Probable/possible human carcinogen	Group 2A/2B	Group B1 (probable; limited evidence from human studies) Group B2 (possible; sufficient evidence from animal studies) Group C (possible; limited evidence from animal studies)	Cannot be determined (possibly "suggestive")
Not classified as to human carcinogenicity	Group 3	Group D	Not likely
Evidence of noncarcinogenicity in humans	—	Group E	—

Note: IARC, International Agency for Research on Cancer; EPA, U.S. Environmental Protection Agency.

The EPA also has proposed to revise the default scaling factor used to extrapolate from animal studies when assessing oral exposures in humans. The new factor scales the daily applied dose (over a lifetime) proportional to the body weight raised to the 0.75 power. This approach is consistent with the current understanding of allometric scaling laws (Sidhu, 1992; West et al., 1997). A different approach has been proposed for inhalation exposures, whereby deposition of particles and gases and the internal doses of gases with different absorption characteristics are separately assessed. These two default approaches differ from the previous application of a single scaling factor based on the body weight to the 0.66 power (U.S. EPA, 1996c).

A better understanding of the underlying mechanisms of carcinogenesis and more progressive agency interpretations have enabled assessors to move beyond the linear, no-threshold dose–response model for certain chemicals. The linear extrapolation-to-zero relationship had been intentionally selected in the absence of better data to reflect a conservatism aimed at reassuring the environmental community that a "plausible" upper bound had been placed on potential health effects. That is, the traditional bias was clearly toward public health protection.

However, overly conservative results benefit neither the individual risk manager nor the policy maker, as they typically lead to inappropriate decisions regarding allocation of limited resources. An example of the impact model selection can have on the risk outcome is shown in Table 2.3. Monies spent on overly conservative environmental clean-ups are unavailable for other needs, such as nutrition programs that could achieve a much greater national benefit in

Table 2.3 Drinking-water guideline corresponding to a 10^{-6} risk level for 1,4-dioxane per different models

Model	Data type	Derived guideline (ppb)	Reference
Linearized multistage	Female mouse liver	2[a]	Sidhu, 1986
Linearized multistage	Rat liver	7	U.S. EPA, 1987
Linearized multistage	Rat nasal turbinate	3	U.S. EPA, 1988
Logit	Rat liver	0.001	E. V. Dhanian, 1993, personal communication
Weibull	Rat liver	0.0001	E. V. Dhanian, 1993, personal communication
Physiologically based pharmacokinetic	Rat liver	3,000	Leung and Paustenbach, 1990

Source: Modified and reprinted with permission from Sidhu and Sidhu (1996; copyright courtesy Professor Dr. Jai Rup Singh). Data type taken from National Cancer Institute (1978).
[a] Using 2.09×10^{-2} $(mg/kg \cdot d)^{-1}$ as the computed oral slope factor (M. C. Martinez, 1986, personal communication).

terms of increased health protection for a fraction of the cost. For example, after more than a billion dollars had been spent on dioxin evaluations (in large part because of public risk perceptions), the head of the EPA office coordinating the dioxin reassessment acknowledged that chloracne was the only demonstrated human health effect for this compound and that the lower estimate of potential carcinogenic risks (especially at environmental levels) was in fact zero.

In responding to this general issue, the EPA's recent draft cancer guidelines establish the mode of action as the centerpiece of the hazard-identification and toxicity-assessment steps (U.S. EPA, 1996c). Although linearity is still the standard default assumption for the dose–response curve, a nonlinear relationship can be applied if supported by other evidence. In this case, a margin-of-exposure analysis is used rather than estimating the probability of effects at low doses, to better reflect biological considerations at environmental levels.

Furthermore, the new cancer guidelines focus on the estimated dose associated with the lower 95% confidence limit (LED_{10}) on the dose with an estimated 10% increased incidence of tumor or relevant nontumor response (ED_{10}) as the general default assumption (Fig. 2.5). This value provides a closer parallel to the benchmark-dose method used to determine reference concentrations and doses for noncarcinogens. It also better accounts for uncertainty in the dose–response data.

Reassessments that capture current experimental data and follow the updated process laid out in the proposed cancer guidelines are currently underway. For example, the EPA has reassessed polychlorinated biphenyls (PCBs) using a nonlinear dose–response curve based on negative genotoxicity tests, which indicates that PCBs act through a different mechanism of action, to arrive at better risk estimates (U.S. EPA, 1996b).

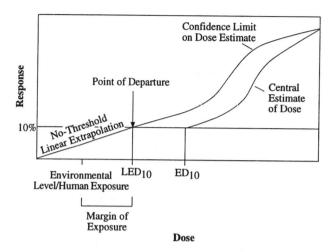

Figure 2.5 Two-part dose–response evaluation: extrapolated and observed ranges. Adapted from U.S. EPA (1996c).

Ecologic Risk Assessment. The framework for the EPA's ecologic risk-assessment process is intentionally general because it must accommodate a range of projects and programs that are widely variable in terms of environmental setting, size of problem area (from localized spills to watersheds), and type of contamination (from relatively benign to biologically persistent and toxic). This general framework is adaptable to the objectives of specific applications, from pesticide management to water quality to Superfund cleanups.

The ecologic risk-assessment process consists of four steps that parallel the human-health assessment, including a quantification option for estimating a hazard quotient. The same "safe concentration" concept applies, as ecotoxicity thresholds and benchmarks have been developed from the available literature to provide insight into potential problems associated with environmental concentrations of chemicals (Opresko et al., 1995; U.S. EPA, 1996a).

As with the human-health assessment, the EPA encourages early external involvement in ecologic risk-analysis activities. This involvement extends from the technical experts in a biological technical assistance group to interested members of the community. Those individuals can be especially helpful in identifying species of local societal value, such as deer.

Of special interest to ecological risk assessors is that many contaminated sites effectively have become wildlife refuges by virtue of restricted human access. In fact, many Federal clean-up sites contain large tracts of land that previously served as buffer zones and now support thriving ecosystems as a result of decades of minimal human disturbance. For example, only about 6% of the 30,000 square miles of land associated with the U.S. DOE environmental-restoration sites is estimated to be contaminated, and much of the remainder serves as home to well-established ecosystems. Thus, active clean-up measures such as large-scale excavation designed to protect against possible future human exposures at these sites can significantly impact ecologic resources. As the ecologic risk-assessment field continues to mature, these effects have begun to be more explicitly included in trade-off analyses with human-health risks. Because ecologic exposures at such sites can be longer and more intense, a number of upcoming decisions are expected to be driven by ecologic risks separate from those that link to the human-health arena via the food ingestion pathway.

Worker Risk Assessment. Risks to workers are a major factor in balancing overall impacts to human health associated with contaminated sites. In the early 1990s, these risks often were addressed qualitatively (U.S. EPA, 1991b) in part because specific data were not available to support quantitative analyses. Another reason was the assumption that compliance with worker-protection regulations mitigated the need for further assessment. However, worker risk estimates are key to informed decisions for contaminated sites, as these represent impacts to real individuals who can be directly exposed to site hazards. This is in contrast to the very hypothetical risks estimated for members of the general public who might possibly be exposed in the future, but not likely at levels as conservatively assumed for purposes of the site risk assessments. The same standard four-step process is applied to assess worker risks as is applied to estimate baseline risks for hypothetical members of the general public, with exposure factors tailored to occupational scenarios.

Weighing trade-offs between likely risks to workers and relatively improbable risks to members of the public remains a difficult risk-management activity. This effort is increasingly supported by comparable health effect estimates, as technical factors combined with a heightened appreciation of worker-exposure issues have led to better quantification of occupational risks. New insights continue to be gained from studies such as focused toxicity tests aimed at developing acute and subchronic toxicity values and from technological advances in real-time environmental monitoring and biomonitoring capabilities and calculation of personal dose–response profiles for individual workers.

In parallel with analytical advances, progress also is being made on the regulatory front as resource constraints have made their mark. Selected highlights follow.

Regulatory Initiatives

Government Performance and Results Act. Over the past several years, the Federal government has been moving toward performance-based versus administrative process–based management systems per the Government Performance and Results Act of 1993. Each Federal agency must prepare a strategic plan and annual reports that identify and status progress against specific performance measures. The EPA is looking at a system with two environmental indicators. The first involves controlling human exposures (i.e., so there will be no unacceptable risks to humans from contaminant releases from a facility), and the second involves controlling groundwater releases (i.e., to achieve no migration across defined boundaries). Additional metrics that include ecologic risks also are being evaluated. Under a parallel strategic planning effort, the DOE performance measures include reducing serious risks at environmental restoration sites first.

In response to this performance-based shift in focus, some stakeholders have expressed concern about less stringent agency oversight of cleanup activities at contaminated sites. They fear that the new process might lead to reduced public participation, wondering if replacing detailed reviews and approvals of project documents such as work plans (which was a very slow process) with performance-based measures will lead to facilities obscuring or avoiding their obligations to involve the community. However, the EPA continues to strongly encourage community outreach as part of the environmental decision-making process for both active facilities and inactive sites.

Hazardous Releases. The EPA's original framework for corrective action that was designed to address hazardous waste problems at operating facilities pursuant to the Resource Conservation and Recovery Act (RCRA) was fairly prescriptive, but it has become somewhat more flexible during the past few years. For example, presumptive remedies are being identified to streamline the compliance process for sites with problems such as volatile organic compounds in soil, contaminated groundwater, and PCBs in soil (forthcoming). In addition, the trend toward more integrated assessments versus single-unit, single-medium analyses continues. Finally, nonresidential land use now is being accepted as a reasonable future scenario; future residential use had been the standard assumption for both the Resource Conservation and Recovery Act and Superfund programs.

Under the Resource Conservation and Recovery Act corrective-action process, action levels typically were set at the 10^{-6} "point of departure" level using conservative exposure assumptions and EPA-approved toxicity values. In acknowledging the progress that has been made in toxicologic research since standard action levels were disseminated in 1990 per extant toxicity values, this point of departure is no longer used as a strict presumption for all final clean-ups such as clean closures. Rather, the level to be attained now also considers the exposure conditions, uncertainties, and evolving data—including toxicity information—along with technical limitations at a given site.

Superfund Soil-Screening Guidance. The EPA (1996g) recently issued guidance for screening site soil concentrations to help identify potential risk problems in a timely manner and focus subsequent assessments. This guidance builds on a similar concentration-based screening approach (1996) and is based on back-calculating the intake-to-risk equations for a residential scenario using standard toxicity values. The results provide concentrations of chemicals in soil at or below which a no-action response generally is warranted. These action levels are distinct from clean-up levels, which are the residual concentrations considered to be safe per anticipated future use. However, if data indicate that action levels are exceeded, further assessment (which often has been interpreted by oversight agencies as clean-up) is warranted.

Some risk managers prefer this "snapshot-in-time" approach, which produces standard action levels by medium based on a static set of exposure assumptions and toxicity values. This is especially attractive for organizations with limited resources, such as state agencies. Many others endorse standardizing the framework without prescribing input values. This more flexible approach would allow ready incorporation of site-specific values, and possibly state-of-the-art toxicity data, and accommodates intersite differences.

Risk-based Corrective Action. The American Society for Testing and Materials (1995) recently developed a tiered methodology for risk-based corrective action at petroleum-release sites that parallels the framework developed by EPA for National Priorities List sites. The overall intent of this process is to ensure that risk information is appropriately incorporated into state programs for corrective action at these sites. This process subsequently has been extrapolated by a number of state agencies to voluntary clean-ups at a variety of industrial properties.

Additional progress has been made on fractionation evaluations, whereby the toxicities of the actual compounds present at a given site are assessed rather than using generic and often unrepresentative group surrogates. For example, if sampling indicates that nonane is the dominant compound present, information for that compound is used together with local environmental-setting data to assess site risks, rather than applying toxicity information for benzene as a default indicator for general petroleum contamination.

Brownfields Redevelopment Initiative. The EPA recently established a brownfields initiative to help communities revitalize abandoned, idle, or underutilized properties typically located in industrial areas. The agency has funded a number of pilot studies aimed at removing administrative and regulatory barriers without sacrificing protectiveness. State agencies have pursued parallel initiatives, typically building on the risk-based corrective action or soil screening–level process or a combination of both. The progress this initiative has achieved is a tribute to innovative risk analysts and agency personnel who are integrating practical risk concepts and engineering measures into constructive land redevelopment.

Such joint creativity typically does not extend to the relaxation of restrictive safety factors that have been incorporated into toxicity values to ensure protectiveness. However, it is interesting to note that in some cases (e.g., within the state of Illinois), the risk-based corrective action guidelines for contaminated sites being addressed under the voluntary remediation program allow carcinogens as well as noncarcinogens to be grouped by endpoint. This expands on the protocol for segregating the health endpoint (hazard index) for noncarcinogens alone in the Superfund risk-assessment process and may be considered for broader application in the future.

SUMMARY AND OUTLOOK

The past several years have been especially productive for the EPA in the area of environmental risk analysis, as the agency has issued a number of guidance reports and proposed rules that reflect improvements in the overall process. These documents address issues ranging from multiple noncancer endpoints and carcinogen reclassification to reduced regulation of low-risk materials. Standard assessment methods are being refined to accommodate the wealth of dose–response and mechanistic data that continues to be generated by toxicologists, and noncancer endpoints are getting more attention. Affected parties are being brought into the decision-making process for environmental actions, and the integrated risk-analysis process is becoming more transparent as scientific, technical, political, economic, social, and other factors are being explicitly incorporated into risk-management decisions.

Over the past 15 years, risk analysis has evolved from a relatively simple box model to a complex system of interrelated steps that reflects our evolving knowledge about human toxicities, risks, and trade-offs. Unparalleled information exchanges that extend to the global level have helped the risk community play a central role in highlighting and enhancing environmental protection. Risk applications also have flourished in areas other than traditional pollution control. Basic principles of risk assessment, management, and communication are being brought to bear on problems ranging from the post–Cold War management of chemical agents and radioactive wastes to the control of environmental pathogens and global warming. A conceptual diagram of an integrated framework that accommodates a range of applications from human to ecological risk assessments for chemical, radiological, and microbial stressors is shown in Figure 2.6.

Risk methods also are being applied to corporate environmental management systems through such frameworks as International Standards Organization 14000, risk-informed prioritization, and life-cycle analyses. Daily newspaper accounts highlight how common risk-informed evaluations have become, as illustrated by the recent scientific and political debate about a continued American presence on the space station Mir.

Risk analysts continue to evaluate the science behind such issues as environmental tobacco smoke, protection of our food supplies, and targeted cancer vaccines. We look forward to further scientific discoveries that will deepen our understanding of the chemical, physical, and biological interactions in our environment and the role of society and technology in solving our problems. Although public policy often lags behind scientific advances, a commitment to continually refine our risk approaches per credible, state-of-the-art information will allow us to best focus our resources and make ever more

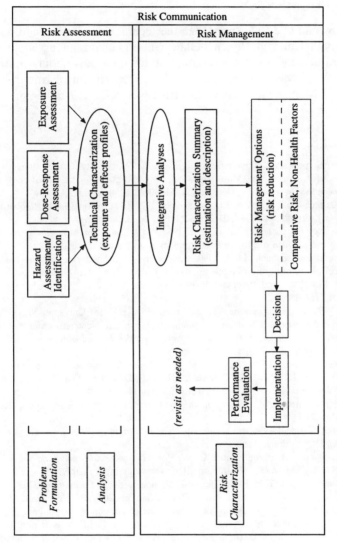

Figure 2.6 Integrated components of multidisciplinary risk-analysis process.

intelligent decisions about protecting human health and the environment as we enter the 21st century.

ACKNOWLEDGMENTS

The authors would like to acknowledge the technical leadership and inspiration of Drs. Harry Salem and Eugene Olajos in organizing an excellent national conference on toxicity in risk assessment and for their outstanding contributions to the field. Work was supported by the U.S. Department of Energy Office of Environmental Management under Contract No. W-31-109-ENG-38.

REFERENCES

American Cancer Society. 1992. *Cancer facts and figures—1992*. Atlanta, GA: Author.
American Society for Testing and Materials. 1995. *Standard guide for risk-based corrective action applied at petroleum release sites*. Designation E1739-95. Philadelphia: Author.
Cotran, R. S., Kumar, V., Robbins, S. L., and Schoen, F. J. 1994. Neoplasia. In *Robbins pathologic basis of disease*, 5th ed., pp. 241–303. Philadelphia: W. B. Saunders.
International Agency for Research on Cancer. 1982. *IARC monographs on the evaluation of the carcinogenic risk of chemicals to humans*, supplement 4. Lyon, France: Author.
Leung, H. W., and Paustenbach, D. J. 1990. Cancer risk assessment for dioxane based upon a physiologically-based pharmacokinetic approach. *Toxicol. Lett.* 51:147–162.
MacDonell, M., Picel, M., and Peterson, J. 1996. Getting it right at Weldon Spring. *RadWaste Magazine*, 3(6):12–18.
Moeller, D. W. 1997. *Environmental health*. Cambridge, MA: Harvard University Press.
Morris, S. C. 1990. *Cancer risk assessment: A quantitative approach*. New York: Marcel Dekker.
National Academy of Sciences. 1986. *Risk assessment in the Federal government: Managing the process*. Washington, DC: National Academy Press.
National Cancer Institute. 1978. *Bioassay of 1,4-dioxane for possible carcinogenicity*. DHEW Publication No. (NIH) 718-1330. Bethesda, MD: U.S. Department of Health, Education and Welfare, Public Health Service, National Institutes of Health.
National Research Council. 1994. *Science and judgment in risk assessment*. Washington, DC: National Academy Press.
National Research Council. 1996. *Understanding risk: Informing decisions in a democratic society*. Washington, DC: National Academy Press.
Opresko, D. M., Sample, B. E., and Suter, G. W. 1995. *Toxicological benchmarks for wildlife: 1995 revision*. ES/ER/TM-86/R1. Washington, DC: Department of Energy.
Pitot, H. C. III, and Dragan, Y. P. 1996. Chemical carcinogenesis. In *Casarett and Doull's toxicology: The basic science of poisons*, 5th ed., ed. C. D. Klaassen, pp. 201–267. New York: McGraw Hill.
Presidential/Congressional Commission on Risk Assessment and Risk Management. 1997. *Framework for environmental risk management, final report*, vols. I,II. Washington, DC: Author.
Sidhu, K. S. 1992. Basis for body weight exponent (0.75) as a scaling factor in energy metabolism and risk assessment. *J. Appl. Toxicol.* 12:309–310.
Sidhu, K. S. 1986. *1,4-Dioxane: Risk assessment*. Lansing, MI: Michigan Department of Public Health.
Sidhu, K. S., Sidhu, J. S. 1996. Risk assessment for environmental carcinogens. In *Current concepts in human genetics: Proceedings of the Second International Symposium on Genetics, Health and Disease*. ed. J. R. Singh, pp. 138–151. Amritsar, India: Guru Nanak Dev University.
Trosko, J. E., Chang, C. C., and Medcalf, A. 1983. Mechanism of tumor promotion: Potential role of intracellular communications. *Cancer Invest.* 1:511–526.

U.S. Department of Energy. 1992a. *Baseline assessment for the chemical plant area of the Weldon Spring site*. DOE/OR/21548-091. St. Charles, MO: DOE Oak Ridge Field Office, Weldon Spring Site Remedial Action Project.

U.S. Department of Energy. 1992b. *Feasibility study for remedial action at the chemical plant area of the Weldon Spring site*, vols. I,II. DOE/OR/21548-148. St. Charles, MO: DOE Oak Ridge Field Office, Weldon Spring Site Remedial Action Project.

U.S. Department of Energy. 1996. *The 1996 baseline environmental management report*. Washington, DC: Office of Environmental Management.

U.S. Environmental Protection Agency. 1986. Guidelines for carcinogen risk assessment. *Fed Regist*. 51:33994–34003.

U.S. Environmental Protection Agency. 1987. *Health advisory: p-Dioxane*. Washington, DC: Author.

U.S. Environmental Protection Agency. 1988. *Integrated Risk Information System database: 1, 4-Dioxane*. Washington, DC: Office of Research and Development.

U.S. Environmental Protection Agency. 1989a. National emissions standards for hazardous air pollutants: Radionuclides, final rule and notice of reconsideration (40 CFR Part 61). *Fed Regist*. 54:51654–51715.

U.S. Environmental Protection Agency. 1989b. *Risk assessment guidance for Superfund, volume I: Human health evaluation manual (part A)*. Interim Final, EPA/540/1-89/002. Washington, DC: Office of Emergency and Remedial Response.

U.S. Environmental Protection Agency. 1989c. *Risk assessment guidance for Superfund, volume II: Environmental evaluation manual (part A)*. Interim Final, EPA/540/1-89/001A (OSWER Directive 9285.7-01). Washington, DC: Office of Emergency and Remedial Response.

U.S. Environmental Protection Agency. 1989d. *Risk assessment methodology, environmental impact statement for NESHAPS radionuclides, volume I, background information document*. EPA/520/1-89/005. Washington, DC: (September 7, 1989d).

U.S. Environmental Protection Agency. 1990. National oil and hazardous substances pollution contingency plan; final rule (40 CFR Part 300). *Fed Regist*. 55:8666–8865 (March 8, 1990).

U.S. Environmental Protection Agency. 1991a. *Human health evaluation manual, supplemental guidance: Standard default exposure factors*. OSWER Directive 9285.6-03. Washington, DC: Office of Solid Waste and Emergency Response.

U.S. Environmental Protection Agency. 1991b. *Risk assessment guidance for Superfund, volume I: Human health evaluation manual (part C, risk evaluation of remedial alternatives)*. Interim Final. EPA/540/R-92/004. Washington, DC: Office of Research and Development.

U.S. Environmental Protection Agency. 1991c *Role of the baseline risk assessment in Superfund remedy selection decisions*. OSWER Directive 9355.0-30. Washington, DC: Author.

U.S. Environmental Protection Agency. 1992. *Dermal exposure assessment: Principles and applications*. EPA/600/8-91/011B. Washington, DC: Office of Research and Development.

U.S. Environmental Protection Agency. 1995a. *Land use in the CERCLA remedy selection process*. Directive No. 9355.7-04. Washington, DC: Office of Solid Waste and Emergency Response.

U.S. Environmental Protection Agency. 1995b. *Proposed guidelines for neurotoxicity risk assessment*. EPA/630/R-95. Washington, DC: Office of Research and Development.

U.S. Environmental Protection Agency. 1996a. *Ecotox thresholds*. EPA/540/F-95/038, ECO Update, Intermittent Bulletin 3(2). Washington, DC: Office of Solid Waste and Emergency Response.

U.S. Environmental Protection Agency. 1996b. *PCBs: Cancer dose–response assessment and application to environmental mixtures*. EPA/600/P-96/001F. Washington, DC: Office of Research and Development.

U.S. Environmental Protection Agency. Proposed guidelines for carcinogen risk assessment: Notice. *Fed Regist*. 61:17960–18011. (April 1996c).

U.S. Environmental Protection Agency. 1996d. *Proposed guidelines for ecological risk assessment*. EPA/630/R-96/001, Washington, DC: Office of Research and Development.

U.S. Environmental Protection Agency. 1996e. *Proposed guidelines for reproductive toxicity assessment*. EPA/630/R-96/009. Washington, DC: Office of Research and Development.

U.S. Environmental Protection Agency. 1996f. *Region IX preliminary remediation goals (PRGs)*. Memorandum from S. J. Smucker, Regional Toxicologist, Technical Support Team, California, to PRG Mailing Table List.

U.S. Environmental Protection Agency. 1996g. *Soil screening guidance: Technical background document*. EPA/530-F-96/128. Washington, DC: Office of Solid Waste and Emergency Response.

U.S. Environmental Protection Agency. 1997. *Guiding principles for Monte Carlo analyses*. EPA/600/R-97/001. Washington, DC: Risk Assessment Forum.

West, G. B., Brown, J. H., and Enquist, B. J. 1997. A general model for the origin of allometric scaling laws in biology. *Science* 276:122126.

Williams, G. M., and Wiseburger, J. H. 1991. Chemical carcinogenesis. In *Casarett and Doull's toxicology: The science of poisons*, 4th ed., ed. M. O. Amdur, J. Doull, and C. D. Klaassen, pp. 127–200. New York: Pergamon Press.

CHAPTER
THREE

HOW TO COMMUNICATE RISK IN A LOW TRUST/HIGH CONCERN ENVIRONMENT

Keith A. Fulton

Fulton Communication, Houston, Texas

I was a chemical plant manager of an 1800-employee plant from October 1985 to November 1991. My senior management encouraged me to spend a significant part of my time in the community. The Bhopal, India, incident had occurred in late 1984, and the chemical industry's public image was in decline regarding safety, health, and environmental issues. My task was to develop an improved dialogue with the Baytown, Texas, community. In some instances, this involved communicating in a low trust/high concern environment. I quickly learned that in this type of environment, communicating risk or other matters concerning our industry requires skill training.

Communicating in a low trust/high concern environment is like riding a bicycle for the first time. In riding a bicycle for the first time, one must do things that seem unnatural, but after sufficient practice, they become automatic. Similarly, one needs new and different methods of communicating from normal communications. In many instances, the normal communication methods feel good yet turn out to be a problem in low trust/high concern environments. With proper skill development, this new communication form becomes relatively easy, just as riding a bicycle does after enough experience.

These skills apply to low trust/high concern environments regardless of the situation. The skills apply to any low trust/high concern situation whether it is with the public regarding an institution, communications within an institution, or communications in one's social life, neighborhood life, with friends, or with family.

People who represent institutions when communicating with the public frequently get into difficulty by focusing mostly on the science, data, and facts. Science, data, and facts are of far less concern in low trust/high concern situations. In these situations, the more important components are people's emotional needs, social needs, and sometimes political needs.

Communicators must realize that the public's perception equals the public's reality, even if that reality is in conflict with the science, data, and facts. The goal for the institutional communicator should be to build trust and credibility. Message testing and case study research by Covello (1989) showed that trust and credibility require four components: empathy, commitment, competence, and honesty. Interestingly, the testing shows that empathy is by far the most important of these four factors. In fact, empathy is 50% of the requirement to build trust and credibility. The other three factors of commitment, competency, and honesty are approximately 17% of the requirement each.

Empathy is not agreement. Empathy is not sympathy. Empathy is simply "walking in the other person's shoes," understanding why he or she feels the way he or she does. If communicators cannot walk in the shoes of someone who does not trust them or has concerns about them, they will be unable to get such people to listen to their science, data, and facts. Therefore, it is appropriate to demonstrate to the listener that one understands where he or she is coming from before beginning a dialogue regarding the facts. This usually can be done fairly quickly but sometimes requires the use of paraphrasing to make sure one understands the underlying concerns.

The other three factors in building trust—commitment, competency, and honesty—are important as well. Commitment in low trust/high concern communications means you will do those things that you told them you would do. Competency means you know what you are talking about, and of course honesty means you are telling the truth. What is interesting about riding the bicycle of low trust/high concern communications is that we are used to focusing on the competency factor first and foremost because that is the biggest factor for effective communications within our institutions. However, if we jump to demonstrating our competency in our low trust/high concern discussion with the public, they will frequently react by not listening and becoming more upset and distrustful. Their view can be, "You don't know what it's like for me and you're putting all your energy into pushing your agenda. You don't care."

Public officials are becoming better skilled at demonstrating the use of empathy to build trust and reduce concern. This was particularly true during the TWA crash off of Long Island in 1996. Shortly after the crash, public officials and TWA officials were besieged with questions from the press about the cause of the accident including numerous questions about missiles and bombs. Rather than discuss what they knew about the crash and what they did not know about the crash, they first expressed sadness about the loss of lives. Their nonverbal communications indicated that they did indeed feel sad.

There are many *traps* in low trust/high concern communications. These are not traps in normal communications. However, they can result in significant barriers in low trust/high concern communications. There are many such traps, but just five are covered here: *humor*, *negatives*, *guarantees*, *jargon*, and *worst-case scenarios*.

Humor is appropriate in most conversations. After-dinner speakers frequently start their speeches with humor. In low trust/high concern conversations, humor can be deadly and should never be used. For example, one should never start a public meeting with, "A funny thing happened on the way over here." Some of the people in that public may have serious concerns about their safety, health, and environment and may want the institution to address those concerns. Use of humor by that representative will be interpreted as condescending, a put-down, and not taking their concerns seriously. In our public meetings, we were trained not to even smile at what we thought might be a preposterous question: "Do you have mutants in your chemical plant because of the toxic chemicals you produce?" Our assumption had to be that question was serious to the person asking the question.

The use of *negative phrases* or *terms* should be minimized. Negative terms are more vivid and more memorable. So, if someone asks the question, "Why are you lying to us tonight?" the answer should not be, "We are not lying," a sentence that contains two negative words: *not* and *lying*. A more appropriate answer should be, "We are telling the truth, and let us tell you the truth about..."

A *guarantee* question is a trap. For example, someone may ask, "Will you guarantee us that there is absolutely no health risk?" or "Will you guarantee us that something will never happen?" In riding this low trust/high concern bicycle for the first time, the tendency would be to answer the question, "No, I can't guarantee that," or to say, "There is only a one in a million chance that..." Once one has responded in this way, most people will perceive a high probability of the incident occurring. In the case of the one-in-a-million response, the focus is on the numerator, not the denominator, no matter how many zeroes are in it. The guarantee question should be responded to with a *sense of the commitment* you are making to assure the risk is not likely to happen. Generally, that is the underlying concern of the questioner, not the probabilities. So, an appropriate response to the guarantee question would be something like, "That would be a very serious matter, that's why we're doing everything possible to ensure it doesn't happen. Let me give you two of the activities that we are doing to make sure that doesn't happen."

A fourth trap is the use of *jargon*. The use of jargon, which makes perfect sense for communicating within institutions, frequently is seen by someone in a low trust/high concern posture as intentionally confusing, a purposeful put-down, or arrogance. Even though this is not the intent, that is the way it is perceived. Therefore, the use of technical terms and the use of acronyms should be eliminated. Even a term like "groundwater" has been interpreted in a public meeting to mean "puddles." So, telling the public that the groundwater is safe to drink may not work. An audience once interpreted 10^{-6} as 4. If a technical term like groundwater must be used, explain what you mean by groundwater at the beginning of these discussion to avoid these negative consequences.

A fifth trap is explaining *worst-case scenarios*. You do not want to leave the receiver with a vivid picture of the worst-case scenario. This can multiply in his or her mind the probability of this incident occurring by several orders of magnitude. The better response is to tell people all the things one is doing to prevent this from happening. Prevention is the key message.

The use of *nonverbal communications* is critical in low trust/high concern communications. Nonverbal communications include body language, voice changes, dress, and barriers between the speaker and receiver. Nonverbal communications are more important or as important as verbal communications in low trust/high concern situations. If people do not trust you, they are not going to believe your words until they have scanned you for clues as to whether you are telling the truth or not. People judge whether you are telling the truth on your nonverbal clues and not your words. That is why, for example, you cannot fake empathy. Empathy is "walking in another person's shoes," understanding where they are coming from. You cannot say, "I understand why you are concerned based on what you've told me" and meanwhile feel irritated towards that individual. Your irritation or any other negative emotion towards that individual will be given away by your nonverbal communication: your eyes, posture, voice tone, eye contact, space, and so forth.

Six basic suggestions for good nonverbal body language are (1) maintaining eye contact while speaking and listening, (2) keeping arms and hands open, (3) squaring up the body, (4) leaning in slightly, (5) being relaxed, and (6) having no physical barriers such as tables and podiums between the speaker and the audience. Most people maintain good eye contact when listening, and not so good when speaking. Imagine the response of someone listening to you after asking you a question that deeply concerns them, and you are looking away more than half the time. Although you may be sincere, they may judge you as being uncertain, insincere, guilty, or arrogant. A lot of that also depends on exactly where you are looking: up, down, or sideways.

Space is also an important factor in one-on-one or small-group circumstances. Generally, you want to mirror the space between you and the listeners that seems comfortable for them. They will indicate this to you very quickly based on how they approach you, or how they move relative to your movements.

Dress is another important nonverbal factor. Generally, you do not want to overdress or underdress. However, it is better to err on the overdressed rather than the underdressed side.

The field of nonverbal communications is extensive and requires good training for anyone who must communication in low trust/high concern situations. Nonverbal communications reflect your emotional state. If in any way you feel negatively towards the people with whom you are talking, you will give it away. The essential thing is not to take any of their comments personally. That is, do not internalize their comments. You should always maintain an attitude that this is not about you personally, that your job is to first understand them and then open up the doors for a dialogue so that they can better understand your knowledge.

In summary, low trust/high concern communications require skills building if one is to be effective in developing a good two-way dialogue.

REFERENCE

Covello, V. T. 1989. Communicating right-to-know information on chemical risks. *Environ. Sci. Technol.* 23:1444–1449.

CHAPTER
FOUR

VALUES AND ETHICAL CHOICES THAT UNDERLIE TOXICOLOGIC AND RISK-ANALYSIS DECISIONS

C. Richard Cothern

University of Maryland (University College), College Park, Maryland; and The George Washington University, Washington, DC

Values and ethics are seldom considered in risk assessment, and then they are thought to be only part of the risk-management section of risk analysis; most think that they do not enter the process in the science or technology of risk assessment. (Cothern, 1996) We should acknowledge this fact and act accordingly.

The generally accepted risk-analysis model is one that separates risk assessment from risk management. By implication values and ethics are thought to be included in the nonrisk, social, and political parts of the risk-management process. It is here contended that the use of values and ethics permeates all stages of the risk-analysis process including risk assessment, risk management, and especially risk communication. Values and ethics blend into the risk-analysis sequence and generally are not separated from it. Although we have known for some time that values in ethics are involved in these decisions, we have thought of them separately simply because that is the way we have done things.

No structured assessment, whether political, economic, or scientific, is normatively neutral. All analytical processes involved in risk analysis at every step contain values and ethics. It is often said that the key that opens the gates to heaven also opens the gates of hell. Thus most decisions can result in serious negative or positive consequences. Decisions are made throughout the risk-assessment process that can have significant effects on the conclusions reached.

Discussed here are the many steps involved in risk assessment and how values and ethical decisions are part of the process. The toxicologist, scientist, or researcher in these fields has to make daily decisions in the face of uncertainty and missing data that turn out often to be based on values and ethics.

VALUES IN TOXICOLOGY

Consider the development of animal bioassays. The first question is which contaminants to test. Should we test the contaminants of interest to the public, political leaders, scientists, or the media? The choice likely is based on one's values. What dose should we test? The general procedure is to start exposures at a dose that is just below one half the maximum tolerated dose. Why choose that dose? Toxicologists and others know this has to do with the amount of money available for the testing. The value here is to spend as little as possible on any one contaminant so that we can test for more contaminants. Which animal species and strain should we test for? The value here is consistency as well as saving funds. How many different doses should we test? The values involved here concern probability, statistics, and cost. How long should the study grow? Should it be for the lifetime of the animal or 90 days or 30 days? Again consistency and cost enter. Which endpoints should we look for? We value the concern of the public for cancer, and thus often we neglect the endpoints of neurotoxicology, immunotoxicology, and developmental toxicology, arguing that we have limited funds and the political pressure is to focus on cancer.

Another variable in which values are involved is the kind of exposure. Should we use oral inhalation or a dermal or gavage route of exposure in a test? In many cases this is determined by the value of who is paying for the test. If the test is required in the development of a drinking-water standard, for example, then inhalation and dermal exposure routes may not be considered.

One of the main questions in exposure analysis is what actually gets to the organ to do the damage. This is a complex question. All too often the value of cost enters, and it is assumed (another default decision) that what enters the body gets to the organ of interest. Mechanisms such as metabolism, excretion, and storage are too often ignored. Techniques such as toxicokinetics and toxicodynamics often are used to analyze the situation. But all too often there are not enough data to justify this level of sophistication. For consistency and cost reasons we assume that it all gets to the final site. If exposure to all sources including air, water, soil, dust, and food are considered, there may be too many data, and they may be too difficult to sort out. Unless a great deal care is taken, the sampling likely will be biased because of nonrepresentative collection. These biases generally reveal the values involved in deciding which data to collect. All too often there is a lack of quality assurance resulting from ignorance, concern for saving money, and the organizational characteristic or location of the quality-control officer. Another variable is the rate of exposure. This is generally assumed to be unimportant, usually because of lack of data.

Consider animal dose−response study data. As seen in Figure 4.1 data must be extrapolated into the unknown. The two stars in the upper righthand corner are the actual data. The curves on the graph show fits to that data for four well-known models. Upper error bars show the upper 95% confidence limit on these model estimates. The vertical dotted line intersects these estimates over a range of six orders of magnitude. It is most likely that the actual value is in this

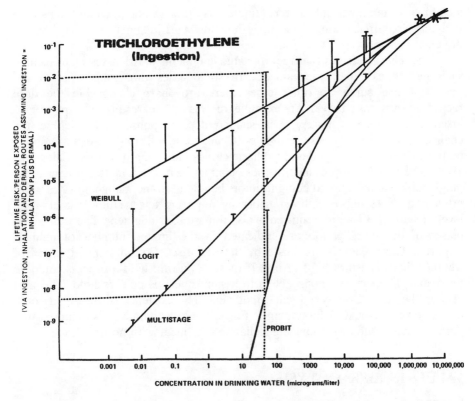

Figure 4.1 Typical dose–response curve. This curve is for drinking-water exposure of mice to trichloroethylene. The actual data are the two stars in the upper righthand corner. The lines are the most likely values from fits using the "models" indicated. The upper 95% confidence limits are shown as error bars.

large range; however, it could be outside this range. The real value could be 0, as the concentration shown could be below a threshold. Extrapolating so many orders of magnitude into the unknown is not statistically allowed, is risky, and could lead to erroneous conclusions.. Assumptions have to be made in order even to produce this figure. However the development of public policy based on extrapolation such as shown in Figure 4.1 is done without questioning the validity of such a procedure. The value involved is that we do know something and cannot afford to ignore even the limited data that are available. This reveals biases in values relating to responsibility. Another unknown is whether what happens to animals also happens to humans. The lifetimes of each are clearly different. In converting from animal to human data weight must be considered. There is not agreement as to whether this should be on the basis of body weight or surface area. Animals and humans even have different physiologies, for example the zymbal gland. Alpha-2u-globulin and peroxisome proliferators are characteristic contaminants that are different for different sexes. What does it mean if a contaminant only affects female rats? It is a value judgment to assume that this also affects female and male humans. This judgment is usually value-driven.

Other characteristics that require value judgments in risk assessment include such factors as repair mechanisms. In some cases thresholds exist in the dose–response curve. In other cases there are sharp changes in the dose recovered–response curve. An example of this is the results of exposure to arsenic, for which a hockey stick–shaped dose–response curve significantly changes the dose–response estimate (Chappell et al. 1997). Also becoming better known are U-shaped and byphasic curves indicating hormesis (Calabrese, 1994). The relative importance of these characteristics is a matter for scientific judgment in values. Should benign tumors be added to the malignant ones? This often is done to improve the statistics by requiring fewer study animals. The level of statistical validity required is also a matter of judgment. The values and biases of the investigation are indicated in the limited number of animals required. These choices are made by the scientists. Consider the situation of whether there is a threshold or not. If there is no threshold a process could be reversible. The simplest approach is to assume there is no threshold. This also errs on the side of safety—a value judgment. The existence of threshold could be based on surrogate contaminants. For example, generally it is assumed that dose–response curves for ionizing radiation are linear with no threshold.

VALUES IN RISK ANALYSIS

General

Seldom do we have scientific fact. Usually because of incomplete data and uncertainty, what are required to complete the analysis are scientific judgments and policies. For example, the assumption of a linear no-threshold dose–response curve for ionizing radiation is not based on scientific fact. It cannot be shown that such a curve does or does not exist. This policy is based on the value of safety. The idea is that a linear, no-threshold dose–response curve is probably the one that gives the highest risk. Thus, assumption of this worst-case scenario errs, if it errs, on the side of safety. Because of our ethical concerns about testing humans, we use animal data and assume that it mimics human reactions.

What about values that are involved in comparative quantitative risk assessment? How do we relate different and multiple endpoints? What is the relative importance of cancer, brain damage, immune-system problems, and developmental problems? What is the relative importance of mortality and morbidity? How do we relate one early fatality to 5000 cases of diarrhea? How do we compare effects on human beings and on the ecological system? Who cares if a fish gets diarrhea? These questions are answered by the risk analyst, sometimes with default assumptions and sometimes with value-based judgements. Seldom are they answered by scientific fact.

In general we are exposed to many different contaminants, and this variety involves potential synergisms and antagonisms. How do we combine the effects of these mixtures? Generally, it is assumed that they add up linearly. We know that in a few cases this is not true. For example, radon and cigarette smoke and asbestos and cigarette smoke have known synergistic interactions. There are a few other examples for which nonadditive effects are known. However, in general these effects are not clearly known and are not included in analyses. The default assumption of linear addition of the components of a mixture is based on ignorance.

How to avoid surprises like thalidomide? All too often there is a triumph of hope over reality in assuming that effects not tested for will not likely happen.

Decisions about what to test and when to test often involve perceptions. For example, is the contaminant natural or manmade? Many people have a dread fear of nuclear power plants. The same people are relatively unconcerned about radon, likely because it is natural in origin. Another perception or characteristic is voluntary versus involuntary. Fluoride is considered beneficial to health of teeth if applied voluntarily but can be detrimental if the exposure is involuntary, as for drinking water. Other important perception characteristics include ordinary versus catastrophic, immediate versus delayed, continuous versus delayed, controllable versus uncontrollable, old versus new, clear versus unclear, and necessary versus luxury. These values often determine what is to be tested.

In comparing risks it often is argued that one cannot compare apples and oranges. The argument goes that the risks from global climate, lead, radon, and cryptosproidium cannot be compared because they are completely different things with nothing in common. As noted in a recent *New Yorker* cartoon, apples and oranges have many similar characteristics. They are edible; have warm colors, round shapes, and similar sizes; contain seeds; grow on trees; are good for juice; have names beginning with a vowel; require similar pesticide treatment; and are unsuitable for most sports. To compare risks, however, involves judgments concerning values and ethics such as relative importance of the substances to the audience being considered and their relative knowledge of the risk being compared.

Some scientific values that are important include honesty, rationality, tolerance of diversity, freedom of inquiry, cooperation, and open communications. These values can cloud the mind of a scientist and lead to decisions about which contaminants to test, which endpoint to consider, and many of the other factors involved in a risk analysis and assessment.

Nonrisk Judgment

Ethical considerations enter risk analysis. These considerations involve determining what is right or good. For example, what is the relative value of the individual versus the group? Is it important to save just one life? Ethics has moved out of the halls of academe and now is well known to the public in such areas as abortion, clothing, animal treatment, behavior of public officials, capital punishment, and overseas killings. It is also part of risk analysis.

Uncertainty raises ethical questions that no amount of science can answer. The classical transcientific question is whether the dose–response curve for ionizing radiation is linear and has no threshold. The ethical question is what to do until science provides certainty. In considering stratospheric ozone it was decided to ban chlorofluorocarbons in spray cans long before it was known what their effects were. Currently the established causes of global climate changes are being challenged because there is not complete scientific certainty. This question has an ethical dimension. What if the earth is warming and we wait too long to do something about it?

If there is great uncertainty about the science, the social and political values have a great influence on the dose–response model or paradigm. (Sagan, 1993). For example, what should we do if there is no demonstrated causal link between a contaminant and a health endpoint being considered. For example, it only recently has been shown that there is a causal link between contaminants in tobacco smoke and lung cancer. Also, what do we do if scientists disagree? Managers often request "one-handed" scientists (who do not say, "On the other hand..."). The choices in the face of uncertainty are value-based ones. We tend to accept the scientific judgment of those we trust the most. What are some other values that we use in risk assessment that are important to us as Westerners? Some examples include democracy, equity, fairness, freedom, individual life, justice, responsibility, safety, stewardship, and trust. These all color our risk-assessment decisions.

Comparative risk analysis does not consider a number of factors. For instance the values, ethics, and perceptions of the public are not included. The uncertainty of risk and which lives are saved is not included. That we are allowed to pollute up to a given standard is not the consideration. We accept that a concentration just below the standard is safe. And who has the burden of proof is not clear.

What are some perceptions of the public that bias or color the thinking of scientists? Many fear plutonium because it has a half life of billions of years. However, all metals have an infinite half life. The public is apathetic about radon, likely because it is natural and cannot be sensed. Superfund was born because people could smell contaminants in their basements and assumed this was bad. We have abandoned the use of nuclear power in the United States because of our dread fear. We hear that dioxin is the most toxic chemical known to man. However, it is not necessarily the most toxic chemical to humans. Several years ago there was a scare about the use of alar. We stopped eating apples and apple sauce because of our concern for our children. We consider pesticides to be helpful and useful, even to the extent of thinking that if we double the application we will get twice the value. There is a perception that electromagnetic fields are dangerous, but it is unclear this time whether that is true scientifically.

An ethical issue is ignorance of science tempered by unreasoned fear. We need to consider emotions, perceptions, values, and ethical dimensions of decisions we make in the scientific arena that influence public policy.

Each of us responds in a different way to questions about risk. We are each an analyst of our own risk. The individual member of the public asks the question, is it safe? The government regulator or enforcer asks the question, what is the number? A lay person responds to risk assessments with the statement that they are only estimates. The economist or businessman asks, how much does it cost? The reporter or representative of the media asks about business news. A local government official may ask, is it feasible? A politician likely asks how does this help me? Someone interested in the broader picture or the ecological viewpoint may ask, how about the other living things? The environmentalist may ask, will one person be affected? No one seems to ask how to these risks relate to people. Thus, there is a range of views and values depending on our viewpoint.

The policy of the linear, no-threshold dose–response curve for ionizing radiation is based on the value of safety. In mandating zero discharge, the value we have used is the sanctity of the individual. Our concern for wetlands is based on our value of stewardship. Our concerns for sustainability and the importance of future generations rest on the value of responsibility. Feelings enter these questions, such as our fear of nuclear power.

CONCLUSIONS

Perhaps the most important response we can have to the knowledge that values and ethics are involved throughout the risk-assessment process is to acknowledge their presence. In our daily work we should continue to look for values and ethical decisions and consider their biasing effect on decisions, rather than either ignoring them or thinking that they are scientific.

We all should participate in discussions of values and ethics. They affect us all and are involved in many of our decisions—especially those that we make as scientists. In this regard we are as well equipped as anyone to enter this discussion.

One value that is important to consider is trust. If we can learn how to develop trust, we can be much more comfortable and open about considering the place of values and ethics in risk assessments (Fukuyama, 1995).

REFERENCES

Calabrese, E. J., ed. 1994. *Biological effects of low level exposures: Dose–response relationships*. Boca Raton, FL: Lewis Publishers.

Chappell, W. R., Beck, B. D., Brown, K. G., Chaney, R., Cothern, C. R., Irgolic, K. J., North, D. W., Thornton, I., and Tsongas, T. A. 1997. Inorganic arsenic: A need and an opportunity to improve risk assessment. *Environ. Health Perspect.* 105:1060–1067.

Cothern, C. R., ed. *Handbook for environmental risk decision-making: Values, perceptions and ethics*. Boca Raton, FL: Lewis Publishers. 1996.

Fukuyama, F. 1995. *Trust: the social virtues and creation of prosperity*. New York: The Free Press.

Sagan, L. 1994. Dose–response relationships. In *Biological effects of low level exposures*, ed. E. J. Calabrese. Boca Raton, FL: Lewis Publishers.

CHAPTER
FIVE

IMPROVING THE RISK-ASSESSMENT PROCESS

Leo G. Abood*

*Department of Pharmacology and Physiology, University of Rochester Medical Center,
Rochester, New York*

The primary objective of this book on risk assessment is to consider the interaction of nonchemical with chemical factors in the risk-assessment process. The procedure in risk assessment is to classify toxic agents with such terms as *neurotoxicants, genotoxicants, carcinogens,* and *immunotoxins.* This classification is based on data derived from dose-related studies in animals and extrapolation to humans, often from lower-level effects observed in animals. Although epidemiologic studies generally are required to establish a relationship of adverse effects to a given toxicant, the attempt is often hampered by confounding and unknown variables. Among the confounding genetic or acquired differences are toxicant sensitivity and variability in such factors as degree of exposure, age, health status, and medications.

The emergence of the so-called Gulf War syndrome, with its diversity of clinical symptoms, has elicited a number of theories attempting to account for this unexplained illness afflicting thousands of military personnel (Health Consequences, 1996). The most common symptoms reported by Persian Gulf veterans include fatigue (20%), skin rash (18%), headache (17%), muscle or joint pain (16%), memory loss (13%), shortness of breath (8%), sleep disturbances (5%), diarrhea and other gastrointestinal symptoms (4%), and chest pain (4%) (VA Persian Gulf Registry). Considering the common occurrence of such symptoms in the urban civilian population along with the environmental, psychosocial, and other factors associated with the disruptive consequences of a large-scale military deployment to a battle zone, attempts to determine the involvement of etiologic factors, particularly toxicologic, have proven difficult.

Such hypotheses include chronic fatigue syndrome, multiple chemical sensitivity (MCS), bacterial mycoplasma, infections, brainstem dysregulation syndrome, organophosphate-induced delayed neuropathy, and somatization disorder, a condition characterized by gastrointestinal, sexual, and pseudo-

*Deceased.

neurological symptoms (American Psychiatric Association, 1994). It is evident from these and many other hypotheses that multiple factors and mechanisms are involved in this unexplained illness.

Over a half century ago the term "psychosomatic medicine" was used to describe a medical discipline utilizing psychotherapy for the treatment of a variety of somatic disorders that were believed to be caused or exacerbated by psychic dysfunction. Although the term is still used and psychotherapeutic methods continue to be used in treating various somatic disorders, a new discipline, psychoneuroimmunology, has emerged whose aim is to understand the neurochemical and physiological mechanisms associated with the interaction of the nervous and immune systems in relation to somatic and psychological dysfunction.

In risk assessment, the autonomic neural state and neurohormonal state of the organism must be taken into account as important modulators of other potential risk factors, such as toxins or infectious agents. Noradrenergic and peptidergic nerve fibers, which abundantly innervate the parenchyma of both primary (bone marrow) and secondary (spleen, lymph nodes) lymphoid organs, have been implicated in the bidirectional neural immune signaling controlling the release and synthesis of lymphocytes, macrophages, and other immunocytes (Felten et al., 1993; Madden et al., 1994). Denervation or pharmacological manipulation of these neurotransmitters can profoundly alter immunological reactivity at the individual cellular level, at the level of complex multicellular interactions (such as antibody response, cytokine production, and cytotoxic T-lymphocyte activity), and at the level of host response to a disease-producing challenge. In addition to neurotransmitters and neuropeptides, lymphoid cells can secrete and synthesize neurohormones and cytokines, and stressors that act through the sympathetic nervous system and the hypothalamic–pituitary–adrenal axis can profoundly alter the course of such immune-mediated challenges as bacterial, viral, and autoimmune challenges and natural killer cell–induced tumoregenesis. The synergistic action of neurotransmitters, neurohormones, cytokines, and cytokine stimulating factors with each other suggests that a simple linear model is inadequate. Future efforts need to be directed towards discovering molecular mechanisms underlying such actions and their role in the etiology of pathology.

Among the important factors to be considered in neurotoxic risk assessment are neurobehavioral mechanisms involved in sensitivity to chemicals. The problem becomes particularly acute in dealing with humans, whose ability to function may have become compromised but who may display no definitive overt signs characteristic of a specific neurotoxic agent. In Chapter 8, Weiss discusses the issues involved in neurobehavioral testing in animals and humans exposed to neurotoxicants. Performance testing must be considered in context, taking into account such factors as changes in the shapes of distribution in an exposed population; the pattern of toxicant exposure, resulting in behavioral sensitization or tolerance; and the shortcomings of reliance on brief performance test batteries to detect delayed or more subtle adverse effects.

The term *multiple chemical sensitivity* has been used to describe a syndrome characterized by such symptoms as asthma, headaches, and depression following exposure of sensitive individuals to environmental chemicals (Overstreet et al., 1996). Although MCS may result from exposure to a broad spectrum of environmental chemicals with various toxic endpoints, the predominance of neurobehavioral symptoms observed would suggest that neurochemical and neurophysiological mechanisms are involved in the etiology of the syndrome. A number of presentations on multiple factors in risk assessment have referred to possible mechanisms for MCS. The Flinders Line rats, which were developed in Australia with increased sensitivity to diisopropyl fluorophosphate and subsequently found to be more sensitive to muscarinic agonists as well as a variety of other drugs, may serve as an experimental model for studying MCS. Because patients appear to have a greater incidence of depression both before and after onset of their chemical sensitivities, Overstreet and coworkers have postulated that cholinergic supersensitivity may be a state predisposing individuals to depressive disorders and MCS.

From results of prechallenge and postchallenge pulmonary-function tests and carbon dioxide pressure, oxygen pressure, and oxygen-saturation measurement in patients manifesting symptoms characteristic of MCS and challenged with their triggering substances, it was concluded that MCS is a manifestation of an anxiety syndrome triggered by their perceptions of environmental insult, exhibiting at least some of the symptoms induced by hyperventilation (Leznoff, 1997). Such a finding reemphasizes the need to consider psychosomatic factors and their mechanisms in MCS.

Mechanisms that have been proposed to account for the symptoms and neurobehavioral dysfunction associated with MCS and long-term potentiation, or chemical kindling, and long-term depression, which are bidirectional neurophysiological mechanisms associated with learning, memory, and seizure activity, have been shown to be involved in the action of many neurotropic drugs and neurotoxicological agents. The neurotoxicity of the anticholinesterase pesticides is discussed in terms of multiple mechanisms including those underlying long-term potentiation and depression.

Among the factors overlooked in determining the reference dose for noncarcinogenic toxic substances is the chemically induced beneficial effects resulting from low-level exposure to them. Among the factors to be considered in order to incorporate beneficial responses into the reference dose process is the dosage range over which the beneficial effects are observed; proximity of the optimal beneficial response dosage to the no-observed-adverse-effects level; and the intraspecies uncertainty factor. In contrast to the current Environmental Protection Agency practices of employing a 10-fold uncertainty factor for intraspecies variation in animal model–based RfD derivation, an uncertainty factor of 5 was more appropriate for predicting adverse effects and optimizing an agent's possible beneficial effects (Calabrese, 1996).

In order to deal with the many variables involved in risk assessment and management, computer technology and software have become indispensable and are being developed to support analysis of decisions pertaining to environmental management. Decision-support systems are computer-based systems that facilitate the use of data, models, and structured decision processes in decisions pertaining to environmental risk management. In Chapter 12, Sullivan et al. describe one such system, decision-support software, which attempts to integrate, analyze, and present environmental information for cost-effective benefit–risk characterization and assessment as well as clean-up strategies.

The chapters in this book attempt to address some the key factors that need to be considered in the development of more comprehensive, integrative methodologies to deal with the complex issues of risk assessment.

REFERENCES

American Psychiatric Association. 1994. *Diagnostic and statistical manual of mental disorders*, 4th ed. Washington, DC: Author.

Calabrese, E. J. 1996. Expanding the reference dose concept to incorporate and optimize beneficial effects while preventing toxic responses from nonessential toxicants. *Regul. Toxicol. Pharmacol.* 24:S68–75.

Health consequences of service during the Persian Gulf War: Recommendations for research and information systems. Washington, DC: National Academy Press 1997.

Leznoff, A. 1997. Provocative challenges in patients with multiple chemical sensitivity. *J. Allergy Clin. Immunol.* 99:438–442.

Overstreet, D. H., Miller, C. S., Janowsky, D. S., and Russell, R. W. 1996. Potential animal model of multiple chemical sensitivity with cholinergic supersensitivity. *Toxicology* 111:119–134.

Felten, D. L., Felten, S. Y., Bellinger, D. L., and Madden, K. S. 1993. Fundamental aspects of neural-immune signaling. *Psychother. Psychosom.* 60:46–56.

Madden, K. S., Felten, S. Y., Felten, D. L., Hardy, C. A., and Livnat, S. 1994. Sympathetic nervous system modulation of the immune system: II. Induction of lymphocyte proliferation and migration in vivo by chemical sympathectomy. *J. Neuroimmunol.* 49:67–75.

CHAPTER
SIX

IMPROVING RISK CHARACTERIZATION AT THE U.S. ENVIRONMENTAL PROTECTION AGENCY

Edward V. Ohanian

U.S. Environmental Protection Agency, Office of Water, Washington, DC

Many environmental policy decisions are based on the results of risk assessment, an analysis of scientific data on existing and projected risks to human health and the environment. Risk assessment makes use of many different kinds of scientific concepts and data, which are used to "characterize" the expected risk associated with a particular agent or action in a particular environmental context. Informed use of reliable scientific information from many different sources is a central feature of the risk-assessment process. Reliable information may or may not be available for many aspects of a risk assessment. Scientific uncertainty is a fact of life for the risk-assessment process, and risk managers must make decisions using assessments that are not as definite in all important areas as would be desirable. Therefore, they need to understand the strengths and limitations of each assessment, and to communicate this information to all participants and the public.

The 1994 National Research Council report addressed the U.S. Environmental Protection Agency's (EPA's) approach to risk assessment. According to the statement accompanying the report, "EPA's overall approach to assessing risks is fundamentally sound despite often-heard criticisms, but the Agency must more clearly establish the scientific and policy basis for risk estimates and better describe the uncertainties in its estimates of risk."

Several stakeholders in environmental issues want enough information to allow them to independently assess and make judgments about the significance of environmental risks and the reasonableness of the agency's risk reduction actions. If the EPA is to succeed and build its credibility and stature as a leader in environmental protection for the next century, it must be responsive and resolve to more openly and fully communicate to the public the complexities and challenges of environmental decision making in the face of scientific uncertainty.

The views expressed in this paper are those of the author and do not necessarily reflect the views and policies of the U.S. Environmental Protection Agency.

On March 21, 1995, EPA Administrator Carol M. Browner issued the EPA Risk Characterization Policy and Guidance addressing certain fundamental principles (U.S. EPA, 1995, 1996; Ohanian, 1995). Specifically, the agency must adopt, as values, transparency in its decision-making process and clarity in communication among all programs and with the public regarding environmental risk and the uncertainties associated with assessments of environmental risk. Also, because transparency in decision making and clarity in communication likely will lead to more external questioning of the agency's assumptions and science policies, the agency must be more vigilant about ensuring that its core assumptions and science policies are consistent and comparable across the program, are well grounded in science, and fall within a "zone of reasonableness." Each program office and each region is asked to develop program- and region-specific policies and procedures for risk characterization consistent with the core principles of transparency, clarity, consistency, and reasonableness. There have been several other activities that have emphasized and supported the EPA's risk-characterization policy by emphasizing the essential role of risk assessment and characterization in an informed decision-making process (National Research Council, 1994, 1996; American Industrial Health Council, 1995; Risk Assessment Advisory Committee, 1996; Commission on Risk Assessment and Risk Management, 1997).

RISK CHARACTERIZATION AND ENVIRONMENTAL REGULATIONS

Risk characterization is the last step in risk assessment and is also the starting point for risk-management considerations and the formulation for regulatory decision making, but it is only one of several important components in such decisions. As the last step in risk assessment, the risk characterization identifies and highlights the important risk conclusions and related uncertainties. Each environmental law administered by the EPA calls for consideration of other factors at various stages in the regulatory process. As required by different statutes, decision makers evaluate technical feasibility (e.g., treatability, detection limits) and economic, social, political, and legal factors as parts of the analysis of whether or not to regulate and, if so, to what extent. Thus, regulatory decisions usually are based on a combination of the technical analysis used to develop the risk assessment and information from other fields. For this reason, risk assessors and risk managers should understand that the regulatory decision usually is not determined solely by the outcome of the risk assessment. For decision makers, societal considerations (e.g., costs and benefits), along with the risk assessment, shape the regulatory decision and should be described as fully as the scientific information set forth in the risk characterization. Information on data sources and analyses, their strengths and limitations, confidence in the assessment, uncertainties, and alternative analyses is as important as is information on the scientific components of the regulatory decision. Decision makers should be able to expect, for example, the same level of rigor from the economic analysis as they receive from the risk assessment. Risk-management decisions involve numerous assumptions and uncertainties regarding technology, economics, and social factors, which need to be explicitly identified for the decision makers and the public.

There are two requirements for full risk characterization. First, the characterization should address qualitative and quantitative features of the assessment. Second, it should identify the important strengths and uncertainties in the assessment as part of a discussion of the confidence in the assessment. This emphasis on a full description of all elements of the assessment draws attention to the importance of qualitative, as well as quantitative, dimensions of the assessment. Particularly critical to full characterization of risk is a frank and open discussion of the uncertainty in the overall assessment and in each of its components. A discussion of uncertainty requires comment on such issues as the quality and quantity of available data, gaps in the database for specific chemicals, quality of the measured data, use of default assumptions, incomplete understanding of general biologic phenomena, and scientific judgments or science policy positions that were employed to bridge information gaps.

The risk-assessment process calls for identifying and highlighting significant risk conclusions and related uncertainties, partly to assure full communication among risk assessors and partly to assure that decision makers are fully informed. Issues are identified by acknowledging noteworthy qualitative and quantitative factors that make a difference in the overall assessment of environmental hazard and risk, and hence in the ultimate environmental regulatory decision. Information that significantly influences the analysis should be noted explicitly in all presentations of the risk assessment and in the related decision. Uncertainties and assumptions that strongly influence confidence in the risk estimate also require special attention. Numerical estimates for risk should not be separated from the descriptive information that is integral to risk characterization.

EPA RISK-CHARACTERIZATION POLICY IMPLEMENTATION EFFORTS

The 1995 EPA Risk Characterization Policy and Guidance applies to risk assessments prepared by the EPA and to risk assessments prepared by others that are used in support of EPA decisions. Assistant administrators and regional administrators are responsible for implementation of this policy within their organizational units by developing office- and region-specific policies and procedures for risk characterization that are consistent with this policy and the associated guidance. Also, Administrator Browner directed the agency's Science Policy Council (SPC) to organize agency-wide implementation activities to promote consistent interpretation of the policy, to assess the progress of implementation, and to recommend revisions to the policy, if necessary. The

SPC established an interoffice implementation team to begin the task of converting the core principles of risk-characterization policy into office- and region-specific guidance for agency risk assessors and managers. To begin to address some of the specific issues, the SPC convened a series of internal colloquia and roundtables on risk characterization. These colloquia and roundtables, held from September 1995 through September 1996, involved all levels of agency personnel in all program offices and several regions in a technical and policy dialogue about the nature and role of risk characterization at the EPA.

In addition to identifying risk-characterization issues generally, a main goal of the colloquia and roundtables was to determine whether the preliminary implementation plans were specific enough to guide the development of good risk characterizations, flexible enough to allow for differences in detail, complete enough to allow objective judgment of compliance, and organized in a way that was useful to the office or region. The colloquia and roundtables brought together multidisciplinary groups, including risk assessors and risk managers, whose different perspectives and opinions illuminated important issues involved in using the draft implementation plans. Presently, the SPC is organizing activities to follow up on suggestions that colloquia participants made to advance agency-wide implementation of the risk-characterization policy. These ongoing activities have included development of training programs for risk assessors and risk managers, preparation of model case studies illustrating the core principles, refinement of the agency's approach to implementation plans, and development of policy and guidance on the use of probabilistic analysis in risk assessments and risk characterizations.

CONCLUSION

There are a number of principles that form the basis for a risk characterization:

- Risk assessments should be transparent, in that the conclusions drawn from the science are identified separately from policy judgments, and the use of default values or methods and the use of assumptions in the risk assessment are clearly articulated.
- Risk characterization should include a summary of the key issues and conclusions of each of the other components of the risk assessment, as well as describe the likelihood of risk. The summary should include a description of the overall strengths and limitations (including uncertainties) of the assessment and conclusions.
- Risk characterization should be consistent in general format but recognize the unique characteristics of each specific situation.
- Risk characterization should include, at least in a qualitative sense, a discussion of how a specific risk and its context compares with other risks. The discussion should highlight the limitations of such comparisons.

- Risk characterization is a key component of risk communication, which is an interactive process involving exchange of information and expert opinion among individuals, groups, and institutions.

REFERENCES

American Industrial Health Council. 1995. *Advances in risk characterization.* Washington, DC: Author.

Commission on Risk Assessment and Risk Management. 1997. *Risk assessment and risk management in regulatory decision-making.* Washington, DC: U.S. Congress.

National Research Council. 1994. *Science and judgment in risk assessment.* Washington, DC: National Academy Press.

National Research Council. 1996. *Understanding risk: Informing decisions in a democratic society.* Washington, DC: National Academy Press.

Ohanian, E.V. 1995. Use of the reference dose in risk characterization of drinking water contaminants. *Human Ecol. Risk Assess.* 1:625–631.

Risk Assessment Advisory Committee. 1996. *A review of the California Environmental Protection Agency's risk assessment practices, policies, and guidelines.* Sacramento, CA: California Environmental Protection Agency, Office of Environmental Health Hazard Assessment.

U.S. Environmental Protection Agency. 1995. *Carol M. Browner's memorandum on EPA risk characterization program, March 21, 1995.* Washington, DC: Author.

U.S. Environmental Protection Agency. 1996. Proposed guidelines for carcinogen risk assessment. *Fed. Reg.* 61:17960–18011.

CHAPTER
SEVEN

MULTIPLE FACTORS IN RISK ASSESSMENT

Leo G. Abood*

Department of Pharmacology and Physiology, University of Rochester Medical Center, Rochester, New York

The aim of this chapter is to consider the interaction of nonchemical with chemical factors in the risk-assessment process, particularly concerning neurotoxicity and the role of psychological factors. The tendency in risk assessment is to classify toxic agents with such terms as *neurotoxicants*, *genotoxicants, carcinogens*, and *immunotoxins*. This classification is based on data derived from dose-related studies in animals and extrapolation to humans, generally from lower-level dose effects observed in animals. Although epidemiologic studies generally are required to establish a relationship of adverse effects to a given toxicant, the attempt often is hampered by confounding and unknown variables. Among such factors are genetic or acquired differences in toxicant sensitivity, variability in degree and conditions of exposure, age, health status, medications and prior toxicant exposure, stress, and demographic factors. The risk-assessment process is further complicated when dealing with multiple chemicals, mechanisms, and toxicologic endpoints.

MULTIPLE MECHANISMS AND FACTORS OF NEUROTOXICANTS

In attempting to characterize and analyze multiple factors in risk assessment, the focus of this chapter is on neurotoxicology. Although neurotoxicants generally are regarded as chemicals whose primary targets are the central and peripheral nervous systems, most toxicants that penetrate the blood–brain barrier are capable of producing neurologic and behavioral symptoms or toxicity. Included in the list of neurotoxicants are pesticides, organic solvents, heavy metals, food-derived toxicants, and combustion products. Pesticides, which make up the major class of neurotoxicants, have been developed to target a key enzyme, such as acetylcholine esterase or aconitase, or a neurotransmitter receptor (e.g.,

*Deceased.

strychnine-inhibiting glycine receptor); the mechanisms of organic solvents, heavy metals, and food-derived and other environmental neurotoxins generally are not well understood. Studies in animals and humans exposed to toxicants affecting the immune system, cell growth and proliferation, endocrine function, and respiration have disclosed the adverse neurobehavioral consequences resulting from broad-spectrum environmental toxicants. Any known chemical capable of producing DNA damage or affecting cell growth and proliferation and able to pass the blood–brain barrier has the potential to affect brain development, neuronal plasticity, memory, emotion, and intelligence. Among the underlying molecular mechanisms for toxicants directly or indirectly affecting neural function are inhibition of respiratory enzymes, alterations in neurotransmitter production and metabolism, changes in the density of pre- and postsynaptic neurotransmitter receptors, alterations in ion-channel density and sensitivity, changes in signal-transduction pathways regulating synaptic transmission and neuronal plasticity, and alterations in DNA and RNA replication leading to neuronal plasticity and degeneration.

By way of example, toxicants such as warfarin and related anticoagulants may affect brain function by diminishing oxygen availability and increased production of porphyrins and other hemoglobin metabolites. Although the fungicide ethylenebisdithiocarbamate has little acute toxicity, chronic exposure to its metabolite, ethylene thiourea, by decreasing thyroid function can adversely affect brain function.

MULTIPLE CHEMICAL SENSITIVITY

In recent years the problems of multiple chemical sensitivity, multiple mechanisms, and nonchemical factors in risk assessment have received considerable attention. Although it is appropriate to utilize traditional risk-assessment methodology in dealing with such toxicologic endpoints as carcinogenicity, genotoxicity, and immunotoxicity, many additional factors have to be considered in dealing with neurotoxicants, particularly at low level concentrations (Weiss, 1994). The term *multiple chemical sensitivity* has been used to describe a syndrome, characterized by such symptoms as asthma, headaches, and depression, that results from exposure of sensitive individuals to environmental chemicals (Miller, 1996). Because it appears to involve a loss of tolerance to low levels of toxic inhalants, as well as drugs and food, following single or multiple exposure to pesticides or other toxicants, the term *toxicant-induced loss of tolerance* is more descriptive. Although multiple chemical sensitivity may result from exposure to a broad spectrum of environmental chemicals with various toxic endpoints, the predominance of neurobehavioral symptoms observed would suggest that neurochemical and neurophysiologic mechanisms are involved in the etiology of the syndrome. One mechanism that has been proposed to account for the symptoms and neurobehavioral dysfunction associated with multiple chemical sensitivity is long-term potentiation (LTP), or chemical kindling (Rossi, 1996).

LONG-TERM POTENTIATION AND LONG-TERM DEPRESSION IN RISK ASSESSMENT

Long-term potentiation and long-term depression (LTD), which are bidirectional neurophysiological mechanisms associated with learning, memory, and seizure activity, have been shown to be involved in the action of many neurotropic drugs and toxicants (Weiss et al., 1995). They also have been invoked as mechanisms in the impairment of hippocampus-dependent memory resulting from psychological stress (Diamond et al., 1996). LTP can be observed experimentally as a persistent electrophysiologic change in such brain regions as the hippocampus, amygdala, and visual cortex following brief high-frequency (60-Hz) electrical stimulation or the administration of subconvulsant doses of convulsant or other drugs. A model for the induction of LTP and LTD in CA3 synapses of the hippocampus is presented in Figure 7.1 (Nakanish, 1996). The LTP cascade is initiated by NMDA (gluaminergic)–receptor activation (Bliss and Collingridge, 1993) and release of intracellular Ca^{2+} followed by activation of a calmodulin-dependent adenylate cyclase (Liedo et al., 1995), leading to the production of cAMP and stimulation of protein kinase A. LTD, which occurs following repetitive low-frequency (1-Hz) stimulation for 10 to 15 min, (Goddard et al., 1969; Weiss et al., 1995, 1997) is under the control of a metabotropic glutaminergic G-protein–coupled receptor negatively regulating cAMP

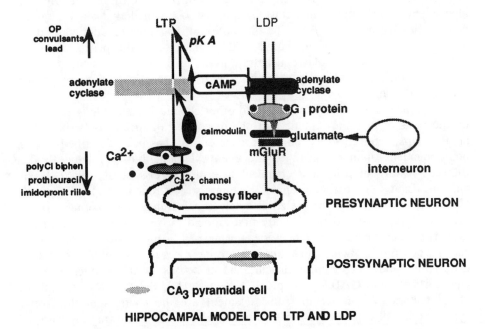

Figure 7.1 A model for long-term potentiation (LTP) and long-term depression (LTD) in the mossy fiber of the hippocampus. *pKA*, phosphoprotein kinase A; mGluR, metabotropic glutaminergic receptor; G_i, G-protein inhibiting adenylate cyclase, OP, organophosphate pesticides.

production (Yokol et al., 1996). Although LTP and LTD primarily involve the amygdala, hippocampus, and other limbic structures, the afterdischarges can spread to cortical and other brain areas, resulting in disverse neurobehavioral changes.

EFFECT OF NEUROTOXIC AGENTS ON LONG-TERM POTENTIATION (KINDLING)

Chronic exposure to neurotoxins may lead to prolonged changes in the excitability of various neural pathways, resulting in brain dysfunction and increased sensitivity to neurotropic agents. Repeated administration of low doses of lindane or endosulfan has been shown to lead to the development of persistent seizures in rats by inducing amygdala LTP (Gilbert and Mack, 1995). Another study revealed that 3-3'-iminodipropionitrile, which disrupts cognitive function and induces astrogliosis in the brain, impairs amygdala kindling (Gilbert and Llorens 1993). Propylthiouracil, which suppresses thyroid along with cognitive function, also has been reported to inhibit LTP (Niemi et al., 1996). LTP in the visual cortex of adult rats also was inhibited following exposure to polychlorinated biphenyls during embryonic development (Altmann et al., 1995). The direct involvement of acetylcholinesterase in LTP was established by demonstrating that the application of acetycholinesterase, but not butyrylcholinesterase, produces LTP in hippocampal neurons. Because this effect could be blocked by a glutamate antagonist it appears to be mediated via excitatory amino acids (Appleyard, 1995). The diminution of cognitive function caused by lead in children has been attributed to LTP blockade in the pyriform cortex, occurring at low micromolar concentrations of lead that were without effect on postsynaptic NMDA-receptor activation or presynaptic calcium responses (Carpenter et al., 1994).

Tolerance or sensitivity to drugs and other chemicals generally is explained on the basis of pharmacokinetic and pharmacodynamic mechanisms; however, another type, referred to as "contingent" tolerance, has been described that is not dependent upon exposure to the chemical alone but is related to the subject's history of drug and chemical exposure (Weiss et al., 1995). If an anticonvulsant (e.g., carbamazepine) is administered repeatedly to amygdala-kindled rats prior to inducing seizures by electrical stimulation, tolerance to the drug develops rapidly. If the rats are first kindled for several days or given the drug after each seizure, tolerance does not develop. Among the neurochemical changes accompanying amygdala kindling are increases in mRNA of enkephalin, dynorphin, and thyrotropin-releasing hormone as well as increases in glucocorticoid and $GABA_A$ receptors (Rosen et al., 1992; Weiss et al., 1995). Other factors to consider in risk assessment are the changes in the liver's concentration of cytochrome P450 caused by alcohol and following exposure to such xenobiotics as pesticides, nitrosamines, polycyclic aromatic hydrocarbons, and halogenated hydrocarbons. Any one toxicant by modulating the expression of cytochrome P450 enzymes can increase the toxicological impact of a variety of other toxic agents (Raucy, 1995).

MULTIPLE MECHANISMS IN THE NEUROTOXICITY OF ORGANOPHOSPHATE INSECTICIDES

Several reports have suggested that exposure to organophosphate pesticides damages the visual system. The prolonged effects of an acute dose of fenthion (dimethyl 3-methyl-4-methylthiophenyl phosphorothionate) were studied on the cholinergic system of the rat retina. Following the administration of a single dose of fenthion to Long-Evans rats, a long-lasting decrease in carbachol-stimulated inositol-phosphate (IP_3) release was observed in the retina, but not in the frontal cortex (Tandon et al., 1994). IP_3 release was depressed at 4 days, and this depression persisted up to 56 days, when the recovery of brain and retinal cholinesterase was almost complete. Fenthion produced 89% inhibition of cholinesterase activity in both tissues at 4 days, and, although there was recovery, slight (15%) inhibition of the enzyme activity was still observed at 56 days in both tissues. Because IP_3 inhibition was observed despite a decrease in the density of muscarinic cholinergic receptor, increased sensitization of cholinergic receptors could not account for the persistent IP_3 inhibition. Thus, this long-lasting perturbation in the retinal cholinergic second-messenger system induced by fenthion may occur independently of depressed cholinesterase activity and down-regulation of muscarinic cholinergic receptor.

The repetitive calcium oscillations associated with neuronal excitability are initiated by phospholipase C–mediated production of IP_3 and generated by a positive feedback mechanism in which calcium potentiates its own release and a negative feedback mechanism terminating calcium release, followed by a slow recovery process between calcium spikes. Possible negative feedback mechanisms accounting for the persistent decrease in IP_3 by fenthion include decreased phospholipase C levels or kinetics as a consequence of decreased tyrosine phosphorylation (Puceat and Vassort, 1996) or degradation of the enzyme by cysteine protease (Wojcikiewicz, 1996). Other mechanisms could involve decreased affinity of the IP_3 receptor resulting from diminished tyrosine phosphorylation (Jayaraman, 1996) or a persistent increase in protein kinase C activity, resulting in inhibition of receptor-evoked IP_3 formation (Willems et al., 1995).

With the use of rat strains that were either hyposensitive or hypersensitive to cholingeric agonists, it was shown that pretreatment with organophosphate pesticides sensitized the hypersenstive rats to treatment with a wide variety of psychotropic agents, including cholinomimetics, caffeine, and cocaine (Overstreet et al., 1996). The use of such strains of rats provides a methodology for investigating the phenomenon of multiple chemical sensitivity.

The spontaneous retinal degeneration occurring in the transgenic mouse has been attributed to the increased turnover of retinal cyclic GMP phosphodiesterase (Farber et al., 1988). It also has been reported that phosphodiesterase inhibitors produce electroretinographic changes in the isolated perfused cat's eye that are similar to changes associated with retinitis (Sandberg et al., 1987). In assessing the visual toxicity of the organophosphate pesticides and other toxicants one needs to consider the systemic effects of a subject's medications. Most classes of drugs are capable of producing toxic effects on striated muscle, secretory–resorption organs, epithelial membranes, retinaganglion, or pigment layers, which can result in morphologic and function visual changes (Fraunfelder and Meyer, 1989). Included in such medications are the antimalarials, antineoplastics, immunosuppressants, antirheumatics, and phenothiazines. Although most of the effects tend to be reversible on discontinuing medication, information on the possible interactions in the visual system of toxicants and various medications is not available.

It has been reported that the administration of 20 mg/kg/d of fenthion for 30 days decreased the number of GABA-positive cells in the lateral geniculate nucleus and pretectal nuclei, a finding that suggests that the reduction of GABA-positive cells may be associated with the abnormal eye movements in human organophosphate-pesticide intoxication (Kojima et al., 1993).

With the use of a cell-cloning assay involving mutants of the *hprt* (hypoxanthine phosphoribosyl transferase) gene, it was reported that exposure of human T lymphocytes to concentrations of malathion ranging from 10 to 600 μg/ml resulted in mutations within specific region of the *hrpt* gene (Pluth et al., 1996). The *hrpt* gene has been used widely for the study of DNA damage induced by cytotoxic agents. Further studies are needed to determine the underlying molecular mechanism for these deletions and how this may relate to agricultural workers' increased risk of cancer.

PSYCHOLOGICAL FACTORS IN RISK ASSESSMENT

In addition to the mechanisms underlying the adverse effects of neurotoxicants, one needs to consider the psychological factors contributing to the symptomatology associated with environmental exposure to chemicals. Over a half century ago the term "psychosomatic medicine" was used to describe a medical discipline utilizing psychotherapy for the treatment of a variety of somatic disorders that were believed to be caused or exacerbated by psychic dysfunction. Although the term still is used in assessing the role of anxiety in somatic disorders (Wientjes and Grossman, 1994) and psychotherapeutic methods continue to be used in treating various somatic disorders, a new discipline, psychoneuroimmunology, has emerged whose aim is to understand the neurochemical and physiological mechanisms associated with the interaction of the nervous and immune systems in relation to somatic and psychological dysfunction (Ader et al., 1995). This new discipline, which is among the topics of this book, promises to provide fresh insights into our understanding of the multiple chemical and mechanistic aspects of risk assessment.

REFERENCES

Ader, R., Cohen, N., and Felten, D. 1995. Psychoneuroimmunology: Interactions between the nervous system and the immune system. *Lancet* 345:99–103.

Altmann, L., Weinand-Haerer, A., Lilienthal, H., and Wiegand, H. 1995. Maternal exposure to polychlorinated biphenyls inhibits long-term potentiation in the visual cortex of adult rats. *Neurosci. Lett.* 202:53–56.

Appleyard, M. E. 1995. Acetylcholinesterase induces long-term potentiation in CA1 pyramidal cells by a mechanism dependent on metabotropic glutamate receptors. *Neurosci. Lett.* 190:25–28.

Bliss, T. V., and Collingridge, G. L. 1993. A synaptic model of memory: Long-term potentiation in the hippocampus. *Nature* 361:31–39.

Carpenter, D. O., Matthews, M. R., Parsons, P. J., and Hori, N. 1994. Long-term potentiation in the piriform cortex is blocked by lead. *Cell Molec. Neurobiol.* 14:723–733.

Diamond, D. M., Fleshner, M., Ingersoll, N., and Rose, G. M. 1996. Psychological stress impairs spatial working memory: Relevance to electrophysiological studies of hippocampal function. *Behav. Neurosci.* 110:661–672.

Farber, D. B., Park, S., Yamashita, C. 1988. Cyclic GMP-phosphdiesterase in *rd* retina. *Exp. Eye Res.* 46:363–374.

Fraunfelder, F. T., and Meyer, S. M. 1989. *Drug-induced ocular side effects and their drug interactions*, 3rd ed. Philadephia: Lea and Febiger.

Gilbert, M. E., and Mack, C. M. 1995. Seizure thresholds in kindled animals are reduced by the pesticides lindane and endosulfan. *Neurotoxicol. Teratol.* 17:143–150.

Gilbert, M. E., and Llorens, J. 1993. Delay in the development of amygdala kindling following treatment with 3, 3'-iminodipropionitrile. *Neurotoxicol. Teratol.* 15:243–250.

Goddard, L. S., Nclntyre, D. C., and Leech, C. K. 1969. A permanent change in brain function resulting from daily electrical stimulation. *Exp. Neurol.* 25:295–300.

Jayaraman, T., Ondrias, K., Ondriasova E., and Marks, A.R. 1996. Regulation of the inositol 1, 4, 5-trisphosphate receptor by tyrosine phosphorylation. *Science* 272:1492–1494.

Kojima, Y., Sekiya, H., and Ishikawa, S. 1993. The effect of organophosphorus pesticide (fenthion) on GABA-cells in the central nuclei. *Nippon Ganka Gakkai Zasshi—Acta Societatis Ophthalmologicae Japonicae* 97:50–57.

Lledo, P. M., Hjelmstad, G. O., Mukherji, S., Soderling, T. R., Malenka, R. C., and Nicoll, R. A. 1995. Calcium/calmodulin-dependent kinase II and long-term potentiation enhance synaptic transmission by the same mechanism. *Proc. Natl. Acad. Sci. U.S.A.* 92:11175–11179.

Miller, C. S. 1996. Chemical sensitivity: Symptom, syndrome or mechanism for disease? *Toxicology* 111:69–86.

Nakanishi, S. 1997. The metabotropic glutamate receptor and hippocampal mossy fiber long term-depression. *IBRO News* 25:6.

Niemi, W. D., Slivinski, K., Audi, J., Rej, R., and Carpenter, D. O. 1996. Propylthiouracil treatment reduces long-term potentiation in area CA1 of neonatal rat hippocampus. *Neurosci. Lett.* 210:127–129.

Overstreet, D. H., Miller, C. S., Janowsky, D. S., and Russell, R. W. 1996. Potential animal model of multiple chemical sensitivity with cholinergic supersensitivity. *Toxicology* 111:119–124.

Pluth, J. M., Nicklas, J. A., O'Neill, J. P., and Albertini, R. J. 1996. Increased frequency of specific genomic deletions resulting from in vitro malathion exposure. *Cancer Res.* 56:2393–2399.

Puceat, M., and Vassort, G. 1996. Purinergic stimulation of rat cardiomyocytes induces tyrosine phosphorylation and membrane association of phospholipase C gamma: A major mechanism for InsP3 generation. *Biochem. J.* 318:723–728.

Raucy, J. L. 1995. Risk assessment: Toxicity from chemical exposure resulting from enhanced expression of CYP2E1. *Toxicology* 105:217–224.

Rosen, J. B., Cain, C. J., Weiss, S. R., and Post, R. M. 1992. Alterations in mRNA of enkephalin, dynorphin and thyrotropin releasing hormone during amygdalakindling: An in situ hybridization study. *Molec. Brain Res.* 15:247–255.

Rossi, J. III 1996. Sensitization induced by kindling and kindling-related phenomena as a model for multiple chemical sensitivity. *Toxicology* 111:87–100.

Sandberg, M. A., Pawlyk, B. S. and Crane, W. G. 1987. Effects of IBMX on the ERgG of the isolated perfuces eye. *Vision Res.* 27:1421.

Tandon, P., Padilla, S., Barone, S., Pope, C. N., and Tilson, H. A. 1994. Fenthion produces a persistent decrease in muscarinic receptor function in the adult rat retina. *Toxicol. Appl. Pharmacol.* 125:271–280.

Weiss, B. 1994. Low-level chemical sensitivity: A perspective from behavioral toxicology. *Toxicol. Ind. Health* 10:605–617.

Weiss, S. R. B., Clark, M., Rosen, J. B., Smith, M. A., and Post, R. M. 1995. Contingent tolerance to the anticonvulsant effects of carbamzepine: Relationship to loss of endogenous adaptive mechanisms. *Brain Res. Rev.* 20:305–325.

Weiss, S. R. B., Kiu-Li, L., Heynen, T., Noguera, E. C., Li, H., and Post, R. M. 1997. Kindling and quenching: Conceptual links to rTMS. *C N S Spectrums* 2:32–40.

Wientjes, C. J., and Grossman, P. 1994. Overreactivity of the psyche or the soma? Interindividual associations between psychosomatic symptoms, anxiety, heart rate, and end-tidal partial carbon dioxide pressure. *Psychosom. Med.* 56:533–540.

Willems, P. H., Smeets, R. L., Bosch, R. R., Garner, K. M., Van Mackelenbergh, M. G., and De Pont, J. J. 1995. Protein kinase C activation inhibits receptor-evoked inositol trisphosphate formation andinduction of cytosolic calcium oscillations by decreasing the affinity-state of the cholecystokinin receptor in pancreatic acinar cells. *Cell Calcium* 18:471–483.

Wojcikiewicz, R. J. H., and Oberdorf, J. A. 1996. Degradation of inositol 1,4,5-trisphosphate receptors during cell stimulation is a specific process mediated by cysteine protease activity. *J. Biol. Chem.* 271:16652–16655.

Yokoi, M., Kobayashi, K., Manabe, T., Takahashi, T., Sakaguchi, I., Katsuura, G., Shigemoto, R., Ohishi, H., Nomura, S., Nakamura, K., Nakao, K., Katsuki, and Nakanishi, S. 1996. Impairment of hippocampal mossy fiber LTD in mice lacking mGluR2. *Science* 273:645–647.

CHAPTER
EIGHT

ENVIRONMENTAL FACTORS MODIFYING SENSITIVITY TO CHEMICALS

Bernard Weiss

Department of Environmental Medicine, University of Rochester School of Medicine and Dentistry,
Rochester, New York

The program of the Society of Toxicology's annual meeting is a huge banquet of topics in almost bewildering variety. A casual observer would find it impossible to discern any unifying theme in all the profusion. Nor can any single toxicologist hope to master more than a small slice of this diverse discipline. Still, toxicology is ruled by an underlying unity because virtually all toxicologists subscribe to a common premise: dose determines response; or, put in more vivid terms, "the dose makes the poison." This principle is the glue that holds the discipline together. Only secondary prominence is accorded a related principle: Organisms vary in their sensitivity to chemicals; or, as we might put it, "the individual defines the response."

This secondary premise is not ignored in toxicology but serves as a kind of background vista. It is embedded in regulatory practices such as the calculation of allowable daily intakes (ADIs) and reference doses (RfDs). These values take explicit account of individual differences by applying safety or uncertainty factors (UFs) designed to embrace wide variations in population sensitivity. For example, a no-observed-adverse-effect level (NOAEL) observed in an animal study may be divided by a UF of 100. A factor of 10 presumably accounts for species differences, and an additional factor of 10 is designed to compensate for individual differences among humans. The implicit assumption, not directly stated, is that these variations are primarily intrinsic to the organism.

Genetic variations in sensitivity have always been accepted and investigated as contributing factors to toxicity. Advances in molecular biology are now prompting a search for more definitive connections; the new Environmental Genome Project of the National Institute of Environmental Health Sciences aims to identify functionally important polymorphisms that modulate the health risks of exposure to environmental agents.

Such presumed congenital variations in sensitivity far overshadow, in scientific visibility, potential environmental determinants. The latter are not trivial: Consider the role of diet in cancer. An emphasis on genetic characteristics need not wholly exclude extrinsic circumstances; the possibility of gene–environment interactions in the determination of toxicity is recognized explicitly in the Human Genome Project. The tenet that genes do not act in isolation is accepted readily in the behavioral sciences, where the relative contributions of genetic and environmental factors to measures such as intelligence quotient (IQ) foster an unending debate. But even those holding antithetical positions in this debate concede that the interplay of these two factors ultimately governs outcome. They simply disagree on the magnitude of each contribution.

Toxicology and risk assessment have not entertained an equivalent debate on any comparable scale. Although none of their practitioners would deny the critical contribution of environmental determinants, in practice they have assigned them a relatively insubstantial role. Neurobehavioral toxicology, however, out of necessity and history, found itself unable to ignore environmental determinants a long time ago. This article examines three examples of how environmental factors regulate the response to toxic challenges: maternal cigarette smoking and offspring intelligence-test scores; behavioral performance in a space vehicle; and the Gulf War syndrome.

DETERMINANTS OF DEVELOPMENTAL NEUROTOXICITY

Intelligence, in the form of IQ scores, is an arena around which much of this argument about the relative influence of environmental and toxic variables has swirled, with lead occupying center stage. After the seminal publication by Needleman et al. (1979) that documented a correlation between dentin lead and IQ in young children, investigators have been compelled to consider all of the other factors, or covariates, that might influence IQ. Some of these are congenital: for example, maternal IQ (although that measure might itself be confounded with earlier maternal exposures). Others are more strictly environmental: for example, family socioeconomic status and the kinds of interactions in which the mother engages with the child. The criteria for selecting and applying covariates have differed among investigators. Especially for the many prospective studies that succeeded Needleman et al., the choice of which possible confounders to include in the multiple regression analyses that typify this literature evokes incessant argument (cf., Bellinger, 1995).

The vehemence of some of these discussions tends to entrap investigators into a kind of statistical paralysis; sometimes the main goal of many analyses seems to be to strip away all conceivable influences other than that of the agent itself. Such a quest for toxic purity cannot be fulfilled. Different environments provide different settings in which toxic properties vary in expression. In common with research on genetic predispositions, different arrays or combinations of environmental variables might govern dose–response functions in ways that are not readily apparent with conventional analyses. One strategy is to appraise them in much the same way we attempt to study combinations of environmental and genetic factors.

Most of the studies conducted to assess the contribution of lead to IQ scores explicitly attend to the setting in which the child is raised. Instruments such as the Home Observation for Measurement of the Environment (HOME) scales are used widely to gauge what are considered to be key factors. The HOME interview protocol evaluates conditions such as how the mother (or caregiver) responds to the child, the kinds of stimulation she provides, the presence of books and other academic materials, and many other aspects of the child's customary environment. Inclusion of HOME scores in multiple regression analyses recognizes that genetic endowment and toxicant exposure alone cannot account for IQ scores completely, and that many external elements wield significant influence.

One question has been mostly ignored so far in this literature: Can it be shown that modifying presumed environmental influences also modifies the expression of toxicity? Bellinger (1995) asks this question in another fashion: What contextual factors are responsible for the response of the "experimental system," namely, the child? Or, stated in another form, should investigators examine how risk factors combine with toxic exposures to determine susceptible populations? In their eagerness to isolate the effects of toxicants, might investigators have thrust aside some crucial synergistic or antagonistic interactions with environmental variables? Has this question has been submerged by the resolve of investigators to quantify the unencumbered, "pure" contribution of agents such as lead, ethanol, polychlorinated biphenyls, and others that alter the process of brain development?

A compelling example of how environmental factors can modify the consequences of toxic exposure comes from research on tobacco. Maternal smoking during pregnancy elevates the risk of mental retardation and attention-deficit hyperactivity disorder in the offspring and tends to lower their IQ scores. Olds et al. (1994) set out originally to assess the effectiveness of intervention in mostly young, unmarried, and poor mothers in a semirural community. Their primary aim was not to study smoking, but to determine if monitoring and education by visiting nurses and expanded medical care might reduce adverse birth outcomes and compensate for the generally unpromising environment in which the children developed.

The sample of about 350 families was assigned to one of four treatments. Two of the the treatments consisted primarily of pediatric screening at 12 and 24 months of age. Two treatments called for home visits by nurses during pregnancy or during both pregnancy and the first 2 years of life. The nurses worked with the mothers to improve health-related behaviors and to obtain various community services.

The children of smoking mothers (10 or more cigarettes per day) who received no or minimal intervention obtained significantly lower (4.35 points) scores on intelligence tests at 3 and 4 years of age than the children of mothers who did not smoke. The children of smoking mothers assigned to intervention

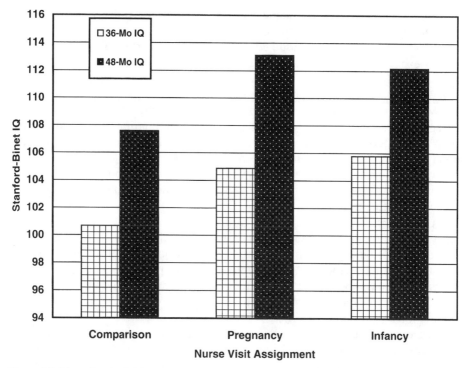

Figure 8.1 Mean Stanford–Binet intelligence quotient (IQ) scores, at 36 and 48 months of age, of children of smoking mothers subjected to different kinds of intervention. The comparison groups received no nurse visits. The other groups received visits either during pregnancy alone or during both pregnancy and the first 2 years of life. Based on data from Olds et al. (1994).

exhibited scores averaging 4.86 points higher than the children of mothers not assigned to nurse visits, bringing them into the nonsmoking range. Figure 8.1, based on Olds et al. (1994), shows how behavioral interventions altered the response to toxicant exposure. The authors speculated that the effects of intervention might have arisen from a variety of causes. Among them they cite some reduction in number of cigarettes smoked and improved nutrition.

Results such as these embody a clear lesson. If we simply investigate, in our usual way, a postulated relationship between a chemical exposure and a single endpoint by clearing away all the possible "confounders," we may lose totally or submerge the most significant guides to risk. Techniques such as path analysis (Dietrich et al., 1997) offer a conduit to the determination of potential intervening variables; for example, lowered birth weights induced by maternal lead exposure helped explain lowered IQ scores in the offspring of mothers with the higher lead levels. But even path analysis is not a sufficient risk-analysis tool if the answers to our questions lie, say, in examining the impact of prenatal lead exposure on children whose families occupy low socioeconomic status and whose

Table 8.1 Hypothetical depression of IQ scores resulting from combinations of maternal smoking and family poverty status

	Poverty status	
	Yes	No
Smoking status		
Yes	High	Medium
No	Medium	Low

parents smoke. Such a deconstruction is possible but rarely attempted. Consider some of the risks to development prevailing in certain environments:

- Toxic chemicals
- Poverty income
- Inadequate schools
- Poor nutrition
- Teen-age pregnancy
- Disrupted family structure
- Poor maternal education
- Maternal smoking
- High violence index

Table 8.1 is a simple, hypothetical representation of this argument. It is designed to show how an observer might rate the potential interactions of maternal smoking and family economic status. The example was chosen because both conditions are known to be associated with lowered IQ scores.

MULTIPLE DETERMINANTS OF PERFORMANCE

A different perspective on the question of environmental context is based on the kind of situation faced by astronauts. In contrast to the chronic health hazards, such as cancer, that dominate terrestrial workplace criteria, space crews have one overriding task: to complete their mission and return safely. The main health hazard is diminished performance. Emergence of a chronic disease 30 years after a mission is not a fear that arouses much apprehension.

Volatile organic solvents such as toluene, a documented neurotoxicant, are one of the potential threats to performance in the space-vehicle environment (Rahill et al., 1996). Toluene has been detected on many space-shuttle missions because it is released from wall panels and other structural components. Workplace standards for solvents, such as threshold limit values (TLVs), are based mostly on neurotoxicity, in fact. Space environments, in contrast to terrestial workplaces, expose the occupants continuously rather than during an

70 TOXICOLOGY IN RISK ASSESSMENT

8-hour day, so that space maximal acceptable concentrations (SMACs) tend to be lower than industrial standards. The space environment also contains many unique and additional challenges to optimal performance. These make it imprudent to try to evaluate the effects of solvents in isolation. A more judicious strategy would be to determine the performance effects of solvents in a setting that mimics features of the space environment.

Figure 8.2 describes what might be termed a *layered risk model*. It is designed to mirror the cumulative impact of some of those elements in a space environment that might diminish performance competence. Solvents in isolation may reduce performance by a small amount. Introduce physical activity, which in essence raises exposure levels (Rahill et al., 1996), and these effects are enhanced. Sleep–wake cycles in space could be radically disrupted, which almost surely adds to or multiplies the baseline effects of solvent exposure. An example of such performance effects is the sharp rise in the incidence of traffic accidents during the period of our diurnal cycle when we customarily are asleep. Respiratory infections, passed from one crew member to another, and consequent immune-system responses may further depress performance; cytokines released by the immune system are well-documented neurotoxicants. Adjustments to microgravity, and drugs taken for motion sickness during certain phases of a mission, inject further possibilities for performance degradation.

In extrapolating to a realistic scenario, experimental research on solvents in isolation provides a rather constricted perspective on what the results could

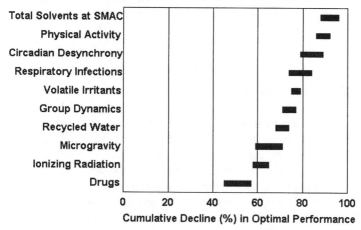

Figure 8.2 Layered risk model of challenges to performance faced by space crews. Each bar represents a range of hypothetically diminished performance imposed by the indicated condition or stressor. Each is positioned to indicate hypothetical overlap with another stressor. SMAC, space maximum acceptable concentration.

mean for a space crew. Low ambient levels of organic solvents in a terrestrial environment might degrade performance slightly or not at all. In combination with sleep disruption and other stresses, even on earth, the joint effects might be considerable; note the potent contribution to traffic accidents of the conjunction of alcohol and sleep disruption. The total setting determines toxicity; weighing its components separately distorts our judgments of risk.

GULF WAR AND OTHER CHEMICAL-SENSITIVITY SYNDROMES

Several thousand veterans of the Persian Gulf War now complain of a collection of health problems labeled as *Gulf War syndrome*. It includes symptoms of fatigue, weakness and malaise, skin rash, headache, respiratory difficulties, and cognitive deficits. Not every veteran with this disorder offers the same complaints to the same degree. Because this group consists mainly of previously healthy males, facile explanations of the type often applied to multiple chemical sensitivity (MCS) such as hysteria, malingering, depression, somatization, or others of the psychiatric labels frequently offered as explanations have not attracted many adherents.

Partial results of a survey comparing deployed and nondeployed troops appear in Figure 8.3 (Centers for Disease Control, 1995). Participating troops from this sample, taken from four different units, showed much higher prevalence rates for these and other symptoms than those not deployed. Of the total of 13 symptoms assayed in the survey, seven referred to nervous-system dysfunction.

Since the original description of the syndrome, many toxic agents have been postulated to explain it. These include fumes and smoke from oil-well fires,

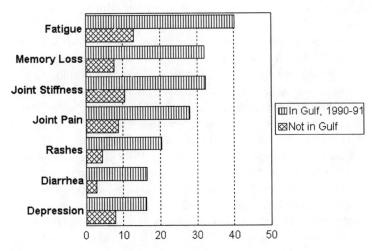

Figure 8.3 Percentage of Gulf War troops reporting chronic health problems, based on a sample size of 3927. Based on Centers for Disease Control (1995).

diesel fumes, toxic paints, pesticides, depleted uranium, vaccines, drugs, microbial infections, anticholinesterase agents, and biological weapons. Anticholinesterase war gases have been more convincingly implicated by recently unearthed reports, but they would account, at most, for only a minority of the veterans with the syndrome. Pyridostigmine, administered as a prophylactic agent, also has been offered as possibility.

Gulf War syndrome also has been conjectured as a form of post–traumatic stress disorder or an immune-system disorder. The evidence for these hypotheses is ambiguous. No single factor or exposure, by itself, currently seems sufficient to carry the entire explanatory load for all veterans claiming to be afflicted. Most observers now seem to accept the conclusion that Gulf War syndrome reflects the actions of multiple factors whose expression varies from individual to individual.

Such diversity can be enveloped by one explanation only by acknowledging multiple etiologies and expression and devising a scheme by which they might be unified in a conceptual model. A quasistatistical model offers a useful perspective.

In their customary environments, both U.S. regular troops and reserves varied widely in their sensitivity to environmental and other stressors even before deployment to the Gulf. In a population that large, some small proportion, even without additional stressors or challenges, would be displaying some adverse symptoms. As a basis for discussion, assume also that the troops displayed a normal (Gaussian) distribution of sensitivity to the environmental agents and other stressors prevailing in those environments. For example, assume that only those individuals beyond 2.5 SDs, from the mean display detectable sensitivity. Suppose, in addition, that the ambient levels of these agents and stressor intensities undergo slight shifts. Assume, for instance, that under these new circumstances the mean distribution of sensitivity is displaced by 0.5 SD. Now, individuals beyond 2.0 SDs fall into the "sensitive" category. Even a slight shift would greatly expand the number of individuals in the sensitive zone, as seen in Figure 8.4. With normal distributions, a shift in the mean exerts a disproportionate effect at the tails of the distribution. In the example here, the proportion of sensitive individuals rises from 0.62% to 2.28%. For a population of 700,000, the number of persons with detectable health problems would increase from 4340 to 15,960 individuals. This kind of statistical explanation could account for the prominence of the Gulf War syndrome. Before deployment, those at the extremes of the sensitivity distribution would have escaped these problems in their accustomed environments. After deployment, they found themselves displaced into the sensitive-responder range because of exposure to higher levels of contaminants and other stressors than they had experienced prior to the Gulf War. As in the space environment, multiple deficits could have accumulated in the kind of cascade modeled by Figure 8.2. None, singly, would have exerted any substantial influence. Should the Gulf War syndrome be primarily immunologic in character, such cumulative

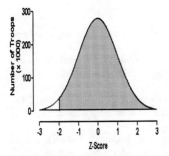 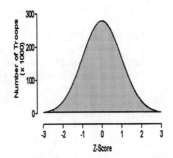

Figure 8.4 The distribution on the right shows the area (light) occupied by individuals who would be labeled as "sensitive" if sensitivity is defined as functioning at a level less than 2.5 SD from the mean. The distribution on the left shows the area that would be occupied by "sensitive" individuals if the mean of the distribution were to be shifted to the left by 0.5 SD.

effects could have shifted enough of the population into the dysfunctional range to account for the phenomenon.

EPILOGUE

Toxicity is more than a reflection of the intrinsic properties of a chemical agent, although we may tend to describe it in such terms. We all recognize that individuals vary in sensitivity and take account of this variability in calculations and regulatory standards. What is not explicitly acknowledged about variations among individuals is the contribution of extrinsic rather than intrinsic determinants. Three examples were discussed: (1) the assessment of developmental neurotoxicity, with outcomes typically calibrated by multiple regression analysis in which covariates are peeled away to reveal a presumably unencumbered measure of toxic potency. Although covariates can act in concert with toxic exposures, analyses of such joint dependencies are usually not performed; (2) a situation in which the integrity of performance is determined by many different factors, both additive and multiplicative, able to modulate the response to a neurotoxicant as a totality; and (3) the Gulf War syndrome, for which explanations might be sought not in specific agents or variables, but in a small shift in the sensitivity of a population. All three examples accentuate how environmental factors, intertwined with individual susceptibility, moderate the response to toxic challenges.

ACKNOWLEDGMENT

Preparation supported in part by NIEHS Center Grants ES01247, ES0819, and ES08958.

REFERENCES

Bellinger, D. C. 1995. Interpreting the literature on lead and child development: The neglected role of the "experimental system." *Neurotoxicol. Teratol.* 17:201–212.

Centers for Disease Control. 1995. Unexplained illness among Persian Gulf War veterans in an Air National Guard unit: Preliminary report—August 1990–March 1995. *MMWR Morb. Mortal. Wkly. Rep.* 44:443–447.

Dietrich, K., Krafft, K., Bornschein, R., Hammond, P., Berger, O., Succop, P., and Bicr, M. 1987. Low-level fetal lead exposure effect on neurobehavioral development in early infancy. *Pediatrics* 80:721–730.

Needleman, H. L., Gunnoe, C., Leviton, A., Peresie, H., Maher, C., and Barret, P. 1979. Deficits in psychological and classroom performance of children with elevated dentine lead levels. *N. Engl. J. Med.* 300:689–695.

Olds, D. L., Henderson, C. R., and Tatelbaum, R. Prevention of intellectual impairment in children of women who smoke cigarettes during pregnancy. *Pediatrics* 93:228–233.

Rahill, A. A., Weiss, B., Morrow, P. E., Frampton, M. W., Cox, C., Gibb, R., Gelein, R., Speers, D., and Utell, M. J. Human performance during exposure to toluene. *Aviat. Space Environ. Med.* 67:640–647.

CHAPTER
NINE

ANIMAL MODEL OF CHEMICAL SENSITIVITY INVOLVING CHOLINERGIC AGENTS

David H. Overstreet, Amir H. Rezvani, Ying Yang, Mani Hamedi, and David S. Janowsky

Skipper Bowles Center for Alcohol Studies and Department of Psychiatry, University of North Carolina School of Medicine, Chapel Hill, North Carolina

In the assessment of risk to individuals exposed to known or potential toxicological agents, there needs to be a consideration of the possibility that especially sensitive populations exist. For example, some individuals have reported side effects after taking pyridostigmine to protect them against potential nerve gas exposure, and others have not. Other individuals have reported increased sensitivity to a variety of chemical agents, usually after a triggering exposure to a specific chemical such as an organophosphate pesticide (e.g., Miller and Mitzel, 1995). The hypothesis that a genetically based cholinergic supersensitivity might underlie the increased sensitivity of these vulnerable human populations is addressed in this chapter by describing in detail the features of an animal model with cholinergic supersensitivity that is also more sensitive to a variety of drugs and other chemical agents and that may, therefore, mimic the human condition labeled multiple chemical sensitivity (MCS). In the final section of this chapter some initial results on the effects of pyridostigmine on this animal model are presented.

The validity of an animal model rests in part on its similarity in structure and function to a target condition in humans. The closer the similarity to the human condition the model is, the greater the probability that manipulations of one will provide information valid for extrapolation to the other. A final proof of validity comes if predictions made from the animal model and applied to the human condition are shown to be accurate. To evaluate the model proposed here, it is important to summarize the observed clinical characteristics of MCS.

MULTIPLE CHEMICAL SENSITIVITY

Multiple chemical sensitivity is a syndrome in which, following acute or repeated exposure to one or more chemicals, most commonly organophosphate pesticides

(OPs), individuals become overly sensitive to a wide variety of chemically unrelated compounds. These can include ethanol, caffeine, and other psychotropic drugs (Ashford and Miller, 1989, 1991; Bell et al., 1992; Cullen, 1987; Miller, 1994). The symptoms of MCS often reported include fatigue, cognitive difficulties, depression, irritability, headaches, dyspnea, digestive problems, musculoskeletal pain, and numbness in the extremities. These conditions often overlap those of common medical illnesses such as depression, somatization disorder, chronic fatigue syndrome, fibromyalgia, asthma, and others. However, a distinguishing feature of MCS is the strong belief of the patients that their symptoms are brought on by common exposures to low levels of volatile organic chemicals such as fragrances, insecticides, traffic exhaust, disinfectants, and perfumes.

Descriptions of MCS have appeared in various journals for more than 40 years. In recent years, occupational-medicine physicians in universities have reported seeing increasing numbers of individuals who appear to have MCS. In addition, there have been three federally sponsored workshops focussed on MCS (Association of Occupational and Environmental Clinics, 1992; National Research Council, 1992; Mitchell and Price, 1994). Sponsoring agencies have included the National Research Council, the Agency for Toxic Substances and Disease Registry, the Environmental Protection Agency, and the National Institute of Environmental Health Sciences. The recommendations from these meetings repeatedly have stressed the need for further research on the condition and the development of animal models.

MCS has been described as a two-step process that is analogous to but different from the process that occurs in allergic diseases (Ashford and Miller, 1991): For both allergies and MCS there is *induction* (initiation, sensitization, or loss of tolerance) as a consequence of an initial chemical exposure or sensitization to bee venom, for example. In both conditions, there is also subsequent *triggering* of symptoms; however, in MCS this may occur from exposure to a wide range of chemically diverse substances, but in allergy antibodies are highly specific and spreading of sensitivities to chemically unrelated substances does not occur.

Patients with MCS most frequently report their condition as being induced by pesticides, especially OPs and carbamates (Ashford and Miller, 1991; Miller and Mitzel, 1995). Significantly, exposures to OP and carbamate agents during the Gulf War included pesticides, pyridostigmine bromide (used as a prophylaxis for nerve agents), and, possibly, low levels of actual nerve agents. Although chemicals in this class can inhibit cholinesterase, rarely have cholinesterase levels been measured in sporadic MCS cases, and frequently symptoms typically associated with cholinesterase inhibition are absent among individuals who report ultimately developing MCS as a consequence of OP exposure. Although acute OP toxicity generally has been considered to be reversible, provided it is not fatal, the toxicology literature contains a variety of examples of individuals who were exposed to these agents and later showed persistent psychological, psychiatric, or neuropsychological deficits (Gershon and Shaw, 1961; Rosenstock et al., 1991; Rowntree at al., 1950; Savage et al., 1988; Tabershaw and Cooper, 1966). To account for these long-lasting effects it has been proposed that OPs may damage cholinergic receptors or in other ways induce injury independent of their ability to inhibit cholinesterase (Gupta and Abou-Donia, 1994; Huff et al., 1994).

Several case reports of individuals developing MCS after exposure to pesticides (Rosenthal and Cameron, 1991; Cone and Sult, 1992) have appeared recently. Even more recently, Miller and Mitzel (1995) surveyed 112 MCS patients, 37 of whom attributed their illness to exposure to an OP or carbamate pesticide and the other 75 to remodeling of a building, a procedure that commonly involves exposures to low levels of mixed solvents emanating from fresh paint, carpeting, glues, and so forth. Following their initial exposure, both groups reported similar symptoms and similar intolerances to chemicals, foods, ethanol, and caffeine. Overall, however, the pesticide-exposed group reported significantly greater symptom severity. The authors interpreted these findings as suggesting a possible common pathway for the development of MCS, despite the fact that the two groups initially experienced exposures to very different classes of chemicals. They hypothesized that the relatively greater neurotoxicity and potency of the cholinesterase inhibitors as compared with mixed low-level solvents might account for the greater symptom severity in the pesticide-exposed individuals.

An important observation in this field is that MCS patients usually report that other individuals simultaneously exposed to similar amounts of pesticides, such as family members, friends, or coworkers, did not develop MCS or even experience transient illness. This observation suggests that a subset or subsets of people may be more vulnerable to developing MCS. Indeed, some (Black et al., 1990; Simon et al., 1990) but not all (Fiedler et al., 1992) researchers have reported greater rates of depression and somatization disorder predating the "initiating" chemical exposure among persons with MCS as compared with controls. Thus, any model must take into account why only some individuals develop MCS after exposures to pesticides or other chemicals.

One such model that is described in the subsequent sections of this article is the Flinders Sensitive Line (FSL) rat. This rat was developed by selective breeding for increased sensitivity to an OP, so it has some etiologic similarity to patients with MCS who were exposed to pesticides.

AN ANIMAL MODEL

The FSL rat model is one with which we have had extensive experience, particularly in research on depressive syndromes (Overstreet, 1993; Overstreet and Janowsky, 1991; Overstreet et al., 1995). Analogies between depressed states and MCS, as well as substance hypersensitivities in FSL rats, first brought our attention to the potential value of this model for experimental studies of MCS, as recently described (Overstreet et al., 1996). Further, because the FSL rats were selectively bred for increased responses to the organophosphate diisopropylfluorophosphate (DFP), it is possible that they may have some special relevance to Gulf War syndrome, commonly reported in individuals exposed to the carbamate, pyridostigmine. Some preliminary findings of our work with pyridostigmine are presented in the final section of this chapter.

Selective Breeding for OP Differences

The FSL rat model arose from a selective breeding program designed to produce two lines of rats, one with high (FSL) and one with low (Flinders Resistant Line [FRL]) sensitivity to the anticholinesterase agent, DFP (Overstreet et al., 1979; Russell et al., 1982). The selective breeding program, which was initiated at Flinders University in Adelaide, Australia, utilized three somatic measures of DFP (Overstreet et al., 1979; Russell et al., 1992). A rank-order system was used to give equal weighting to each of the three variables. Rats that had the lowest average ranks were intermated to establish and maintain the line of more sensitive rats (FSL); rats that had the highest average ranks were intermated to establish and maintain the line of more resistant rats (FRL). Subsequent studies showed that randomly bred Sprague–Dawley rats, from which the lines were originally derived, were not different from the FRL rats. On the other hand, FSL rats were significantly more sensitive to DFP than the other two groups (Overstreet et al., 1979; Russell et al., 1982).

Biochemical Mechanisms

This project was initiated, in part, to develop genetically resistant lines of rats so that the biochemical mechanisms of resistance could be compared with those of tolerance. Early studies ruled out changes in acetylcholinesterase as a mechanism to account for the differential sensitivity of FSL and FRL rats to DFP (Overstreet et al., 1979; Russell and Overstreet, 1987; Sihotang and Overstreet, 1983), just as has been found for tolerance development (see Russell and Overstreet, 1987). Because DFP-tolerant rats were subsensitive to the effects of muscarinic agonists (e.g., Overstreet et al., 1973), the effects of muscarinic agonists on the FSL and FRL rats were examined (Overstreet 1986; Overstreet and Russell, 1982; Overstreet et al., 1986a,b). These studies showed that the FSL rats were more sensitive to pilocarpine, arecoline, and oxotremorine than were the FRL rats; this supersensitivity was seen for a variety of responses, including hypothermia, reduced locomotor activity, and suppression of bar pressing for water reward (Overstreet and Russell, 1982). Thus, FSL rats, developed by selectively breeding for increased sensitivity to DFP, exhibited opposite changes in sensitivity to muscarinic agonists compared with DFP-tolerant rats.

Biochemical studies indicated that the FSL rats exhibited greater numbers of muscarinic receptor-binding sites in the hippocampus and striatum than the FRL rats (Overstreet et al., 1984; Pepe et al., 1988)., but there were no differences in acetylcholine turnover (Overstreet et al., 1984). Thus, once again, the FSL rats appear to represent the converse of DFP-tolerant rats, having increased numbers of receptors rather than reduced numbers (see Russell and Overstreet, 1987). It appears that both tolerance and acute sensitivity to cholinergic agents are related to postsynaptic rather than presynaptic cholinergic mechanisms. Although in both instances there have been detectable changes in the muscarinic receptors themselves, there are some findings, such as the increased sensitivity of FSL rats to noncholinergic agents (see subsequent section), that suggest that postreceptor mechanisms also may contribute.

Behavioral Features of FSL Rats

The FSL and FRL rats differ on a large number of behavioral tasks, as recently summarized in several review papers (Overstreet et al., 1995, 1996). In this section we highlight a number of the key differences. The FSL rats have been reported to have less locomotor activity than the FRL rats under a number of experimental conditions (Bushnell et al., 1995; Overstreet, 1986; Overstreet and Russell, 1982) but not all (Criswell et al., 1994; Rezvani et al., 1994). They are even less active if stressed prior to exposure to the open field (Overstreet, 1986; Overstreet et al., 1989a).

Results from several other behavioral paradigms are consistent with the view that depression-like psychomotor retardation symptoms are more apparent in the FSL rats after exposure to stressors. For example, the FSL rats are impaired in active avoidance paradigms compared with the FRL rats (Overstreet and Measday, 1985; Overstreet et al., 1990a, 1992a). Another stress-oriented paradigm that has provided important information about behavioral differences between FSL and FRL rats is the forced swim test. Upon initial exposure in a cylinder (18–20 cm diameter) of water (25°C), FSL rats are more immobile than the FRL rats (Overstreet, 1986; Overstreet et al., 1986a, Pucilowski and Overstreet, 1993; Schiller et al., 1992). This exaggerated immobility of the FSL rats is counteracted by chronic but not acute treatment with antidepressants (Overstreet, 1993; Pucilowski and Overstreet, 1993; Schiller et al., 1992). These findings provide further support for the contention that the FSL rat is a useful animal model of depression.

There are also differences in reward-related behaviors between the FSL and FRL rats, which are consistent with the proposal that the FSL rats are a model of depression. In operant bar-pressing tasks, the FSL rats bar-pressed at lower rates and had to be maintained at a lower percentage of their free-feeding body weight and have smaller food pellets (37 versus 45 mg) in order to keep their motivation sufficiently high to complete the session (Bushnell et al., 1995; Overstreet and Russell, 1982). Despite these differences in reward-related and stress-related behaviors, there appear to be no differences between the FSL and FRL rats in the ability to perform a matching-to-sample task (Bushnell et al., 1995). However, this test was carried out under normal, unstressed conditions, and it is not clear whether similar findings would be obtained under stressed conditions. For example, FSL and FRL rats have similar amounts of saccharin consumption under baseline conditions, but the FSL rats exhibit greater decreases after exposure to chronic mild stress (Pucilowski et al., 1993).

The FSL rats also have elevated rapid eye movement (REM) sleep and reduced latency time to REM sleep (Shiromani et al., 1988, Benca et al., 1996), as has been reported in human depressives (Benca et al., 1992). Human depressives are also more sensitive to the effects of cholinergic agonists on REM sleep latency (Janowsky et al., 1994), but there are no data in the FSL rats regarding drug effects on sleep.

In sum, the FSL rats and depressed humans exhibit a large number of behavioral and physiological similarities (see Overstreet, 1993; Overstreet et al., 1995, 1996, for more detailed accounts).

Multiple Chemical Sensitivity in FSL Rats

Clinical observations suggest that MCS may be initiated by acute or chronic exposure to a variety of chemical agents (Miller and Mitzel, 1995). Because the FSL rats were bred selectively to have increased responses to the anticholinesterase agent DFP, it should not be surprising that they exhibited increased sensitivity to muscarinic agonists (Daws et al., 1991; Overstreet, 1986; Overstreet and Russell, 1982; Overstreet et al., 1992a; Schiller et al., 1988). It also has been reported that human depressives are more sensitive to directly acting muscarinic agonists (Gann et al., 1992; Gillin et al., 1991) as well as anticholinesterases (Gann et al., 1992; Janowsky and Risch, 1987; Nurnberger et al., 1989; O'Keane et al., 1992; Schreiber et al., 1992; Sitaram et al., 1987). A similar increased sensitivity to anticholinesterases has been observed in patients with MCS (Cone and Sult, 1992; Miller and Mitzel, 1995; Rosenthal and Cameron, 1991), but there are no published data for patients with MCS regarding sensitivity to direct cholinergic agonists. FSL rats are also more sensitive to nicotine, which interacts with nicotinic cholinergic receptors (Schiller and Overstreet, 1993).

The cholinergic system interacts with many other major neurotransmitter systems, including the serotonergic, dopaminergic, GABAergic, and noradrenergic systems. Having animals with clear-cut differences in the cholinergic system afforded us the opportunity to test how the FSL and FRL rats differ in response to drugs interacting with these other neurotransmitter systems. Evidence from various drug-challenge studies, in which relatively selective drugs are given to FSL and FRL rats, have revealed a substantial number of differences between the FSL and FRL rats, as summarized in Table 9.1. FSL rats were found to exhibit a greater degree of hypothermia after a variety of drugs that interact with the serotonin 5-HT1A receptor (Wallis et al., 1988; Overstreet et al., 1992a, 1994). This outcome is consistent with much of the evidence suggesting supersensitive serotonergic mechanisms in depressives (Arango et al., 1990; Arora and Meltzer, 1989; Mikuni et al., 1991), but is not consistent with neuroendocrine studies reporting blunted responses to serotonergic agonists, which suggests serotonergic hyposensitivity (Lesch et al., 1990; Meltzer and Lowy, 1987). There are no data on the effects of selective serotonergic agents in MCS patients, but there is one report of supersensitive responses in individuals with chronic fatigue syndrome, which is related to MCS (Behan et al., 1995).

To date no evidence has been obtained to indicate any differences in responses to noradrenergic agents in the FSL rats (Overstreet, 1989; Overstreet et al, 1989a). In contrast, there are quite a number of differences with regard to dopaminergic agents (Table 9.1). The FSL rats are supersensitive to the hypothermic (Crocker and Overstreet, 1991) and aggression-promoting (Pucilowski et al., 1991a) effects of apomorphine, a mixed D1/D2 agonist, and quinpirole, a selective D2 agonist. On the other hand, the FSL rats were subsensitive to the stereotypy-inducing effects of similar doses of the same compounds, and there were no apparent differences in dopamine D2 receptors between FSL and FRL rats (Crocker and Overstreet, 1991). These opposite changes in sensitivity in the various functions might be related to the type of modulation of these functions by the cholinergic and dopaminergic systems. Stimulation of both cholinergic and dopaminergic systems promotes hypothermic and aggressive responses (Cox et al., 1980; Pucilowski, 1987; Ray et al., 1989), but cholinergic stimulation reduces activity and stereotypy, thereby opposing the effects of dopaminergic stimulation (Fibiger et al., 1970; Klemm, 1989).

The FSL and FRL rats are differentially sensitive to the effects of several pharmacological agents that have modulatory roles at the GABA-A receptor, as summarized in Table 9.1. However, as with the case of dopamine agonists, the differential effects are observed only for some actions of the drugs, not for all. For example, the hypothermic effects of ethanol are significant higher in the FSL rats compared with the FRL rats, but the sedative effects are similar (Overstreet et al., 1990b). Similarly, the behavioral suppressant effects of

Table 9.1 Drug classes to which FSL rats are more sensitive than FRL rats

Drug class	Compound	Responses
Anticholinesterase	Diisopropyl fluorophosphate	Temperature/drinking
	Physostigmine	Temperature/activity
Muscarinic agonist	Oxotremorine	Temperature/activity
	Pilocarpine	Temperature/activity
	Arecoline	Temperature/activity
Nicotinic agonist	Nicotine	Temperature/activity
Dopamine D1/2 agonist	Abomorphine	Temperature
Dopamine D2 agonist	Quinpirole	Temperature
	Raclopride	Catalepsy
5-HT-1B agonist	m-Chlorphenylpiperazine	Temperature/activity
5-HT-1A agonist	8-OH-DPAT	Temperature
	Buspirone	Temperature
Benzodiazepine agonist	Diazepam	Temperature/activity
Multiple (GABA, 5-HT)	Ethanol	Temperature

Note: 5-HT, 5-hydroxytryptamine.

diazepam are significantly greater in the FSL rats (Pepe et al., 1988), but its anxiolytic effects in the two lines are comparable (Schiller et al., 1991). The fact that these two commonly abused psychotropic drugs both modulate GABA function at the GABA-A receptor suggests that there might be differences in GABA-A receptor subtype composition between the two lines, but there is not biochemical evidence for such differences as yet. Furthermore, despite differences in sensitivity to the hypothermic effects of ethanol, the FSL and FRL rats do not differ in their rates of voluntary ethanol consumption (Overstreet et al., 1992a).

In summary, it appears that the FSL rat is more sensitive to a variety of chemical agents in addition to the OP anticholinesterase agent for which they were selectively bred. In this regard, the FSL rat is somewhat analogous to MCS patients who have become more sensitive to a range of agents following exposure to OP anticholinesterases. The extent of the similarity between the FSL rats and MCS patients, on one hand, and human depressives and MCS patients, on the other, is evaluated further in the next section.

FSL RATS RESEMBLE MCS AND DEPRESSED PATIENTS

As Table 9.2 summarizes, the behavioral features of individuals with MCS and those of depressed patients and FSL rats are strikingly similar in regard to weight, appetite, activity and stressability, hedonia, and sleep. There are also some uncertainties in Table 9.2, suggesting several studies that might be carried out in MCS patients to test further the extent of the associations among the three groups. For example, polysomnographic recordings of sleep in asymptomatic MCS patients would be particularly informative, because there is evidence that the REM sleep changes seen in depressed patients may be a trait marker of this disorder (Benca et al., 1992; Janowsky et al., 1994). Because REM

Table 9.2 Comparison of characteristics and behavioral features of patients with multiple chemical sensitivity, FSL rats, and depressed patients

	Patients with multiple chemical sensitivity	FSL rats	Depressed patients
Weight	Up or down	Down	Up or down
Appetite	Up or down	Down	Up or down
Blood pressure	Up or down	Not determined	Up or down
Food craving	++	+	+
Sleep disturbances	+++	++	+++
Loss of drive	+++	+++	+++
Reduced activity	+++	+++	+++
Cognitive disturbance	+++	+/−	+++
Gender ratios (female:male)	4:1	F > M	2:1

Note: +, more affected than controls; −, not different from controls.

sleep alterations also can be related to altered cholinergic mechanisms in general (Shiromani et al., 1987; Janowsky et al., 1994), a finding of REM sleep changes in MCS patients would suggest that altered cholinergic mechanisms might underlie abnormal sensitivity to chemicals. Such a finding also would be consistent with a cholinergic hypothesis as one possible explanation for the similarity between the MCS patients and depressives.

Another similarity between MCS and depressed patients is the ratio of females to males affected: There are many more females than males expressing the symptoms (Table 9.2). In general, twice as many females than males report depressive symptoms (Goodwin and Jamison, 1990). Similarly, the ratio of female to male MCS patients reaches 4:1 in some studies (Miller and Mitzel, 1995). Again, there is some parallel between the rats and humans, because adult female FSL rats are more sensitive to cholinergic agonists than their male counterparts (Netherton and Overstreet, 1983). The possible greater sensitivity of adult females to cholinergic agonists therefore might account partially for the greater incidence of depression (Overstreet et al., 1988) and MCS in women.

Given the behavioral similarities between MCS patients and those who are depressed (Table 9.2), it is likely that depressed patients might be hypersensitive to similar drugs. Unfortunately, as described in Table 9.3, there is very little information about the sensitivity of depressed individuals to the range of drugs reported to cause problems in MCS patients, other than depressives' supersensitivity to anticholinesterases and cholinergic agonists (Janowsky et al., 1994). There is somewhat more evidence for a general increase in sensitivity to drugs in the FSL rats (Tables 9.1, 9.3). It is particularly noteworthy that the FSL rats are more sensitive to both alcohol (Overstreet et al., 1990b) and nicotine (Schiller and Overstreet, 1993). The information on the effects of alcohol and nicotine in depressed patients is more complex, as implied by the question marks in Table 9.3. There are many studies reporting an interaction of depression with primary alcoholism on one hand (e.g., Kendler et al., 1993; Maier et al., 1994; Schuckit, 1986) and an interaction of smoking with depression on the other (Breslau et al., 1991; Glassman, 1993). Indeed, smoking cessation leads to depression in remitted depressives (Glassman, 1993). However, we are not aware of any studies specifically stating that depressed patients report intolerances for alcohol or nicotine.

It should be stressed that FSL rats also may be less sensitive to certain drugs (Crocker and Overstreet, 1991; Pucilowski et al., 1991). Furthermore, depressed patients exhibit blunted hormonal responses to a number of drugs affecting serotonergic and noradrenergic systems (Meltzer and Lowy, 1987). Consequently, more data from depressed individuals and FSL rats must be collected on their sensitivities to a broader range of chemicals. If the cholinergic system supersensitivity is one mechanism underlying MCS, depression, and the behavioral pathology of the FSL rats, then it would be predicted that both FSL rats and depressed individuals would be more sensitive to such drugs. What also are needed are additional data on depressed individuals and FSL rats with respect to the triggering of symptoms by chemical or food exposures (Table 9.3).

Table 9.3 Comparison of drug sensitivity in patients with multiple chemical sensitivity, FSL rats, and depressed patients

Compound	Patients with multiple chemical sensitivity	FSL rats	Depressed patients
Anticholinesterases	+++	+++	+++
Solvents, etc.	+++	Not determined	Not determined
Ethanol	+++	++	+?
Nicotine	+++	++	+?
Xanthines	+++	Not determined	Not determined
Foods	+++	Not determined	Not determined

Note: +, more sensitive than controls; ?, mixed, uncertain data.

Although we have emphasized the strong possibility of a cholinergic link among MCS patients, depressed patients, and FSL rats, other neurotransmitter systems may be involved. Serotonin has been implicated in depression (Meltzer and Lowy, 1987) and recent experiments on the Flinders rats suggest that serotonergic mechanisms may play an important role in some of their altered behaviors (Overstreet et al., 1994). However, there are no data on serotonergic mechanisms in MCS patients.

A somewhat more complex neurotransmitter model proposes that the various neurochemical systems interact with one another and that abnormal behavioral states may arise from an alteration in one system that creates an imbalance in that system's interactions with others. For example, Janowsky et al. (1972) proposed that depression and mania were the consequence of imbalances between the noradrenergic and cholinergic systems, with depression being associated with relative cholinergic overactivity and mania being associated with relative noradrenergic overactivity. An animal parallel to this observation was reported by Fibiger et al. (1970). This model can account for some of the effects observed in the FSL rats following administration of noncholinergic drugs. For example, FSL rats are more sensitive to the hypothermic effects of dopamine agonists, but less sensitive to their sterotypy-inducing effects (Table 9.1; Crocker and Overstreet, 1991). Because dopaminergic and cholinergic systems work in parallel to regulate temperature but in opposition to regulate activity and stereotypy, an overactive cholinergic system could account for the findings with the dopamine agonists (see Overstreet, 1993). A similar argument could be made for chollinergic–serotonergic interactions as underlying depression and MCS.

Another type of mechanism that could underlie MCS, depression, and the behavioral pathology of FSL rats is a change in second messenger rather than neurotransmitter functions. Several investigators have proposed that changes in G proteins, cyclic adenosine monophosphate, or other second messenger systems may be involved in depression (Lesch and Manji, 1992; Avissar and Schreiber, 1993; Wachtel, 1989). Furthermore, it has been argued that the functional muscarinic responses in the FSL and FRL rats are too divergent to be accounted for by the relatively small differences noted in muscarinic receptors (Overstreet, 1993). This "downstream" hypothesis may account more easily for the pervasiveness of the chemical sensitivity described in MCS patients, which involves many classes of chemical compounds besides those having direct effects on neurotransmitter systems. Differences in second messengers could be hereditary or induced by exposure to chemical agents or by the effects of chemical agents on cholinergic or monoaminergic mechanisms. Further study of FSL rats, MCS patients, and depressed patients using diverse approaches is needed to obtain a greater understanding of the mechanisms that may underlie MCS.

PRELIMINARY FINDINGS ON PYRIDOSTIGMINE

We propose that the characteristics of the animal model that we have described are sufficiently analogous to MCS to warrant its use in testing hypotheses about the etiology and mechanisms of action involved in the syndrome. An example of the type of experimental protocols suggested by this review is the study of FSL and FRL rats after exposure to volatile solvents and other chemicals to which MCS patients report intolerance. This could be done with or without preexisting exposure to cholinergic agents. If FSL rats do exhibit increased sensitivity to a wide variety of chemical agents, then treatment approaches could be attempted, for example using antidepressant drugs. It should be emphasized that proposing antidepressant treatment does not presume that depression is the cause of MCS; indeed, quite the reverse might be true. For example, exposure to OPs might augment cholinergic sensitivity, leading to both MCS and depression. The possibility that increased cholinergic sensitivity might underlie both MCS and depression suggests further experiments in these patient groups. Questions that could be explored are whether there is a subset of depressed patients who report intolerance to varied substances, and whether these same patients exhibit a greater sensitivity to cholinergic agents. A further question could be whether this subset of depressed patients would benefit from avoidance of certain drugs and environmental exposures. Finally, it would be of interest to know whether patients with MCS have altered cholinergic responsivity, particularly in light of a recent study that demonstrated that chronic fatigue syndrome, which is related to MCS, is associated with cholinergic supersensitivity (Chaudhuri et al., 1997).

Another research direction that could be taken is to propose that individual differences in cholinergic sensitivity may have accounted in part for the varied responses of Gulf War participants to pyridostigmine and other agents. Given the large differences in cholinergic sensitivity between the FSL and FRL rats, we would predict substantial differences in responses to pyridostigmine in these animals. The remainder of this section summarizes the preliminary results of our findings.

FSL and FRL rats were selected from breeding colonies maintained at the University of North Carolina at Chapel Hill, and randomly bred Sprague–Dawley rats (from which the FSL and FRL rats originally were derived) were obtained to act as a reference group. Both males and females were used. At about 70 days of age the rats were injected intraperitoneally with sodium pentobarbital (35 mg/kg) to induce anesthesia for implanting the telemetry transmitters, which provided continuous monitoring of core body temperature, general activity, and, in some cases, heart rate.

After a 1-week period to allow recovery, the FSL, FRL, and Sprague–Dawley rats were adapted to the home cages for 24 hr and then injected subcutaneously with a mixture of peripherally acting methyl atropine, 2.0 mg/kg, and oxotremorine, 0.2 mg/kg, to determine hypothermic responses. As can be seen in Figure 9.1, the FSL rats exhibited the greatest hypothermic responses to oxotremorine, as expected. However, the randomly bred Sprague–Dawley rats were significantly more hypothermic than the FRL rats, suggesting that both lines have now diverged from control rats.

Approximately three days after the methyl atropine/oxotremorine challenge, the rats were given pyridostigmine (PYR) bromide by gavage. The design called

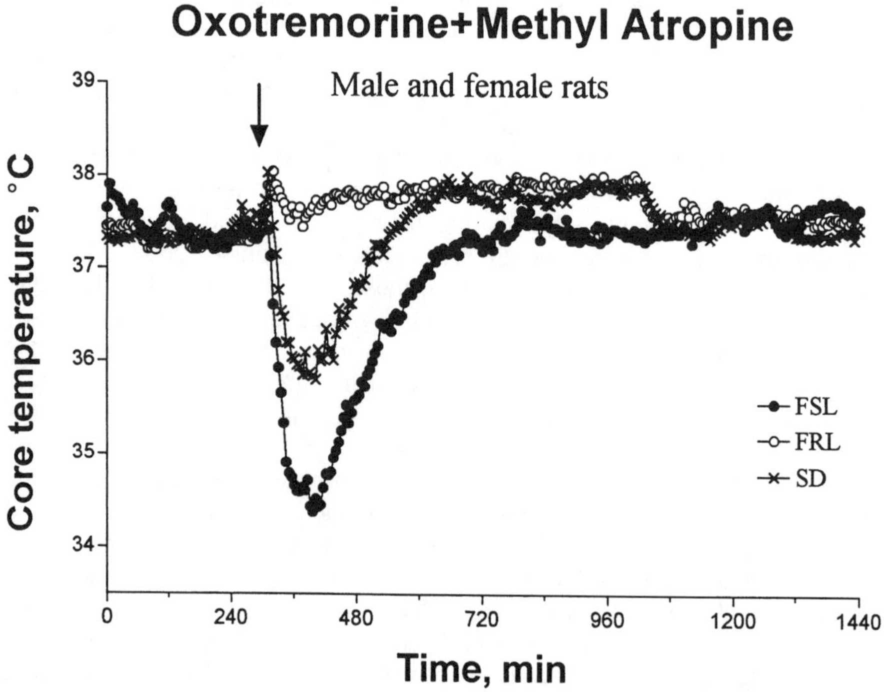

Figure 9.1 Hypothermic effects of oxotremorine in telemetrically monitored FSL, FRL, and Sprague–Dawley rats. The results are the mean temperatures of 10 males and 10 females in each group. Note that the FSL rats exhibit the greatest peak decreases in temperature, and the Sprague–Dawley rats have intermediate responses.

for four groups (vehicle and 4, 12, 36 mg/kg), but only the initial results from the two groups receiving higher doses are reported here. Temperature and activity were continuously recorded for 30 min after the PYR. The rats then were sacrificed by decapitation and blood removed and stored for the later analysis for cholinesterase activity and growth hormone levels. These assays are still in progress, so we report on the physiologic results in this chapter; in addition, because the effects of PYR were not very striking, with little or no evidence of line differences, only the FSL and FRL data are presented.

PYR had relatively few detectable effects on core body temperature at 12 mg/kg (Fig 9.2). There appeared to be a line difference in the females at 36 mg/kg (Fig. 9.3A), but neither the FSL nor the FRL rats exhibited any obvious hypothermia. In contrast, both male FSL and FRL rats exhibited modest but similar hypothermic responses to 36 mg/kg PYR (Fig. 9.3B). There were no detectable line differences in the effects of PYR on activity (data not shown).

These relatively small effects of PYR were not unexpected, because it is a quaternary compound and does not normally get into the brain. However, Friedman et al. (1996) have shown that PYR can penetrate the blood–brain barrier in mice exposed to stressors, so it was thought that the FSL rats, which are more sensitive to stressors (see Overstreet, 1993; Overstreet et al., 1995), might exhibit a hypothermic response to PYR and the FRL rats would not. The fact that both male groups exhibit very similar small responses after 36 mg/kg PYR suggests that they both have intact blood–brain barriers. Experiments on the effects of pyridostigmine in the two lines after exposure to stressors are needed to clarify this issue.

As indicated previously, the growth hormone assays are still in progress. We expect them to be quite revealing, because it has been well documented that PYR, despite its inability to penetrate the blood–brain barrier, significantly increases growth-hormone levels in both rats and humans (Martin et al., 1978; Mazza et al., 1994). In fact, patients with a variety of ailments, such as depression, obsessive-compulsive disorders, and chronic fatigue syndrome, exhibit abnormal responses to PYR (Chaudhuri et al., 1997; Ghigo et al., 1993; Lucey et al., 1993; O'Keane et al., 1992, 1994). Because some of these patient groups exhibit behavioral symptoms overlapping with or similar to those described in Gulf War veterans, it is possible that they too may exhibit abnormal responses, but no such study is available as yet. The FSL and FRL rats thus may represent animal analogs of patient and control groups, respectively, and can be useful in elucidating the mechanism of action of PYR.

ACKNOWLEDGMENTS

The work described in this chapter was supported in part by funding provided by the Australian Research Grants Committee, the National Health and Medical Research Committee of Australia, and the U.S. Army. We express our appreciation to Dawn Forte and Elijah Clark, Jr., for technical support.

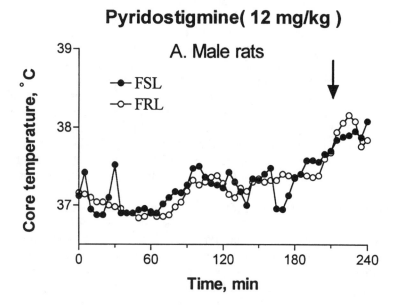
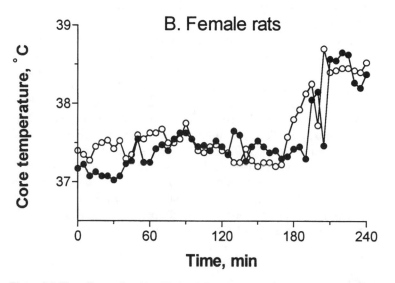

Figure 9.2 The effects of pyridostigmine (12 mg/kg, orally) on core body temperature in male (*A*) and female (*B*) FSL and FRL rats. The results are the mean temperatures of five animals per group.

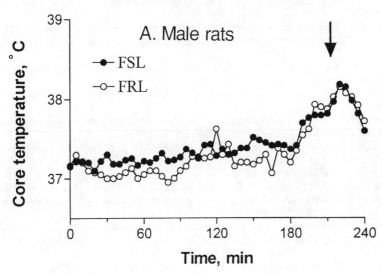
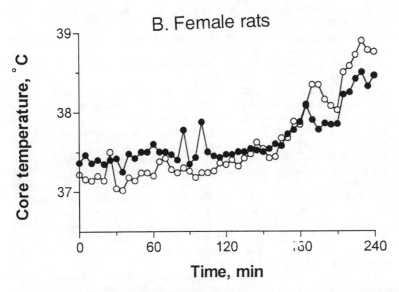

Figure 9.3 The effects of pyridostigmine (36 mg/kg, orally) on core body temperature in male (*A*) and female (*B*) FSL and FRL rats. The results are the mean temperatures of five animals per group.

REFERENCES

Arango, V., Ernsberger, P., Marzuk, P. M., Chen, J. S., Tierney, H., Stanley, M., Reis, D. J., and Mann, J. J. 1990. Autoradiographic demonstration of increased serotonin 5-HT$_2$ and B-adrenergic receptor binding sites in the brain of suicide victims. *Arch. Gen. Psychiatry* 47:1038–1047.

Arora, R. C., and Meltzer, H. Y. 1989. Serotonergic measures in the brains of suicide victims: 5-HT$_2$ binding sites in the frontal cortex of suicide victims and control subjects. *Am. J. Psychiatry* 146:730–736.

Ashford, N. A., and Miller, C. S. 1989. *Chemical sensitivity*. Report to the New Jersey State Department of Health.

Ashford, N. A. and Miller, C. S. 1991. *Chemical exposure: Low levels and high stakes*. New York: Van Nostrand Reinhold.

Association of Occupational and Environmental Clinics. 1992. Advancing the understanding of multiple chemical sensitivity. *Toxicol. Indust. Health* 8:1–257.

Avissar, S., and Schreiber, G. 1989. Muscarinic receptor subclassification and G-proteins: Significance for lithium action in affective disorders and for the treatment of extrapyramidal side effects of neuroleptics. *Biol. Psychiatry* 26:113–130.

Backheit, A. M., Behan, P. O., Dinan T. G., Gray, C. E., and O'Keane, V. 1992. Possible upregulation of hypothalamus 5-hydroxytryptamine receptors in patients with postviral fatigue syndrome. *Br. Med. J.* 304:1010–1012.

Bell, I. R., Miller, C. S., and Schwartz, G. E. 1992. An olfactory-limbic model of multiple chemiccal sensitivity syndrome: Possible relationships to kindling and affective spectrum disorders. *Biol. Psychiatry* 32:218–242.

Benca, R. M., Overstreet, D. H., Gilliland, M. A., Russell, D., Bergmann, B. M., and Obermeyer, W. H. 1996. Increased basal REM sleep but no no difference in dark induction or light suppression of REM sleep in Flinders Rats with cholinergic supersensitivity. *Neuropsychopharmacology* 15:45–51.

Benca, R. M., Obermeyer, W. H. Thisted, R. A., and Gillin, J. C. 1992. Sleep and psychiatric disorders: A meta-analysis. *Arch. Gen. Psychiatry* 49:651–670.

Black, D. W., Rathe, A., and Goldstein, R. B. 1990. Environmental illness. A controlled study of 26 subjects with "20th Century Disease." *JAMA* 264:166–170.

Breslau, N., Kilbey, M. M., and Andreski, P. 1991. Nicotine dependence, major depression and anxiety in young adults. *Arch. Gen. Psychiatry* 48:1061–1074.

Bushnell, P. J., Levin, E. D., and Overstreet, D. H. 1995. Spatial working and reference memory in rats bred for autonomic sensitivity to cholinergic stimulation: Acquisition, accuracy, speed, and effects of cholinergic drugs. *Neurobiol. Learning Mem.* 63:116–132.

Chaudhuri, A., Majeed, T., Dinan, T., and Behan, P. O. 1997. Chronic fatigue syndrome: A disorder of central cholinergic transmission. *J. Chron. Fatigue* 3:3–16.

Cone, J. E., and Sult, T. A. 1992. Acquired intolerance to solvents following pesticide/solvent exposure in a building: A new group of workers at risk for multiple chemical sensitivities? *Toxicol. Indust. Health* 8:29–39.

Cox, B., Kerwin, R. W., Lee, T. F., and Pycock, C. J. 1980. A dopamine-5-hydroxytryptamine link in the hypothalamic pathways which mediate heat loss in the rat. *J. Physiol.* 303:9–21.

Criswell, H. A., Overstreet, D. H., Rezvani, A. H., Johnson, K. B., Simson, P. E., Knapp, D. J., Moy, S. S., and Breese, G. R. 1994. Effects of ethanol, MK-801, and chlordiazepoxide on locomotor activity in different rat lines: Dissociation of locomotor stimulation from ethanol preference. *Alcohol. Clin. Exp. Res.* 18:917–923.

Crocker A. D., and Overstreet, D. H. 1991. Changes in dopamine sensitivity in rats selectively bred for differences in cholinergic function. *Pharmacol. Biochem. Behav.* 38:105–108.

Cullen, M. R. 1987. Workers with multiple chemical sensitivities. *Occup. Med. State Art Rev.* 2:655–806.

Daws, L. C., Schiller, G. D., Overstreet, D. H., and Orbach, J. 1991. Early development of muscarinic supersensitivity in a genetic animal model of depression. *Neuropsychopharmacology* 4:207–217.

Fibiger, H. C., Lytle, L. D., and Campbell, B. A. 1970. Cholinergic modulation of adrenergic arousal in the developing rat. *J. Comp. Physiol. Psychol.* 3:384-389.
Fiedler, N., Maccia, C., and Kipen, H. 1992. Evaluation of chemically sensitive patients. *J. Occup. Med.* 34:529-538.
Friedman, A., Kaufer, D., Shemer, J., Hendler, I., Soreq, H., and Tur-Kaspar, I. 1996. Pyridostigmine brain penetration under stress enhances neuronal excitability and induces immediate transcriptional response *Nature Med.* 2:1382-1385.
Gann, H., Riemann, D., Hohagen, F., Dressing, H., Muller, W. E., and Berger, M. 1992. The sleep structure of patients with anxiety disorders in comparison to that of healthy controls and depressive patients under baseline conditioons and after cholinergic stimulation. *J. Affect. Disord.* 26:179-190.
Gershon, S. and Shaw, F. H. 1961. Psychiatric sequelae of chronic exposure to organophosphorus insecticides. *Lancet* i:1371-1374.
Ghigo, E., Nicolosi, M., Arvat, E., Marcone, A., Danelon, F., Mucci, M., Franceschi, M., Smirne, S., and Camanni, F. 1993. Growth hormone secretion in Alzheimer's disease: Studies with growth hormone-releasing hormone alone and combined with pyridostigmine or arginine. *Dementia* 4:315-320.
Gillin, J. C., Sutton, L., Ruiz, C., Kelsoe, J., Dupont, R. N., Darko, D., Risch, S. C., Golshan, S., and Janowsky, D. 1991. The cholinergic rapid eye movement induction test with arecoline in depression. *Arch. Gen. Psychiatry* 48:264-270.
Glassman, A. H. 1993. Cigarette smoking: Implications for psychiatric illness. *Am. J. Psychiatry* 150:546-553.
Goodwin, F. K., and Jamison, K. R. 1990. *Manic-depressive illness*. New York: Oxford University Press.
Gupta, R. P., and Abou-Donia, M. B. 1994. In vivo and in vitro effects of diisopropyl phosphofluoridate (DFP) on the rate of brain tubulin polymerization. *Neurochem. Res.* 19:435-444.
Huff, R. A., Corcoran, J. J., Anderson, J. K., and Abou-Donia, M. B. 1994. Chlorpyrifos oxon binds directly to muscarinic receptors and inhibits cAMP accumulation in rat striatum. *J. Pharmacol. Exp. Ther.* 269:329-335.
Janowsky, D. S. and Risch, S. C. 1987. Acetylcholine mechanisms in affective disorders. In *Psychopharmacology: The third generation of progress*, ed. H. Y. Meltzer, pp. 527-534. New York: Raven Press.
Janowsky, D. S., El-Yousef, M. K., Davis, J. M., and Sekerke, H. J. 1972. A cholinergic-adrenergic hypothesis of mania and depression. *Lancet* ii:632-635.
Janowsky, D. S., Overstreet, D. H., and Nurnberger J. I. Jr. 1994. Is cholinergic sensitivity a genetic marker for the affective disorders? *Am. J. Med. Genet.* (*Neuropsychiatr. Gen.*) 54:335-344.
Kendler, K. S., Heath, A. C., Neale, M. C., Kessler, R. C., and Eaves, L. J. 1993. Alcoholism and major depression in women: A twin study of the causes of comorbidity. *Arch. Gen. Psychiatry* 50:690-698.
Klemm, W. R. 1989. Drug effects on active immobility responses: What they tell us about neurotransmitter systems and motor function. *Prog. Neurobiol.* 32:403-422.
Kupfer, D. J. 1976. REM latency: A psychobiological marker for primary depressive disease. *Biol. Psychiatry* 11:159-174.
Lesch, K. P. and Manji, H. K. 1992. Signal-transducing G proteins and antidepressant drugs: Evidence for modulation of alpha-subunit gene expression in rat brain. *Biol. Psychiatry* 32:549-579.
Lesch, K. P., Disselkamp-Tietze, J., and Schmidtke, A. 1990. 5-HT1A receptor function in depression: Effect of chronic amitriptyline treatment. *J. Neural Transm.* 80:157-161.
Lucey, J. V., Butcher, G., Clare, A. W., and Dinan, T. G. 1993. Elevated growth hormone responses to pyridostigmine in obsessive-compulsive disorder: Evidence of cholinergic supersensitivity. *Am. J. Psychiatry* 150:961-962.
Maier, W., Lichtermann, D., and Minges, J. 1994. The relationship between alcoholism and unipolar depression: A controlled family study. *J. Psychiatry Res.* 28:303-316.

Martin, J. D., Durand, D., Gurd, W., Faille, G., Audet, J., and Brazeau, P. 1978. Neuropharmacological regulation of episodic growth hormone-releasing hormone release into hypophysial portal blood of conscious sheep. *Endocrinology* 133:1247–1251.

Mazza, E., Ghigo, E., Boffano, G., Valeto, M., Naccarioi, M., Arvat, D., Bellone, J., Procopio, M., Muller, E. E., and Camanni, F. 1994. Effects of direct and indirect acetylcholine receptor agonists on growth hormone secretion in humans. *Eur. J. Pharmacol.* 254:17–20.

Meltzer, H. Y., and Lowy, M. T. 1987. The serotonin hypothesis of depression. In *Psychopharmacology: The third generation of progress*, ed. H. Y. Meltzer, pp. 513–526. New York: Raven Press.

Mikuni, M., Kusumi, I., Kagaya, A., Kuroda, Y., Mori, H., and Takahashi, K. 1991. Increased 5-HT-2 receptor function as measured by serotonin-stimulated phosphoinositide hydrolysis in platelets of depressed patients. *Prog. Neuro-Psychopharmacol. Biol. Psychiatry* 15:49–62.

Miller, C. S. 1994. White paper: Chemical sensitivity. History and phenomenology. *Toxicol. Indust. Health* 10:253–276.

Miller, C. S. and Mitzel, H. C. 1995. Chemical sensitivity attributed to pesticide exposure versus remodeling. *Arch. Env. Health* 50:119–129.

Mitchell, F. L. and Price, P. 1994. Proceeding of the conference on low-level exposure to chemicals and neurobiologic sensitivity. *Toxicol. Indust. Health* 10:1–300.

National Research Council 1992. *Multiple chemical sensitivities: Addendum to biologic markers in immunotoxicology*. Washington, DC: National Academy Press.

Netherton, R. A. and Overstreet, D. H. 1983. Genetic and sex differences in the cholinergic modulation of thermoregulation. In *Environment, drugs and thermoregulation*, ed. P. Lomax and E. Schonbaum, pp. 74–77. Basel: Karger.

Nurnberger, J. I. Jr., Berrettini, W., Mendelson, W., Sack, D., and Gershon, E. S. 1989. Measuring cholinergic sensitivity: I. Arecoline effects in bipolar patients. *Biol. Psychiatry* 25:610–617.

O'Keane, V., O'Flynn, K., Lucey, J., and Dinan, T. G. 1992. Pyridostigmine-induced growth hormone responses in healthy and depressed subjects: Evidence for cholinergic supersensitivity in depression. *Psychol. Med.* 22:55–60.

O'Keane, V., Abel, K. and Murray, R. M. 1994. Growth hormone responses to pyridostigmine in schizophrenia: Evidence for cholinergic dysfunction. *Biol. Psychiatry* 36:582–586.

Overstreet, D. H. 1986. Selective breeding for increased cholinergic function: Development of a new animal model of depression. *Biol. Psychiatry* 21:49–58.

Overstreet D. H. 1989. *Correlations of ethanol-induced hypothermia in FSL and FRL rats with hypothermia induced by other drugs*. Presented at 13th Annual Symposium of the North Carolina Alcoholism Research Authority, Raleigh, NC.

Overstreet, D. H. 1993. The Flinders Sensitive Line rats: A genetic animal model of depression. *Neurosci. Biobehav. Rev.* 17:51–68.

Overstreet, D. H., and Janowsky, D. S. 1991. A cholinergic supersensitivity model of depression. In *Neuromethods*, vol. 19, ed. A. Boulton, G. Baker, and M. Martin-Iverson, pp. 81–114. Clifton, NJ: Humana Press.

Overstreet, D. H., and Measday, M. 1985. Impaired active avoidance performance in rats with cholinergic supersensitivity: Its reversal with chronic imipramine. Presented at 4th International Congress of Biological Psychiatry, Philadelphia, PA.

Overstreet, D. H., and Russell, R. W. 1982. Selective breeding for sensitivity to DFP: Effects of cholinergic agonists and antagonists. *Psychopharmacology* 78:150–154.

Overstreet, D. H., Kozar, M. D., and Lynch, G. D. 1973. Reduced hypothermic effects of cholinomimetic agents following chronic anticholinesterase treatment. *Neuropharmacology* 12:1017–1032.

Overstreet, D. H., Russell, R. W., Helps, S. C., and Messenger, M. 1979. Selective breeding for sensitivity to the anticholinesterase, DFP. *Psychopharmacology* 65:15–20.

Overstreet, D. H., Russell, R. W., Crocker, A. D., and Schiller, G. D. 1984. Selective breeding for differences in cholinergic function: Pre- and Post-synaptic mechanisms involved in sensitivity to the anticholinesterase, DFP. *Brain Res.* 294:327–332.

Overstreet, D. H., Booth, R., Dana, R., Risch, S. C., and Janowsky, D. S. 1986a. Enhanced elevation of corticosterone following arecoline administration to rats selectively bred for increased cholinergic function. *Psychopharmacology* 88:129–130.

Overstreet, D. H., Janowsky, D. S., Gillin, J. C., Shiromani, P., and Sutin, E. L. 1986b. Stress-induced immobility in rats with cholinergic supersensitivity. *Biol. Psychiatry* 21:657–664.

Overstreet, D. H., Russell, R. W., Crocker, A. D., Gillin, J. C., and Janowsky, D. S. 1988. Genetic and pharmacological models of cholinergic supersensitivity and affective disorders. *Experientia* 44:465–472.

Overstreet, D. H., Double, K., and Schiller, G. D. 1989a. Antidepressant effects of rolipram in a genetic animal model of depression: Cholinergic supersensitivity and weight gain. *Pharmacol. Biochem. Behav.* 34:691–696.

Overstreet, D. H., Janowsky, D. H., and Rezvani, A. H. 1990a. Impaired active avoidance responding in rats selectively bred for increased cholinergic function. *Physiol. Behav.* 47:787–788.

Overstreet, D. H., Rezvani, A. H., and Janowsky, D. S. 1990b. Increased hypothermic responses to ethanol in rats selectively bred for cholinergic supersensitivity. *Alcohol Alcohol* 25:59–65.

Overstreet, D. H., Rezvani, A. H., and Janowsky, D. S. 1992. Genetic animal models of depression and ethanol preference provide support for cholinergic and serotonergic involvement in depression and alcoholism. *Biol. Psychiatry* 31:919–936.

Overstreet, D. H., Janowsky, D. S., Pucilowski, O., and Rezvani, A. H. 1994. Swim test immobility cosegregates with serotonergic but not cholinergic sensitivity in cross breeds of Flinders Line rats. *Psychiatr. Genet.* 4:101–107.

Overstreet, D. H., Pucilowski, O., Rezvani, A. H., and Jaowsky, D. S. 1995. Administration of antidepressants, diazepam and psychomotor stimulants further confirms the utility of Flinders Sensitive Line rats as an animal model of depression. *Psychopharmacology* 121:27–37.

Overstreet, D. H., Miller, C. M., Janowsky, D. S., Russell, R. W. 1996. A potential animal model of multiple chemical sensitivity with cholinergic supersensitivity. *Toxicology* 111:119–134.

Pepe, S., Overstreet, D. H., and Crocker, A. D. 1988. Enhanced benzodiazepine responsiveness in rats with increased cholinergic function. *Pharmacol. Biochem. Behav.* 31:15–20.

Pucilowski, O. 1987. Monoaminergic control of affective aggression. *Acta Neurobiol. Exp.* 47:25–50.

Pucilowski, O. and Overstreet, D. H. 1993. Effect of chronic antidepressant treatment on responses to apomorphine in selectively bred rat strains. *Pharmacol. Biochem. Behav.* 32:471–475.

Pucilowski, O., Danysz, W., Overstreet, D. H., Rezvani, A. H., Eichelman, B., and Janowsky, D. S. 1991a. Decreased hyperthermic effect of MK-801 in selectively bred hypercholinergic rats. *Brain Res. Bull.* 26:621–525.

Pucilowski, O., Overstreet, D. H., Rezvani, A. H., and Janowsky, D. S. 1993. Chronic mild stress-induced anhedonia: Greater effect in a genetic rat model of depression. *Physiol. Behav.* 54:1215–1220.

Ray, A., Sen, P., and Alkondon, M. 1989. Biochemical and pharmacological evidence for central cholinergic regulation of shock-induced aggression. *Pharmacol. Biochem. Behav.* 32:867–871.

Rezvani, A. H., Overstreet, D. H., Ejantkar, A., and Gordon, C. J. 1994. Autonomic and behavioral responses of selectively bred hypercholinergic rats to oxotremorine and diisopropyl fluorophosphate. *Pharmacol. Biochem. Behav.* 48:703–707.

Rosenstock, L., Keifer, M., Daniell, W., McConnell, R., and Claypoole, K. 1991. Chronic central nervous system effects of acute organophosphate pesticide intoxication. *Lancet* 338:223–227.

Rosenthal, N. and Cameron, C. L. 1991. Exaggerated sensitivity to an organophosphate pesticide [letter]. *Am. J. Psychiatry* 148:270.

Rowntree, D. W., Neven, S., and Wilson, A. 1950. The effect of diisopropylfluorophosphonate in schizophrenia and manic depressive psychosis. *J. Neurol. Neurosurg. Psychiat.* 13:47–62.

Russell, R. W. and Overstreet, D. H. 1987. Mechanisms underlying sensitivity to organophosphorus anticholinesterase agents. *Prog. Neurobiol.* 28:97–129.

Russell, R. W., Overstreet, D. H., Messenger, M., and Helps, S. C. Selective breeding for sensitivity to DFP. Generalization of effects beyond criterion variables. *Pharmacol. Biochem. Behav.* 17:885–891, 1982.

Savage, E. P., Keefe, T. J., and Mounce, L. M. 1988. Chronic neurological sequelae of acute organophosphate pesticide poisoning. *Arch. Environ. Health* 43:38–45.

Schiller, G. D., and Overstreet, D. H. 1993. Selective breeding for increased cholinergic function: Preliminary study of nicotinic mechanisms. *Medic. Chem. Res.* 2:578–583.

Schiller, G. D., Orbach, J., and Overstreet, D. H. 1988, December. Effects of intracerebroventricular administration of site selective muscarinic drugs in rats genetically selected for differing cholinergic sensitivity. Presented at meeting of Australasian Society for Clinical and Experimental Pharmacology, Adelaide.

Schiller, G. D., Daws, L. C., Overstreet, D. H., Orbach, J. 1991. Absence of anxiety in an animal model of depression with cholinergic supersensitivity. *Brain Res. Bull.* 26:443–447.

Schiller, G. D., Pucilowski, O., Wienicke, C., and Overstreet, D. H. 1992. Immobility-reducing effect of antidepressants in a genetic animal model of depression. *Brain Res. Bull.* 28:821–823.

Schreiber, W., Lauer, C. J., Krumrey, K., Holsboer, F., and Krieg, J. C. 1992. Cholinergic REM sleep induction test in subjects at high risk for psychiatric disorders. *Biol. Psychiatry* 32:79–90.

Schuckit, M. A. 1986. Genetic and clinical implications of alcoholism and affective disorders. *Am. J. Psychiatry* 143:140–147.

Shiromani, P. J., Gillin, J. C., and Hendrickson, P. 1987. Acetylcholine and the regulation of REM sleep: Basic mechanisms and clinical implications for affective illness and narcolepsy. *Annu. Rev. Pharmacol. Toxicol.* 27:137–156.

Shiromani, P. J., Overstreet, D. H., Levy, D., Goodrich, C. A., Campbell, S. S., and Gillin, J. C. 1988. Increased REM sleep in rats selectively bred for cholinergic hyperactivity. *Neuropsychopharmacology* 1:127–133

Sihotang, K., and Overstreet, D. H. 1983. Studies on the possible relationship of brain proteins to behavioral sensitivity to DFP. *Life Sci.* 32:413–420.

Simon, G. E., Katon, W. J., and Sparks, P. J. 1990. Allergic to life: Psychological factors in environmental illness. *Am. J. Psychiatry* 147:901–906.

Sitaram, N., Jones, D., Dube, S., Keshavan, M., Bell, J., Davies, A., and Reynal, P. 1987. The association of supersensitive cholinergic-REM induction and affective illness within pedigrees. *J. Psychiatry Res.* 21:487–497.

Tabershaw, I. R. and Cooper, C. 1966. Sequelae of acute organic phosphate poisoning. *J. Occup. Med.* 8:5–20.

Wachtel, H. 1989. Dysbalance of neuronal second messenger function in aetiology of affective disorders: A pathophysiological concept hypothesizing defects beyond first messenger receptors. *J. Neural Transm.* 75:21–29.

Wallis, E., Overstreet, D. H., and Crocker, A. D. 1988. Selective breeding for increased cholinergic function: Increased serotonergic sensitivity. *Pharmacol. Biochem. Behav.* 31:345–350.

CHAPTER
TEN

APPLICATION OF CHEMICAL HORMESIS CONCEPT TO RISK ASSESSMENT: REPRODUCTIVE TOXICITY AS AN EXAMPLE

Edward J. Calabrese and Linda A. Baldwin

Environmental Health Sciences Department, School of Public Health, University of Massachusetts, Amherst, Massachusetts

During the recent development of a chemical hormesis database (Calabrese and Baldwin, 1997), numerous studies involving reproductive endpoints were identified that satisfied a weight-of-evidence conclusion for evidence of hormesis. The defintion of hormesis used in this research is low-dose stimulation followed by higher-dose inhibition, with the most common form of hormesis following the widely recognized β-curve (Fig. 10.1) (Stebbing, 1982). The use of the β-curve follows from the widespread use of growth as a principal endpoint in hormesis research. The term *U-shaped*, emphasized by Davis and Svensgaard (1990), is applied most appropriately if the endpoint relates to a traditional toxicologically based health endpoint such as cancer that displays a background incidence greater than 0.0. For the purposes of this chapter, the occurrence of chemical hormesis was restricted to those dose–response relationships most conforming to the β- or U-shaped curves.

Selection of studies for review was based primarily on the nature of the study design, quality of data, phylogenetic diversity, and range of reproductive processes and endpoints. Evaluation of the hormetic response was based on (1) magnitude of the low dose stimulatory response, (2) the number of doses establishing reliability of the β-curve, (3) statistical power, and (4) reproducibility of the data.

Within the broad categories of chemical agents, studies demonstrating evidence of chemical hormesis in reproductive toxicity data are presented by model species.

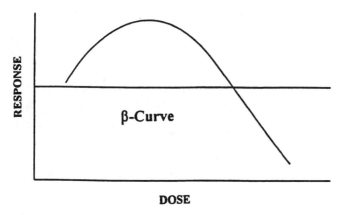

Figure 10.1 The most common dose–response curve showing hormesis, the β-curve.

HEAVY METALS

Daphnids

The phenomenon of reported stimulatory effects of very low concentrations of cadmium on reproductive endpoints in *Daphnia magna* (Elnabarawy et al., 1986) was investigated by Bodar et al. (1988) for its consistency with hormesis. A broad range of Cd concentrations (0.5, 1, 5, 10, 20, and 50 ppb) was used to assess the effects on number of neonates per female, neonate size, and time to first brood (Bodar et al., 1988). Significant increases (25%–45% depending on concentration) in number of neonates per female were observed at the lower Cd concentrations (0.5, 1, and 5 ppb); adverse effects on reproduction occurred at 10 ppb or more. Days to first brood displayed a nonsignificant shortening at 0.5 and 1 ppb. Analysis of neonate size revealed that although the low-dose groups produced more neonates, their average length was reduced. If transformed into dry weight values, however, the average neonate biomass per female indicated that the low-dose (0.5 and 1 ppb) females produced considerably more biomass than the control. Within the context of reproductive strategy, the authors speculated that the low-dose Cd-induced response was nonspecific (i.e., hormesis) based on the increased biomass data.

Fathead Minnow

Enhancement of egg production in the fathead minnow (*Pimephales promales*) exposed to low doses of Cd was reported by Pickering and Gast (1972). The authors noted that this marked increase in egg production (two- to three-fold over control), observed in replicate experiments, was unexpected. Higher doses of Cd inhibited egg production.

Polychaete Worms

A broad dose range (range depending upon species and metal), including six doses plus control, was used to assess the effects of heavy metals on fecundity in two species of polychaete worms (Reish and Carr, 1978). Low-dose stimulation of fecundity compared with control was observed with Cd (28.5%), copper (50%), and mercury (15%) in *Ctenodrilus serratus*, and with Cd (26%), copper (11%), lead (76%), mercury (62%), and zinc (16%) in *Ophryotrocha diedema*. Reproduction was markedly inhibited at high doses for all metals in both species.

Hydra

Asexual reproduction (i.e., bud production) was stimulated in hydra following exposure to subtoxic doses of one of two inorganic lead compounds, lead nitrate or lead chloride (Browne and Davis, 1977). This temporary increase in bud production was observed after treatments lasting from 5 min to 1 hr. A comparable enhancement of bud production was observed in hydra (*Hydra littoralis*) exposed to copper (Stebbing and Pomroy, 1977). These authors hypothesized that the low-dose effects were caused by a stimulatory counterresponse to the inhibitory effect of the copper (i.e., response compensation). They also suggested that this hypothesis might account for the observations of Browne and Davis with lead.

Mice

Analysis of data compiled and presented by Daston et al. (1991) revealed an enhancement of several reproductive endpoints in CD1 mice exposed to cadmium chloride ($CdCl_2$). Six different dosages of $CdCl_2$ ranging from 0.25 to 8.0 mg/kg/d were administered orally to groups of mice. Apparent hormetic relationships were observed for the number of implants, number of live fetuses per litter, and maternal weight gain compared with untreated controls (Calabrese and Baldwin, 1993).

Sea Urchins

The use of sea urchins as a biologic test system to assess reproductive effects of environmental contaminants has long been recognized (Kobayashi, 1971; Stebbing, 1980). Of particular interest to the study of hormesis has been a series of reports by Pagano and associates (Giordano et al., 1983; Pagano et al., 1982, 1986) concerning the effects of selected inorganic agents (i.e., selenium, cadmium, copper, and zinc) on a range of reproductive endpoints in two species of sea urchins (i.e., *Paracentrotus lividus*—eggs and sperm; and *Echinus esculentus*—sperm).

Experiments involved pretreatment of sperm in vitro following 0.10% suspension of concentrated sperm into filtered sea water to which various contaminants were added. Exposure was followed by insemination of untreated eggs from an individual female. The experiment was designed to test sperm inactivation and was used to assess fertilization success and quality of offspring. Dose–response trends in fertilization rates were related to agent levels and exposure lengths and termed *promotion index*.

In the sperm-inactivation tests, offspring quality based on cytological evaluation was not affected up to spermiotoxic levels regardless of the duration of the exposure (1 min to several hours). However, fertilization success with both species displayed clear dose-dependency. The fertilization success of *E. esculentus* sperm was increased by Cd levels ranging from 10^{-7} to 10^{-6} kmol/m^3 then suppressed by higher Cd concentrations. A similar low-dose enhancement of fertilization success also was seen with zinc. Similar experiments in *P. lividus* also revealed a comparable low-dose stimulatory, high-dose inhibitory response with Cd. Experiments with Zn in *P. lividus* revealed a dose-dependent (10^{-7}–10^{-5} kmol/m^3) increase and no inhibitory response.

Other experiments with *P. lividus* revealed that copper affected fertilization, displaying a dose–response relationship that closely resembled that of Cd with its close conformity to the β-curve. More specifically, low concentrations of Cu (10^{-9}–10^{-7} kmol/m^3) enhanced fertilization success, but higher doses were inhibitory, with the values falling to zero at 10^{-6} kmol/m^3 or more. Observations of low-dose increases in fertilization rates by Cd and Cu occurred at about 10^{-10} kmol/m^3 and about 10^{-7} kmol/m^3, respectively. Consequently, the stimulatory responses occurred at concentrations that are in the approximate natural background.

The joint effects of both Cd and Zn and Cd and Cu were assessed over the range of stimulatory and inhibitory concentrations. In the case of Cd and Zn with *E. esculentus* at 10^{-7} kmol/m^3, in which Cd and Zn had promotion indexes of about +130 and +60, respectively, the response was a −20 promotion index. These findings suggest that the joint exposure of multiple agents in hormetic areas may lead to a net negative response. Similar experiments with *P. lividus* did not display what would appear to be either an antagonistic relationship or simply a type of "dose-additivity" if the response was in the toxic range. The striking response with *E. esculentus* was not seen in comparable joint chemical exposures with *P. lividus*. Based on experiments with doses causing hormetic responses with Cd and Cu, the responses were comparable to those reported for either agent alone. In the cases of Cd and Zn, it appears that a decrease (slight to moderate) in the magnitude of the hormetic response occurred. The principal point is that the joint exposure at individually hormetic doses still displayed an apparent hormetic response.

These studies represent an attempt to advance current understandings of hormetic dose–response relationships, because the experiments provided exposures that encompassed ambient concentrations, joint exposures, and related exposure conditions to hormetic responses. The fact that hormetic responses were observed with Cd, Cu, Se, and Zn for fertilization success in *E. esculentus* or *P. lividus* supports that generalizability of these responses. However, a strikingly different response with joint exposures in the hormetic zone between the two species suggests that this phenomenon requires considerable follow-up investigation.

PESTICIDES

It is well documented in the field of insect control that repeat administration of most broad-spectrum foliar pesticides frequently affects resurgences in populations of other species. Proposed explanations for this phenomenon include (1) eradication of predator species (De Bach, 1946; Radcliffe, 1972); (2) removal of competitive species (Ripper, 1956); (3) change in plant-nutrient balance (Chapman and Allen, 1948); (4) physical alteration of leaf surface promoting colonization (DeBach, 1946; van Emden, 1966); (5) selection of genetically resistant species that reproduce more rapidly (Hrdy, 1979; Eggers-Schumacher, 1983); and (6) direct physiologic stimulation of reproduction (Gordon and McEwen, 1984; Huffaker and Spitzer, 1950). Of relevance to the current report is the hypothesis that the pesticidal treatment results in a direct physiologic enhancement of reproductive endpoints.

Green Peach Aphid

Observations of green peach aphid population increases following application of the insecticide azinphosmethyl (Founk, and McClanahan, 1970; Ritcey et al., 1982) provided the basis for laboratory and field investigations. Gordon and McEwen (1984) reported that first-generation aphids derived from mothers that had been confined to cabbage leaves dipped in azinphosmethyl produced more offspring during each of the first three days of reproduction compared with controls. Seven replicated field studies with green peach aphids on azinphosmethyl-treated potato foliage revealed that aphids continuously exposed to insecticide produced 20% to 30% more offspring than the unexposed controls (Lowery and Sears, 1986b). Subsequent laboratory trials with five concentrations ranging from 110 to 1650 ppm azinphosmethyl showed increased responses at all concentrations, with significant enhancement only at the intermediate concentration of 550 ppm (Lowery and Sears, 1986a). However, the maximum increase observed in the laboratory was only 10% compared with 28% in the field. The authors concluded that laboratory experiments may not accurately reflect the magnitude of the response seen in the field, because laboratory conditions are optimized and may not permit sufficient opportunity for gain in the system.

Cotton Stainer

Reproduction studies with dieldrin and the cotton stainer (*Dysedercus fasciatus*) revealed a hormetic-like dose–response curve for total number of eggs produced

(Hodjat, 1971). This study employed a dose range from 0.2 to 10 μg per individual with nine treatments and a control. Egg production was significantly enhanced at 0.2, 0.4, and 0.6 μg/individual, with increases of 16.1%, 17.5%, and 8.5%, respectively. Significant decreases (30.0%–98.7%) in egg production were observed at the higher doses.

Mites

Numerous observations that severe outbreaks of spider mites typically followed the application of dichlorodiphenyltrichloroethane (DDT) led Huffaker and Spitzer (1950) to hypothesize that "some of the results were consistent with the idea of a physiological stimulus to reproduction under DDT influence." Hueck et al. (1952) conducted two field and two laboratory experiments to test this hypothesis. In general, DDT treatment in the field and laboratory stimulated egg production in the fruit tree red spider mite (*Metatetranychus ulmi koch*) by about 50% to 60%. Data from the laboratory study revealed a β-curve dose–response relationship, suggesting a hormetic relationship. Rodriguez et al. (1957), using nine doses (5 to 2000 ppm) plus control, likewise reported that DDT enhanced mite populations on cotton at low doses (10 ppm was the maximum response concentration), but not at higher doses. Low doses of DDT also were shown to enhance the number of offspring (by 20% compared with controls) produced by the European spider mite, a species very susceptible to DDT-induced death (Kuenen, 1958). However, at the highest doses the number of adults that emerged was reduced by nearly 50%. The author suggested that the low-dose stimulatory effect was offset by the concomitant susceptibility to death at the highest doses and put forth the argument that the less-susceptible an arthropod species is to DDT (e.g., the fruit tree red spider mite), the greater the possibility that reproductive stimulation will occur.

The effects of dimethoate on reproduction in the soil mite *Hypoaspis aculeifer* was investigated by Folker-Hansen et al. (1996). Twenty-four neonate juveniles were exposed to each of four conconcentrations of dimethoate (0.230, 0.333, 0.483, and 0.700 mg/kg soil) plus a control. A significant increase in egg production was observed at 0.333 mg/kg and a significant decrease at the highest concentration (0.700 mg/kg). A similar stimulative effect of dimethoate on number of offspring of *H. aculeifer* also was reported by Krogh (1995) at the same concentration range.

Egyptian Cotton Leafworm

Enhanced egg production was observed in the Egyptian cotton leafworm (*Prodenia littura* F.) following treatment with carbaryl (Essac et al., 1972). The magnitude of the response was highly dependent upon the dose administered and the larval instar stage exposed, with the sixth instar stage the most consistent and profoundly affected. It is interesting to note that the doses that stimulated egg production in this model were high (i.e., LD_{10}, LD_{25}, LD_{50}, LD_{70}).

Western Corn Rootworm

Carbaryl treatment also was shown to enhance egg production in the corn rootworm at doses ranging from 0.28% to 0.95% of the LD_{50} (Ball and Su, 1979). Similar stimulatory responses were reported in the same study for carbufuran, but at much lower doses (i.e., 0.0033% and 0.0046% of the LD_{50}).

Confused Flour Beetle

The effect of sublethal doses of sodium fluoride (NaF) on reproduction in the confused flour beetle (*Trifolium confusum* Duval) was investigated by Johansson (1947). The fecundity of beetles raised from eggs exposed to four different concentrations of NaF (0.0001%, 0.001%, 0.01%, and 0.1%) plus a control was determined. Egg production was notably higher for beetles reared on 0.01% NaF compared with controls. At the lower concentrations (0.0001% and 0.001%) only a slight increase compared with controls was observed. A replicate experiment strongly supported the initial findings with respect to the nature of the dose–response relationship.

Mosquito

Reproduction in the mosquito (*Aedes aegypti* L.) was evaluated following exposure to sublethal concentrations of DDT or dieldrin (Sutherland et al., 1967). The doses selected were the same for both insecticides (0.00025, 0.0005, 0.001, and 0.002 ppm), with the range extending from 0.25 to 2 times the $LC_{0.1}$. The number of basal follicles, which is generally equivalent to the ovariole number unless the ovariole is underdeveloped, was the reproductive endpoint chosen for analysis. Both DDT and dieldrin increased the number of basal follicles in a progressive fashion at all concentrations up to 10% and 20% at 0.001 and 0.002 ppm, respectively, compared with controls. Follow-up experiments confirmed these stimulatory effects. The authors concluded that short sublethal exposures of DDT or dieldrin may be sufficient to indirectly stimulate egg production in the mosquito. It should be noted that ethanol, the insecticidal solvent, also stimulated the production of basal follicles, but the authors were able to separate the solvent effect from the effect of the insecticides.

Citrus Thrips

The effect of four pesticides (dicofol, esfenvalerate, formetanate, and malathion) on citrus thrip fecundity was investigated (Morse and Zareh, 1991). Four treatment groups per pesticide were selected encompassing a range of 0.001% to 10% mortality rate ($LC_{0.001}$ to LC_{10}) calculated by probit analysis of acute toxicity data. An increase in mean number of offspring per female compared with controls was observed for each pesticide. The maximum increase was two- to three-fold at the calculated $LC_{0.01}$ of dicofol, 1.75-fold at the $LC_{0.1}$ of esfenvalerate, 2.8-fold at the $LC_{0.1}$ of formetanate, and three-fold at the $LC_{0.1}$ of malathion. The authors concluded that the increase in fecundity was caused by a direct hormetic effect on the insect rather than a response to chemical-induced changes in the leaf, because the thrips were placed on detached, untreated leaves hours after spraying.

Mice

Analysis of data compiled and presented by Daston et al. (1991) revealed an enhancement of several reproductive endpoints in CD1 mice exposed to dinocap (Calabrese and Baldwin, 1993). Mice administered dinocap orally at six different dosages (5 to 120 mg/kg/d) showed low-dose enhancement in both maternal weight gain and number of implants per litter.

MISCELLANEOUS CHEMICALS

In addition to the data presented on $CdCl_2$ and dinocap with mice, apparent hormetic relationships also were revealed for three other chemicals in the analysis of data presented by Daston et al. (1991; Calabrese and Baldwin, 1993). Mice administered p.o. six different dosages of bromodeoxyuridine ranging from 10 to 750 mg/kg/d showed enhanced low-dose responses in maternal weight gain, number of implants per litter, and number of live fetuses per litter compared with controls. Likewise, diphenylhydantoin, administered to mice p.o. at five different dosages (5 to 90 mg/kg/d), and trypan blue, administered p.o. at six different dosages (2.5 to 80 mg/kg/d), displayed apparent hormetic relationships for the same three endpoints.

DISCUSSION

Although chemical hormesis is assessed predominantly in terms of growth endpoints (e.g., root or shoot lengths), a relatively small, but nonetheless impressive, body of work exists displaying reproductive endpoints in apparent hormetic relationships (Table 10.1). These dose–response relationships were consistent with criteria previously developed for the evaluation of evidence of hormesis (e.g., magnitude of response and relationship to the no-observed-adverse-effect level) (Calabrese and Baldwin, 1997). Most notable with respect to these findings is the diverse phylogenetic range of species demonstrating low-dose enhancement of reproductive endpoints within the β-curve framework. Evidence of chemical hormesis was observed in experiments with arachnids (mites), crustaceans (daphnids), insects, hydrozoans (hydra), annelids (polychaete worms), and rodents. It should be noted that similar findings have been reported

Table 10.1 Summary of organisms demonstrating low-dose stimulation of reproduction organized by chemical agent

Agent	Model	Endpoint	References
Heavy metals			
Cadmium	Dapnids	Number of neonates	Elnabarawy et al., 1986; Bodar et al., 1988
	Fathead minnow	Egg production	Pickering and Gast, 1972
	Polychaetes	Fecundity	Reish and Carr, 1978
	Mice	Number of implants, number of live fetuses, maternal weight gain	Daston et al., 1991
Copper	Polychaetes	Fecundity	Reish and Carr, 1978
	Hydra	Bud production	Stebbing and Pomroy, 1977
Mercury	Polychaetes	Fecundity	Reish and Carr, 1978
Zinc	Polychaetes	Fecundity	Reish and Carr, 1978
Lead	Polychaetes	Fecundity	Reish and Carr, 1978
	Hydra	Bud production	Browne and Davis, 1977
Pesticides			
Azinphosmethyl	Aphids	Number of offspring	Gordon and McEwen, 1984; Founk and McClanahan, 1970; Ritcey et al., 1982; Lowery and Sears, 1986a, b
Dieldrin	Cotton stainer	Egg production	Hodjat, 1971
	Mosquito	Number of basal follicles	Sutherland et al., 1967
DDT	Mites	Egg production	Hueck et al., 1952
	Mites	Number of offspring	Kuenen, 1958
	Mites	Number of offspring	Rodriguez et al., 1957
	Mosquito	Number of basal follicles	Sutherland et al., 1967
Carbaryl	Leafworm	Egg production	Essac et al., 1972
	Rootworm	Egg production	Ball and Su, 1979
Carbufuran	Rootworm	Egg production	Ball and Su, 1979
Dimethoate	Mites	Egg production	Folker-Hansen et al., 1996
Sodium fluoride	Beetle	Egg production	Johansson, 1947
Dicofol	Citrus thrips	Number of offspring	Morse and Zareh, 1991
Esfenvalerate	Citrus thrips	Number of offspring	Morse and Zareh, 1991
Formetanate	Citrus thrips	Number of offspring	Morse and Zareh, 1991
Malathion	Citrus thrips	Number of offspring	Morse and Zareh, 1991
Dinocap	Mice	Maternal weight gain, number of implants	Daston et al., 1991
Miscellaneous			
BRDU	Mice	Number of implants, number of live fetuses, maternal weight gain	Daston et al., 1991
DPH	Mice	Number of implants, number of live fetuses, maternal weight gain	Daston et al., 1991
Trypan blue	Mice	Number of implants, number of live fetuses, maternal weight gain	Daston et al., 1991

Note: BRDU, bromodeoxyuridine; DPH, diphenylhydantoin.

in bacteria (Welch et al., 1946) and fungi (Cambell and Saslaw, 1949) with respect to reproduction following exposure to antibiotics.

The range of endpoints showing low-dose enhancement typically included number of offspring, egg production, number of basal follicles, maternal weight, number of implants, and number of live fetuses per litter. The range of chemicals was limited primarily to metals and insecticides.

It is interesting that recognition of the occurrence of low-dose stimulation is not necessarily a controversial concept. For example, ecologists and applied entomologists have long recognized the fact that insect outbreaks often follow pesticidal applications. Although this often has been attributed to elimination of predator or competitive species, the hypothesis has been put forth for a role of hormetic-like physiologic stimulation based on supportive field and laboratory data. The principal issue is not whether low doses directly enhance reproduction, but the overall significance of the phenomenon of insect outbreaks. If hormesis as a concept is viewed not simply in biologic terms, the question of whether it is beneficial or not is often contextual.

ACKNOWLEDGMENT

This chapter was sponsored in part by an award to the University of Massachusetts (Edward J. Calabrese, Principal Investigator) by the Texas Institute for Advancement of Chemical Technology, Inc.

REFERENCES

Ball, H. J., and Su, P. P. 1979. Effect of sublethal dosages of carbofuran and carbaryl on fecundity and longevity of the female western corn rootworm. *J. Econ. Entomol.* 72:873–876.

Bodar, C. W. M., Van Leeuwen, C. J., Voogt, P.A., and Zandee, D. I. 1988. Effect of cadmium on the reproduction strategy of *Daphnia magna*. *Aquatic Toxicol.* 12:301–310.

Browne, C. L., and Davis, L. E. 1977. Cellular mechanisms of stimulation of bud production in *Hydra* by low levels of inorganic lead compounds. *Cell. Tiss. Res.* 177:555–570.

Calabrese, E. J., and Baldwin, L. A. 1993. Possible examples of chemical hormesis in a previously published study. *J. Appl. Toxicol.* 13:169–172.

Calabrese, E. J., and Baldwin, L. A. 1997. The dose determines the stimulation (and poison): Development of a chemical hormesis database. *Int. J. Toxicol.* 16:545–549.

Campbell, C. C., and Saslaw, S. 1949. Enhancement of growth of certain fungi by streptomycin. *Soc. Exp. Biol. Med. Proc.* 70:562–563.

Chapman, R. K., and Allen, T. C. 1948. Stimulation and suppression of some vegetable plants by DDT. *J. Econ. Entomol* 41:616–623.

Daston, G. P., Rogers, J. M., Versteeg, D. J., Sabourin, T. D., Baines, D., and Marsh, S. S. 1991. Interspecies comparisons of A/D ratios: A/D ratios are not constant across species. *Fundam. Appl. Toxicol.* 17:696–722.

Davis, J. M., and Svensgaard, D. J. 1990. U-shaped dose-response curves: Their occurrence and implications for risk assessment. *J. Toxic. Environ. Health* 30:71–83.

DeBach, P. 1946. An insecticidal check method for measuring the efficacy of entomophagous insects. *J. Econ. Entomol.* 39:695–697.

Eggers-Schumacher, H. A. 1983. A comparison of the reproduction performance of insecticide-resistant and susceptible clones of *Myzus persicae*, the green peach aphid (Homoptera: Aphididae). *Can. J. Entomol.* 116:783-784.

Elnabarawy, M. T., Welter, A. N., and Robideau, R. R. 1986. Relative sensitivity of three daphnid species to selected organic and inorganic chemicals. *Environ. Toxicol. Chem.* 5:393-398.

Essac, E. G., El-Gogary, S., Abdel-Fatah, M. S., and Ali, A. M. 1972. Effect of carbaryl, methyl parathion, and endrin on egg production and percent pupation of the Egyptian cotton leafworm, *Spodoptera littoralis* (Boisd.). *Zeits. Angew. Entomol.* 71:203-270.

Folker-Hansen, P., Krogh, P. H., and Holmstrup, M. 1996. Effect of dimethoate on body growth of representatives of the soil living mesofauna. *Ecotoxicol. Environ. Safety* 33:207-216.

Founk, J., and McClanahan, R. J. 1970. Foliar potato insect control. *C.C.P.U.A. Res. Rep.*, pp. 122-123.

Giordano, G. G., Pagano, G., Calicchio, G., de Angelis, M., Esposito, A., Malgieri, F., Rota, A., Malgieri, F., Rota, A., Vamvakinos, E., Saward, D., and Sabbioni, E. 1983. EEC Commission Contract Report ENV/554/I-(S). Brussels: EEC Commission.

Gordon, P. L., and McEwen, F. L. 1984. Insecticide-stimulated reproduction of *Myzus persicae*, the green peach aphid (Homoptera: Aphididae). *Can. J. Entomol.* 116:783-784.

Hodjat, H. 1971. Effects of sublethal doses of insecticides and of diet and crowding on *Dysdercus fasciatus* Sign. (Hem., Pyrrhocoridae). *Bull. Entomol. Res.* 60:367-378.

Hrdy, I. 1979. Insecticide resistance in aphids. In *Proceedings of the IX International Congress on Plant Protection*, vol. 1:*Plant protection and fundamental aspects*, ed. T. Kommendahl. College Park, MD: Entomological Society of America.

Hueck, H. J., Kuenen, D. J., Den Boer, P. J., and Jaeger-Draafsel, E. 1952. The increase of egg production of the fruit tree red spider mite (*Metatetranychus ulmi koch*) under influence of DDT. *Physiol. Comp.* 2:371-377.

Huffaker, C. B., and Spitzer, C. H. 1950. Some factors affecting Red Mite populations on pears in California. *J. Econ. Entomol.* 43:819-831.

Johansson, T. S. K. 1947. Some physiological effects of sublethal doses of sodium fluoride on the confused flour beetle (*Tribolium confusum* Duval). Thesis, University of Wisconsin.

Kobayashi. N. 1971. *Publication of Seto Marine Biology Laboratory* 18:379-406.

Krogh, P. G. 1995. Effects of pesticides on the reproduction of *Hypoaspis aculeifer* (Gamasida: Laelapidae) in the laboratory. *Acta Zool. Fennica* 196:333-337.

Kuenen, D. J. 1958. Influence of sublethal doses of DDT upon the multiplication rate of *Sitophilus granarius* (Coleopt. Curculionidae). *Entomol. Exp. Appl.* 1:147-152.

Lowery, D. T., and Sears, M. K. 1986a. Effect of exposure to the insecticide azinphosmethyl on reproduction of green peach aphid (Homoptera: Aphididae). *J. Econ. Entomol.* 79:1534-1538.

Lowery, D. T., and Sears, M. K. 1986b. Stimulation of reproduction of the green peach aphid (Homoptera: Aphididae) by azinphosmethyl applied to potatoes. *J. Econ. Entomol.* 79:1530-1533.

Morse, J. G., and Zareh, N. 1991. Pesticide-induced hormoligosis of citrus thrips (Thysanoptera: Thripidae) fecundity. *J. Econ. Entomol.* 84:1169-1174.

Pagano, G., Cipollaro, M., Corsale, G., Esposito, A., Ragucci, E., Giordano, G. G., and Trieff, N. M. 1986. The sea urchin: Bioassay for the assessment of damage from environmental contaminants. In *Community toxicity testing, ASTM STP 920*, ed. pp. 66-92. J. Cairns, Jr., Philadelphia: American Society for Testing and Materials.

Pagano, G., Esposito, A., and Giodano, G. G. 1982. Fertilization and larval development in sea urchins following exposure of gametes and embryos to cadmium. *Arch. Environ. Contam. Toxicol.* 11:47-55.

Pickering, Q. H., and Gast, M. H. 1972. Acute and chronic toxicity of cadmium to the fathead minnow (*Pimephales promelas*). *J. Fish. Res. Bd. Can.* 29:1099-1106.

Radcliffe, E. B. 1972. Population responses of green peach aphid in Minnesota on potatoes treated with various insecticides. *Proc. North Cent. Branch Entomol. Soc. Am.* 27:103-105.

Reish, D. J., and Carr, R. S. 1978. The effect of heavy metals on the survival, reproduction, development, and life cycles for two species of polychaetous annelids. *Mar. Poll. Bull.* 9:24-27.

Ripper, W. E. 1956. Effect of pesticides on the balance of arthropod populations. *Annu. Rev. Entomol.* 1:403–438.

Ritcey, G., McGraw, R., and McEwen, F. L. 1982. Insect control on potatoes in Ontario from 1973 to 1982. *Proc. Entomol. Soc. Ont.* 113:1–6.

Rodriguez, J. G., Chen, H. H., and Smith, W. T. Jr. 1957. Effects of soil insecticides on beans, soybeans and cotton and resulting effect on mite nutrition. *J. Econ. Entomol.* 50:587–593.

Stebbing, A. R. D. 1980. Increase in gonozooid frequency as an adaptive response to stress in *Campanularia flexuosa*. In *Developmental and cellular biology of coelenterates*, ed. P. Tardent, and R. Tardent, pp. 27–32. Amsterdam: Elsevier.

Stebbing, A. R. D. 1982. Hormesis: The stimulation of growth by low levels of inhibitors. *Sci. Total Environ.* 22:213–234.

Stebbing, A. R. D., and Pomroy, A. J. 1977. A sublethal technique for assessing the effects of contaminants using *Hydra littoralis*. *Water Res.* 12:631–635.

Sutherland, D. J., Beam, F. D., and Gupta, A. P. 1967. The effects on mosquitoes of sublethal exposure to insecticides. I DDT, dieldrin, malathion and the basal follicles of *Aedes aegypti* (L). *Mosquito News* 27:316–323.

van Emden, H. F. 1966. Studies on the relations of insect and host plant: III. A comparison of the reproduction of *Brevicoryne brassicae* and *Myzus persicae* (Hemiptera: Aphididae) on brussels sprout plants supplied with different rates of nitrogen and potassium. *Entomol. Exp. Appl.* 9:444–460.

Welch, H., Price, C. W., and Randall, W. A. 1946. Increase in fatality rate of *E. typhosa* for white mice by streptomycin. *J. Am. Pharm. Assoc.* 35:155–158.

CHAPTER
ELEVEN

TRENDS IN TOXICOLOGY MODELING FOR RISK ASSESSMENT

Shayne C. Gad

Gad Consulting Services, Raleigh, North Carolina

The broad realm of risk assessment (as it applies to toxicology) is based on assembling a number of known facts (primarily exposure routes and levels on one hand and biologic responses on the other) and then somehow melding these two to produce an estimate of the quantity or incidence of risk inherent in given real or potential situations. The biologic-response end of experimental results usually is obtained in a nonhuman species at some relatively high dose or exposure level, from which an attempt is made to predict the level of impact in humans at much lower levels. The means of bridging the gaps from what we know to where we are concerned is the domain of risk assessment. If this is done in a manner that attempts to develop or employ logical, quantitative means, modeling is employed.

In this chapter, we examine the assumptions involved in both the risk-assessment and modeling undertakings. In doing so, we take a critical look at the steps involved in low-dose extrapolation models and methods, present the framework on which risk assessment is based (including more recent approaches such as the benchmark dose), and describe the ways in which modeling has been done and is being done and how it continually influences the risk-assessment process (Hallenbeck, 1993; Haimes, 1998).

RISK ASSESSMENT

Risk assessment in toxicology is not limited to carcinogenesis. Rather, it may be applied to all the possible toxicologic consequences of exposure to chemicals or agents that can be determined objectively to have happened in exposed individuals. It is a yet more difficult process if the effects are delayed relative to point of exposure in occurence. Because the consequences of toxic events of concern are extreme yet may be distanced from the actual cause (exposure) by time (unlike with exposure to an acutely lethal agent, such as carbon monoxide), society is willing to accept only a low level of risk while maintaining the benefits of use of the agent. Though the most familiar (and, to date, best developed) case is that of carcinogenesis, much of what is presented for risk assessment also may be applied to the other endpoints of concern.

Mutagens generally are not conceded to have thresholds, but the human health concern of those that are not established as carcinogens or teratogens is conjectural. Certainly materials identified as mutagens in an in vivo mammalian system (such as a dominant lethal study in mice or in vivo sister chromatid exchange in rabbits or rats) should be treated more conservatively than those whose mutagenicity has been established only in bacterial or biochemical test systems. The U.S. Environmental Protection Agency (EPA) (1984a) has proposed a regulatory process for the assessment of risks from mutagens that is not noticeably different from their approach to carcinogens, and that utilizes dose–response data from many test systems (even biochemical) as a starting point.

Developmental toxicants now are clearly established to have dose–response relationships that are subject to both time and quantity-of-dose thresholds (Jusko, 1972). The exposure of the fertilized ovum must occur within a time window in which the ovum is susceptible. Likewise, the dose must be sufficient to cause an effect and yet not so great as to cause a spontaneous abortion of the embryo or fetus. Rai and Van Ryzin (1985) have proposed a dose–response model for developmental toxicity that includes two approaches to low-dose extrapolation based on a one-hit model. This model is also useful for mammalian dominant lethal data, which can be considered a subset of either developmental or reproductive toxicity data. Kimmel et al. (1990) have developed and proposed the benchmark dose approach for the same area, and Leroux et al. (1996) have put forward a biologically based model for dose–response in developmental toxicity.

Reproductive toxicants are a whole new wide world to worry about. Though Gross et al. (1970) suggested caution in evaluating data that might be improperly suggestive of a nontoxic threshold level, there is a clear consensus that there are thresholds below which reproductive agents are inactive. The difficulty is that such a wide variety of biochemical and physiologic processes are involved in the successful operation of the reproductive process that we do not yet have adequate experimental methods to detect and quantitate all possible effects. Dixon and Nadolney (1985) and Roberts (1989) have presented brief overviews of the problems involved in going from our present state of knowledge in this area to the performance of meaningful risk assessments.

Though some of the fine points may vary, one should expect that the risk-assessment process for any irreversible toxicant will follow the general form and steps presented in this chapter, and such assessment should be undertaken with full knowledge of the involved uncertainties, weaknesses, and difficulties.

Quantitation of Exposure

The remaining problem (or step) in performing a risk assessment is quantitating the exposure of the human population, both in terms of how many people are exposed by what routes (or means) and to what quantities of an agent they are exposed, and adjusting for any special sensitivities or susceptibility factors of a group that is of specific concern (such as children or the elderly).

This process of identifying and quantitating exposure groups within the human population is beyond the scope of this text, except for some key points. Classification methods are again the key tool for identifying and properly delimiting human populations at risk. An investigator must first understand the process involved in making, shipping, using, and disposing of a material. The EPA has proposed guidelines for such identification and exposure quantitation (U.S. EPA, 1984b). The exposure groups can be very large or relatively small subpopulations, each with a markedly different potential for exposure. For di-(2-ethyl-hexyl)phthalate, for example, the following at-risk populations have been identified:

IV route: 3,000,000 receiving blood transfusions (50 mg/yr)
            50,000 dialysis patients (4500 mg/yr)
            10,000 hemophiliacs (760 mg/yr)
Oral route: 10,000,000 children under 3 years of age (434 mg/yr)
            220,000,000 adults (dietary contamination (1.1 mg/yr)

Not quantitated were possible inhalation and dermal exposure.

All such estimates of exposure in humans (and of the number of humans exposed) are subject to a large degree of uncertainty. Additionally, the way in which total doses are divided in their delivery is well established as being significant (Wilson and Holland, 1982).

An alternative approach to achieving society's objective for the entire risk-assessment procedure—protecting the human population from unacceptable levels of known risks—is the classical approach of using safety factors. In 1972, Weil summarized this approach as follows:

> In summary, for the evaluation of safety for man, it is necessary to: (1) design and conduct appropriate toxicologic tests, (2) statistically compare the data from treated and control animals, (3) delineate the minimum effect and maximum no ill-effect levels (NIEL) for these animals, and (4) if the material is to be used, apply an appropriate safety factor, e.g., (a) 1/100 (NIEL) or 1/500 (NIEL) for some effects or (b) 1/500 (NIEL), if the effect was a significant increase in cancer in an appropriate test.

This approach has served society reasonably well over the years, once the experimental work identified potential hazards and quantitated observable dose–response relationships. Until such time as the more elegant risk-assessment procedures can install greater public confidence, the use of the safety-factor approach should not be abandoned.

Low-dose Extrapolation

Risk assessment, in the sense in which we consider it in this book, and as it is performed by toxicologists, involves a number of separate steps, each of which involves some form of mathematical model to bridge gaps in biological knowledge. In a very crude sense, these steps can be categorized as answers to one of three problems:

1. Given knowledge of what happens at relatively high doses in one or more animal species, we must predict what would happen in the same species at much lower dose levels.
2. We must estimate what actual human exposures are. This means identifying groups or classes of exposed people and estimating "lifetime exposure."
3. Given the dose–response estimation made (for animals from step 1) and exposure estimates for classes of people (from step 2), we must finally couple the two by some model that translates "mice to men." That is, we must perform a species-to-species extrapolation.

The second and third steps are addressed separately in the final section of this chapter. The first step, known as *low-dose extrapolation*, is addressed here.

Threshold

The process of low-dose extrapolation, no matter which method is used, consists of three distinct steps. First, the actual dose–response data points available (which, for reasons discussed previously, are invariably in the high-dose or high-response region) are identified, providing a starting point. Second, a mathematical method is selected and employed to extend the dose–response relationship from the known region to the regions of interest or concern. Third, we make a basic assumption about the nature of the dose–response relationship in the extreme low-dose or response region and then proceed to develop a model specific to the compound of interest.

A basic assumption about the extreme low-dose region concerns the question of threshold. For all biologic phenomena except perhaps carcinogenesis and mutagenesis, it is a basic principle of biology that there is a dose level (threshold) below which no response evolves (Dinman, 1972). But there remains a controversy as to applicability of the concept of a threshold for carcinogenesis and mutagenesis (Albert et al., 1979), though there are good cases for no-effect levels for even these (see Table 11.1). This has led to a number of very conservative measures in applicable regulatory risk-assessment approaches:

1. Use of upper confidence limits on the estimated virtually safe dose (VSD) instead of on the VSD itself
2. Use of the most sensitive animal species
3. Use of the most sensitive sex of that species

Table 11.1 Estimated no-effect quantities of some potent carcinogens and toxic agents

Agent	Molecular weight	Calculated no-effect level (g/kg body weight)	Molarity	Molecules per kilogram body weight
Aflatoxim	312	5×10^{-9}	1.6×10^{-11}	9.6×10^{12}
1,2,5,6-dibenzanthracene (subcutaneous)	278	2.5×10^{-4}	9×10^{-7}	5.4×10^{17}
1,2,5,6-dibenzanthracene (subcutaneous)	278	2.5×10^{-5}	9×10^{-8}	5.4×10^{16}
3-Methylcholanthrene (subcutaneous)	268	2.5×10^{-5}	9.3×10^{-8}	5.6×10^{16}
2,4-Benz-a-pyrene (skin)	252	2.5×10^{-6}	1×10^{-8}	6×10^{16}
Aramite	335	1×10^{-1}	3×10^{-4}	1.8×10^{20}
Tetrachlorodibenzodioxin	320	6×10^{-8}	1.9×10^{-10}	1.1×10^{14}
Botulinum toxin (mouse)	900,000	6.5×10^{-11}	7×10^{-17}	4.2×10^{7}

Sources: Freidman, 1973; Carlberg (1979a, b).

4. Use of the most sensitive strain within a species
5. Expression of dosage given on a dietary concentration basis rather than on a body-weight basis when extrapolating from animals to humans; this results in about a 15-fold lower acceptable exposure for humans as compared with the mouse.
6. The slope of unity found using Mantel–Bryan (a model for low-dose extrapolation to be discussed later) is almost always less than the observed data, thereby resulting in lower acceptable exposure (Mantel, 1963).

The arguments for the existence of the threshold are as numerous and tend to be more mechanistic. These are summarized as follows:

1. Most (if not all) carcinogens and mutagens exhibit a dose–response relationship, resulting in an apparent or effective threshold for at least some agents. This is the classical toxicology argument, coming from the general case of all other toxic actions and finding no reason or data to support these actions being different (Klaassen and Doull, 1980). Theoretic analysis of the process of carcinogenesis as understood for radiation (the case in which we have the most human data) likewise suggests a lack of linearity at very low doses (Arlcy, 1961).

2. Toxicity, including carcinogenesis, is a dynamic process that includes absorption of an agent into the body, distribution to various tissues, reversible or irreversible reactions with cellular components, adaptation and repair by molecular and cellular components of the body, and ultimately clearance from the body by metabolism or excretion. Such pharmacokinetic processes are generally linear only within prescribed ranges. Gehring and Blau (1977) have proposed that such pharmacokinetic processes provide a conceptual basis for understanding how metabolic thresholds may lead to a disproportionate increase in toxicity, including carcinogenesis, above certain dose levels. They also have conducted and presented work on vinyl chloride carcinogenesis and pharmacokinetic data to support this proposal.

Because an organism as large as either a mouse or a man has a tremendous number of cells, a large number of defense mechanisms of high efficiency, and low probability of a "hit"—a carcinogen being effective in initiating or promoting a neoplasm—there is a biologic threshold based on just stochastic or probabilistic grounds. The last aspect (low probability of a "meaningful" reaction) arises from consideration of the fact that the vast majority of molecules with which a carcinogen comes in contact (and reacts) in a multicellular organism cannot then contribute to the development of a neoplasm—they are, in effect, a multitude of "dummies" acting to block the assassin's shot.

Cross-species Extrapolation

Having investigated the methods that are available to extrapolate the risk of an irreversible event from a high dose range to a low dose range in the same animal species, we must now address the question of a means to extrapolate from an animal species to humans. This extrapolation has both qualitative aspects (to be discussed here) and quantitative aspects (called scaling, to be discussed later).

The qualitative aspects of species-to-species extrapolations are best addressed by a form of classification analysis tailored to the exact problem at hand. This approach identifies the physiologic, metabolic, and other factors that may be involved in the risk-producing process in the model species (for example, the carcinogenesis process in test mice), establishes the similarities and differences between these factors and those in humans, and comes up with means to bridge the gaps between these two (or to identify the fact that there is no possible bridge).

Tomatis (1979) has provided an excellent evaluation of the comparability of carcinogenicity findings between rodents and man, in general finding the former to be good predictors of the endpoint in the latter. However, in his 1984 Stokinger lecture, Weil pointed out that the model species should respond biologically to the material as similarly as possible to man; that the routes of exposure (actual and possible) should be the same; and that there are known wide variations in response to carcinogens. Diechmann (1975) for example, has reviewed studies demonstrating that 2-naphthylamine is a human and dog carcinogen but not active in the mouse, rat, guinea pig or rabbit.

Smith (1974) discussed interspecies variations of response to carcinogens, including N-2-fluorenyl-acetamide, which is potent for the dog, rabbit, hamster, and rat (believed to result from formation of an active metabolite by N-hydroxylation), but not in the guinea pig or steppe lemming, which do not form this metabolic derivative.

Table 11.2 represents an overview of the classes of factors that should be considered in the first step of a species extrapolation. Examples of such actual differences that can be classified as among these factors are almost endless.

The absorption of compounds from the gastrointestinal tract and from the lungs is comparable among vertebrate and mammalian species. There are, however, differences between herbivorous animals and omnivorous animals resulting from differences in stomach structure. The problem of distribution within the body probably relates less to species than to size and is discussed under scaling. Metabolism, xenobiotic metabolism of foreign compounds, metabolic activation, or toxification or detoxification mechanisms (by whatever name) is perhaps the critical factor, and this can differ widely from species to species. The increasing realization that the original compound administered is not necessarily the ultimate carcinogen makes the further study of these metabolic patterns critical.

Table 11.2 Classes of factors to be considered in species-to-species extrapolations in risk assessment

Sensitivity of model animal (relative to humans)	Relative population differences	Differences between test and real world environment
Pharmacologic	Size	Physical (temperature, humidity, etc.)
Receptor	Heterogeneity	
Life span	Selected "high class"	Chemical
Size	nature of test	Nutritional
Metabolic function	population	
Physiologic		
Anatomic		
Nutritional requirements		
Reproductive and developmental processes		
Diet		
Critical reflex and behavioral responses (as emetic reflex)		
Behavioral		
Rate of cell division		
Other defense mechanisms		

In terms of excretory rates, the differences between the species are not very great; small animals tend to excrete compounds more rapidly than large ones in a rather systematic way. The various cellular and intercellular barriers seem to be surprisingly constant throughout the vertebrate phylum. In addition it is beginning to be appreciated that the receptors, such as DNAs, are comparable throughout the mammalian species.

There are life-span (or temporal) differences that have not been considered adequately, either now or in the past. It takes time to develop a tumor, and at least some of that time may be taken up by the actual cell-division process. Cell-division rates appear to be significantly higher in smaller animals. Mouse and rat cells turn over faster than human cells—perhaps at twice the rate. On the other hand, the latent period for development of tumors is much shorter in small animals than in large ones (Hammond et al., 1978).

Another problem is that the life span of man is about 35 times that of the mouse or rat; thus there is a much longer time for a tumor to appear. These sorts of temporal considerations are of considerable importance.

Body size, irrespective of species, seems to be important in the rate of distribution of foreign compounds throughout the body. A simple example of this is that the cardiac output of the mouse is on the order of 1 mL/min, and the mouse has a blood volume of about 1 mL. The mouse is turning its blood volume over every minute. In man, the cardiac output per minute is only 1/20 of the blood volume. So the mouse turns its blood over and distributes whatever is in the blood or collects excretory products over 20 times faster than man.

Another aspect of the size difference that should be considered is that the large animal has a very much greater number of susceptible cells that may interact with potential carcinogenic agents, though there is also a proportionately increased number of "dummy" cells.

Rall (1977, 1979) and Borzelleca (1984) have published articles reviewing such factors, and Calabrese (1983) and Gad and Chengelis (1988) have published excellent books on the subject.

Having delineated and quantified species differences (even if only having factored in comparative body weights and food consumption rates), we can proceed to some form of quantitative extrapolation. This process is called *scaling*.

There are currently three major approaches to scaling in risk assessment. These are by fraction of diet, by body weight, and by body surface area (Calabrese, 1983; Schmidt-Nielsen, 1984).

The "fraction-of-diet" method is based on converting the results in the experimental animal model to man on a milligram (of test substance) per kilogram (diet) per day basis. If the experimental model is the mouse, this leads to an extrapolation factor that is six-fold lower than on a body-weight (mg/kg) basis (Association Food and Drug Officials, 1959). Fraction-of-diet factors are not considered accurate indices of actual dosages, because the latter are influenced not only by voluntary food intake, as affected by palatability and caloric density of the diet and by single or multiple caging, but more particularly by the age of the animal. During the early stages of life, anatomic, physiologic, metabolic, and immunologic capabilities are not fully developed. Moreover, the potential for toxic effect in an animal is a function of the dose ingested, and ultimately of the number of active molecules reaching the target cell. Additionally, many agents of concern do not have ingestion as the major route of intake in man. Both the Environmental Protection Agency (EPA) and the Consumer Product Safety Commission frequently employ a fraction-of-diet scaling factor.

Human diets are generally assumed to be 600 to 700 g/d; in mice they are 4 g/d and in rats 25 g/d (the equivalent of 50 g/kg/d).

There are several ways to perform a scaling operation on a body weight basis. The most common is to simply calculate a conversion factor (K) as

$$\frac{\text{Weight of human (70 kg)}}{\text{Weight of test animal (0.4 kg for rat)}} = K$$

More exotic methods for doing this, such as that based on a form of linear regression, are reviewed by Calabrese (1983), who believes that the body-weight method is preferable.

A difficulty with this approach is that the body weights of both animals and man change throughout life. An "ideal man" or "ideal rat" weight is therefore utilized.

Finally, there are the body surface area methods, which attempt to factor in differences in metabolic rates based on the principle that these change in proportion with body-surface area (because as the ratio of body-surface area to body weight increases, more energy is required to maintain constant body temperature). There are several methods for doing this, each having a ratio of dose to the animal's body weight (in milligrams per kilogram) as a starting point, resulting in a conversion factor with milligrams per square meter as the unit.

The EPA version generally is calculated as:

$$(M_{\text{human}}/M_{\text{animal}})^{1/3} = \text{surface factor}$$

where M is mass in kilograms. Another form is calculated based on constants that have been developed for a multitude of species of animals by actual surface area measurements (Spector, 1956). The resulting formula for this is:

$$A = KW^{2/3}$$

where A is the surface area in square centimeters, K is constant, specific for each species, and W is weight in grams. A scaling factor then is calculated simply as a ratio of the surface area of man over that of the model species.

The "best" scaling factor is not generally agreed upon. Though the majority opinion is that surface area is preferable if a metabolic activation or deactivation is known to be both critical to the risk-producing process and present in both the model species and man, these assumptions may not always be valid. Table 11.3 presents a comparison of the weight and surface area extrapolation methods for eight species.

Table 11.3 Extrapolation of a dose of 100 mg/kg in the mouse to other species

			Extrapolated dose (mg)		
Species	Weight (g)	Surface area (cm^3)^a	Body weight (A)	Body surface area (B)	Ratio A/B
Mouse	20	46.4	2	2	1.0
Rat	400	516.7	40	22.3	1.79
Guinea Pig	400	564.5	40	24.3	1.65
Rabbit	1500	1272.0	150	54.8	2.74
Dog	12000	5766.0	1200	248.5	4.83
Cat	2000	1381.0	200	59.5	3.46
Monkey	4000	2975.0	400	128.2	3.12
Human	70000	18000.0	7000	775.8	9.02

^{a}Surface area (except in case of man) calculated from formula: Surface area (cm^2) − K(W$^{2/3}$), where K is a constant for each species and W is body weight (values of K and surface area of man taken from Spector [1956]).

Schneiderman et al. (1975) and Dixon (1976) have published comparisons of these methods, but Schmidt-Nielsen (1984) should be considered the primary source on scaling in interspecies comparisons.

Susceptibility Factors

Of increasing concern in recent years is the realization that not all exposed populations are equally at risk. Although experimental data in animals are generated primarily using healthy young adult animals, these are not necessarily representative of the entire populations that are exposed.

In particular, children, the elderly, and individuals with compromised health should at least be considered in exposure and risk assessments. The entire list of factors to potentially consider, however, is much longer (see Table 10.2). Such populations may have greater degrees of susceptibility because of a range of factors (Guzelian et al., 1992; and Perera, 1997). Both the EPA (for pesticides) and the Food and Drug Administration (FDA) recently have taken steps that make risk assessment more conservative in the cases in which children may be an exposed population.

MODELING

Modeling is the means by which we attempt to understand (at least quantitatively) the relationships between the available data and the outcome (biologic response) of interest.

In conducting any analysis and in the modeling of complex toxicologic phenomena, a set of operating assumptions must be adopted to allow for as precise an analysis or model as possible. These are defined by the specific problem at hand and can be either simple or complex (Gad, 1998). Some general assumptions include:

- A model should be based upon the single defined endpoint as above.
- There is no operative high-dose to low-dose linearity. However, there is linearity within the low-dose region of interest (less than about 16%).
- Both cumulative and peak exposure matter (Yanyshev and Antomonov, 1998; Gad and Chengelis, 1997).
- Human data via the route of likely exposure is the most desirable for use in any modeling efforts and always should take precedence over animal data (or human data via a different route of exposure) if the two conflict. Nonhuman primate data, though less desirable than human data, is more desirable than other animal data. As previously discussed in the risk-assessment section, there are a wide range of available methodologies for extrapolating from animal data to human effects (also see Gad and Chengelis, 1988), but each such extrapolation (be it species-to-species or route-to-route or from one time interval to another) contributes further to the uncertainty associated with the process.
- Though best recognized in the case of carcinogenesis (Guess and Hoel, 1977; Littlefield et al., 1980; Ljinsky et al., 1981), the relationship between dose and response is much more complex than that the higher the dose, the greater the incidence of response in the exposed population. The response portion of the concept also covers both severity of response and time to response (the greater the dose, the sooner the response or effect occurs or is expressed).
- Any model must provide confidence intervals and an envelope of validity. Any predictive number without an estimate of the uncertainty associated with it (in the dimension of interest—for our purposes, either concentration or time) is of suspect validity and minimal utility.
- Predicted values for all currently employed models are generally for healthy males and the general populations. Sensitive populations would require application of further safety factors. Whether the values produced out of these evaluation also can be used for healthy females (or those that are young or old or have compromised health) is unknown and requires additional evaluation to determine.

As it was determined in initial trials and evaluations that slopes and curves in the central region of the response range (that is, from 16% up through 50% and beyond) were not representative of those in the region of interest for this effort, modeling was restrained to the lower end of the exposure range. Focusing on the range of responses at 16% or less, it was found that a modification of the nonlinear response method and the use of weighted measures performed acceptably. This modification (and any other meaningful model) requires that specific calculations be performed for alterations in either agent or response—it is not possible to produce a general model across either of these "dimensions of interest" (that is, for either all agents of a class or all effects of a single agent) without sacrificing significant degrees of precision in predictive accuracy.

It should be noted that the model does not specify slope—no model will. Rather, the data set utilized in performing calculations determines the derived slope.

Furthermore, complex integrative (organism level) responses (such as lethality) are very different than any of the single physiologic/functional endpoints and cannot be used to predict functional endpoints. In fact, lethality data (and any slope derived from them) from the center of the response range (that is, in the "stable" region surrounding the median lethal dose (LD_{50}), with responses in the range of about 16%–84%) does not provide a meaningful basis for the estimation of lower limit lethality, as both mechanisms and subject populations are different.

The result is not truly a "hockey stick," but rather for any one endpoint a curve with a sharp discontinuity (change in slope) as lower exposure regions are reached, particularly as cumulative exposures are spread over more time. This "break" or discontinuity in the curve occurs at or about the 16% response region. It is likely that this location is a reflection as much of the (underlying) probit methodology as of a difference in biologic mechanisms or affected populations, but this does not change the utility of the approach.

In a very real sense, the model in the central or statistically stable response region (that is, within a standard deviation of the 50% response point) is independent from that in the asymptotic (lower and upper) response regions. In this central region, the confidence regions tend to be less broad and to have smoother borders.

Traditional dose- and time–response tables serve to present answers to focused questions of interest. However, it should be kept in mind that the data of interest are usually multidimensional. Both time (length of exposure) and dose (total cumulative and peak) are major determinants of response, and response (expressed as an incidence or percent proportion of those exposed expressing a response) itself is a variable. As a result, the most accurate graphic representation of model outputs are distinct response surface plots. Actual data points also are plotted, to allow the reader to gain a feeling for the relationship among response curves, their associated confidence intervals, and the actual available data.

Physiologically Based Pharmacokinetic

Pharmacokinetic modeling is the process of developing mathematical explanations of absorption, distribution, metabolism, and excretion of chemicals in organisms. Two commonly used types of compartmental pharmacokinetic models are data-based and physiologically based. The data-based pharmacokinetic models correspond to mathematical descriptions of the temporal change in the blood–tissue level of a xenobiotic in the animal species of interest. This procedure considers the organism as a single homogeneous compartment or as a multicompartmental system with elimination occurring in specific compartments of the model. The number, behavior, and volume of these hypothetical compartments are estimated by the type of equation chosen to describe the data, and not necessarily by the physiologic characteristics of the model species in which the blood–tissue concentration data were acquired.

Although these data-based pharmacokinetic models can be used for interpolation, they should not be used for extrapolation outside the range of doses, dose routes, and species used in the study on which they were based. In order to use the data-based models to describe the pharmacokinetic behavior of a chemical administered at various doses by different routes, extensive animal experimentation would be required to generate similar blood–time course data under respective conditions. Even within the same species of animal, the time-dependent nature of critical biologic determinants of the disposition (e.g., tissue glutathione depletion and resynthesis) cannot easily be included or evaluated with the data-based pharmacokinetic modeling approach. Further, because of the lack of actual anatomic, physiologic, and biochemical realism, these data-based compartmental models cannot be used easily in interspecies extrapolation, particularly to predict pharmacokinetic behavior of chemicals in humans. These various extrapolations, which are essential for the conduct of dose–response assessment of chemicals, can be performed more confidently with a physiologically based pharmacokinetic (PBPK) modeling approach. This chapter presents the principles and methods of PBPK modeling as applied to the study of toxicologically important chemicals.

PBPK modeling is the development of mathematical descriptions of the uptake and disposition of chemicals based on quantitative interrelationships among the critical biologic determinants of these processes. These determinants include partition coefficients, rates of biochemical reactions, and physiological characteristics of the animal species. The biologic and mechanistic basis of the PBPK models enable them to be used, with limited animal experimentation, for extrapolation of the kinetic behavior of chemicals from high dose to low dose, from one exposure route to another, and from test animal species to people.

The development of PBPK models is performed in four interconnected steps: model representation, model parameterization, model stimulation, and model validation. Model representation involves the development of conceptual, functional, and computational descriptions of the relevant compartments of the animal as well as the exposure and metabolic pathways of the chemical. Model parameterization involves obtaining independent measures of the mechanistic determinants, such as physiologic, physicochemical, and biochemical parameters, which are included in one or more of the PBPK model equations. Model simulation involves the prediction of the uptake and disposition of a chemical for defined exposure scenarios, using a numerical integration algorithm, simulation software, and a computer. Finally, the model validation step involves the comparison of the a priori predictions of the PBPK model with experimental data to refute, validate, or refine the model description, and the characterization of the sensitivity of tissue dose to changes in model parameter values. PBPK models after appropriate testing and validation can be used to conduct extrapolations of the pharmacokinetic behavior of chemicals from one exposure route or scenario to another, from high dose to low dose, and from one species to another.

The PBPK model development for a chemical is preceded by the definition of the problem, which in toxicology often is related to the apparent complex nature of toxicity. Examples of such apparent complex toxic responses include nonlinearity in dose–response, sex or species differences in tissue response, differential response of tissues to chemical exposure, qualitatively or quantitatively different responses for the same cumulative dose administered by different route or scenarios, and so forth. In these instances, PBPK modeling studies can be utilized to evaluate the pharmacokinetic basis of the apparent complex nature of toxicity induced by the chemical. One of the values of PBPK modeling, in fact, is that accurate description of target tissue dose often resolves behavior that appears complex at the administered dose level.

The principal application of PBPK models is in the prediction of the target tissue dose of the toxic parent chemical or its reactive metabolite. Use of the target tissue dose of the toxic moiety of a chemical in risk-assessment calculations provides a better basis of relating to the observed toxic effects than the external or exposure concentration of the parent chemical. Because PBPK models facilitate the prediction of target tissue dose for various exposure scenarios, routes, doses, and species, they can help reduce the uncertainty associated with the conventional extrapolation approaches. Direct application of modeling includes:

- High-dose/low-dose extrapolation
- Route–route extrapolation
- Exposure-scenario extrapolation
- Interspecies extrapolation

Risk-assessment Models

There are at least nine different major models for extrapolating a line or curve across the entire range from a high-dose region to a low-dose region. In this section we examine each of these models and compare them in terms of characteristics and outcome. Some of these models are such that they handle only quantal (also called dichotomous) data, others also accommodate time-to-tumor information.

In these models, certain standard symbols are used. Most of these models express the probability of a response, P, as a function, f, of dosage, D, so that $P = f(D)$ and the models differ only with respect to choice of function. The nonthreshold models assume that if proporation p of control animals respond to a dose that $f(D) = p$ only for D equal to zero, and that for any nonzero $D, f(D)p > 0$ (that is, there is a response). Threshold models assume the existence of a D_0 such that for all $D < D_0$, $f(D) = p$ (that is, that there is some dose below which there is no response). If safety is defined as zero increase over control response, then a nonthreshold model would require that any nonzero dosage be associated with some finite risk.

One hit. The one-hit model is based on the assumption that cancer initiates from a single cell as a result of a random occurrence or "hit" that causes an irreversible alteration in the DNA of a susceptible cell type. It is also assumed that the likelihood of this hit is proportional to the level of carcinogen exposure. This suggests a direct linear dose response such that if one is to diminish the risk from 10^{-2} to 10^{-8}, then the dose should be divided by 10^6.

Accordingly, the one-hit model is also called the *linear model*, though a number of the other models also behave in a linear manner at lower doses. Based on the concept that a single receptor molecule of some form responds after an animal has been exposed to some single unit of an agent, the probability of tumor induction by exposure to the agent is then

$$P(d) = 1 - \exp(-1\lambda)D$$

where

$$D\chi 0, 0 \alpha P(D) \alpha_1$$

λ is an unknown rate constant (or slope) and D is the expected number of hits at dose level D. "Dose" is used in a very general sense. It may mean the total accumulated dose or the dosage rate in terms of body weight, surface-area approximations, or concentration in the diet. Computing the one-hit model in terms of the exponential series gives

$$P(D) = \frac{\lambda D}{1} \frac{(\lambda D)^2}{1 \cdot 2} + \frac{(\lambda D)}{1 \cdot 2 \cdot 3} \cdots$$

which, for small values of P(D), is well approximated by

$$P(D) = \lambda D$$

Though Hoel et al. (1975) have argued that this model is consistent with reasonable biologic assumptions, there is now almost universal agreement that the model is excessively conservative. The concept of a hit is a metaphor for a variety of possible elementary biochemical events, and the model must be considered phenomenologic rather than molecular. This model is essentially equivalent to assuming that the dose–response curve is linear in the low-dose region. Thus, the slope of the one-hit curve at dose D is $\Sigma[1 - P(D)]$ and for dose levels at which P(D) < .05 varies by less than 5%, that is, is essentially constant and equal to Σ. The linear model is one of two models, the other being the probit model, specified by the U.S. EPA (1976) in its interim guidelines for assessment of the health risk of suspected carcinogens. The assumption of low-dose linearity generally leads to a very low VSD, so low as to lead the FDA Advisory Committee (1971) to remark that assuming linearity "would lead to few conflicts with the result of applying the Delaney clause." The one-hit model, having only one disposable parameter, Σ, often fails to provide a satisfactory fit to dose–response data in the observable range. Other models described here, by introducing additional parameters, often lead to reasonable fits in the observable range.

An additional degree of conservatism is introduced by extrapolating back to zero from the upper confidence limit (UCL) for the net excess tumor rate (treated minus control rate). The linear model assumes that the tumor rate is proportional to dose, or that $P(D) = \Sigma D$. The upper confidence limit for the slope is UCL divided by experimental dosage. Thus an estimate of an upper limit for the proportion of tumor bearing animals, P_u, for a given dose D is

$$P_u = \frac{UCL \cdot D}{D_e}$$

where D_e is the experimental dosage. Conversely, the dose D for a given P_u is

$$D = \frac{P_u D_e}{UCL}$$

The linear model may serve as a conservative upper boundary for probit dose–response curves. This upper boundary on the proportion of tumor-bearing animals may not be as conservative as one might imagine. Crump et al. (1976), Peto (1978), and Guess et al. (1977) have shown that the curvilinear dose–response curve resulting from the multistage model is well approximated by the linear model at low dose levels. Gross et al. (1970) discussed the statistical aspects of a linear model for extrapolation.

Probit model. This model assumes that the log tolerances have a normal distribution with mean T and standard deviation σ. The proportion of individuals responding to dose D, say $P(D)$, is then simply

$$P(D) = \Phi[(\log D - \mu)/\sigma] = \Phi(\alpha + \beta \log D)$$

where $\Phi(x)$ is the standard normal integral from $-X$ to X, $\alpha = -\mu \neq \sigma$ and $\beta = 1\sigma$. This dose–response curve has $P(D)$ near zero if D is near zero and $P(D)$ increasing to unity as dose increases. A plot of a typical probit dose–response is given by an S-shaped (sigmoid) curve. The quantity above is referred to as the slope of the probit line, where

$$Y = \Phi^{-1}[P(D)] = \alpha + \beta \log D$$

and $Y + 5$ is the probit of P. This is the same model we presented earlier in this chapter for linearizing a special case of quantal response, the data for LD_{50}s. Despite its nonthreshold assumption it is a characteristic of the probit curve that as dose decreases, zero response is approached very rapidly, more rapidly than any power of dose. Other curves to be considered approach zero response more slowly than the probit.

An alternative derivation of the probit model that relates it to time to response has been given by Chand and Hoel (1974) using the Druckrey (1967) observation that median time to tumor, T, is related to dose, D, by the equation $Dt^n = C$, where n and C are constants unrelated to D. Combining this relation with an assumed log-normal distribution of response time then gives the $P(D)$ as probability of response to any given time, T_o, where I and ϑ are simple function of n, CT_o, and the standard deviation of the distribution of response times.

The actual method that has the probit model as its basis is the Mantel–Bryan procedure. As originally proposed, this procedure used the probit model but with a preassigned slope of unity. The rationale for this slope was that all observed probit slopes at the time of the proposal exceeded that value, the procedure therefore being considered conservative. An additional conservative feature involves use of the 99% UCL of the proportion responding at a dose level, rather than the observed proportion. The procedure then extrapolates downward to a response level of 10^{-8}, using each separate dose level in the experiment, or combinations, taking as the VSD the highest of the values obtained. A conservative method of taking account of the response of the control group also was given. An improved version of the procedure, which included several sets of independent data and better methods of handling background response rates and responses at multiple doses, has since been published (Mantel et al., 1975).

A dosage D_o is said to be virtually safe if

$$f(D_o) < p + (1 - p)P_o$$

where P_o is some near-zero lifetime risk, such as 10^{-8}, the value proposed by Mantel and Bryan, or 10^{-6}, the value adopted by the FDA. The VSD then is calculated as $f^{-1}[(1 - p)P_o]$. The calculation thus requires choosing a model, f, determining the value of its disposable constants from observations in the observable range, and extrapolating down to the unobservable elevation in response, P_o, to determine the VSD.

One of the advantages of the Mantel–Bryan procedure is that it rewards a larger experiment by reducing the UCL, which results in a larger dose for a selected proportion of tumor-bearing animals. Table 11.4 shows some dosages for a series of sample sizes; all yield observed tumor rates of 4%, with no tumors in the controls for a predicted tumor probability of less than one in a million.

Some situations, such as cigarette smoking in man and diethylstilbestrol in mice, have indicated slopes on the order of 1. Thus one must be careful to establish that the slope of the dose–response curve is sufficiently large before applying the Mantel–Bryan procedure, indicating the desirability of multiple-dose experiments.

According to Mantel and Schneiderman (1975) the Mantel–Bryan methodology has several advantages:

1. It does not need an experimental estimate of the slope.
2. Statistical significance is not needed.

Table 11.4 Mantel–Bryan dosages for various sample sizes with the same proportion of experimental animals with tumors

Sample size	No. of animals with tumors	Upper 99% confidence limit	Dosage (fraction of experimental dosage)
50	2	0.158	1/5630
100	4	0.112	1/3430
200	8	0.085	1/2400
400	16	0.069	1/1860

Note: Predicted tumor probability $< 10^{-6}$.

3. It takes into account a nonzero spontaneous background tumor incidence.
4. It considers multiple-dose studies.
5. Any arbitrary acceptable risk can be calculated.
6. It avoids categorizing a substance in absolute terms.
7. It permits the investigator flexibility in study design.

Mantel and Bryan (1961) provided an example of an actual study in which the carcinogen 3-methylcholanthrene was given to mice as a single injection, with 12 different dose levels used. Table 11.5 provides the methodology and findings of the Mantel–Bryan procedure.

Table 11.5 Illustration of methodology for determining the "safe" dose from results at several dose levels

Dose per Mouse (mg) (1)	Log dose (2)	Result (no. of tumors/ no. of mice) (3)	Combined result (no. of tumors/ no. of mice) (4)	Maximum p value 99% assurance (5)	Corresponding normal deviate (6)	Calculated "safe" (1/100 million) log dose [(2)–(6) – 5.612] (7)
0.000244	6.388^{-10}	0/79	0/158	0.0288	−1.899	2.675^{-10}
0.000975	6.990^{-10}	0/41	0/79	0.0566	−1.584	2.962^{-10}
0.00195	7.291^{-10}	0/19	0/38	0.1141	−1.205	2.884^{-10}
0.0039	7.592^{-10}	0/19	0/19	0.2152	−0.789	2.769^{-10}
0.0078	7.893^{-10}	3/17	3/17	0.480	−0.050	2.331^{-10}
0.0156	8.194^{-10}	6/18	6/18	0.729	+0.610	1.972^{-10}
0.0312	8.495^{-10}	13/20	13/20	0.871	+1.131	1.752^{-10}
0.0625	8.796^{-10}	17/21	17/21	0.958	+1.728	1.456^{-10}
0.125	9.097^{-10}	21/21	—	—	—	—
0.25	9.398^{-10}	21/21	—	—	—	—
0.50	9.699^{-10}	21/21	—	—	—	—
1.0	10.000^{-10}	20/20	—	—	—	—

Source: Mantel and Bryan, 1961.

Some criticisms of the Mantel Bryan procedure are:

1. The normal distribution may not offer as accurate a description in the tails of the distribution as it does in the central parts, especially if one proceeds out to 10^{-6} or 10^{-8}.
2. The use of the arbitrarily low slope of unity for downward extrapolation has been criticized because of the lack of observational support.
3. The argument does not incorporate any of the present understandings of the process of carcinogenesis.
4. The model is insufficiently conservative, because the extrapolated probability approaches zero with decreasing dose more rapidly than any polynomial function of dose, and, in particular, more rapidly than a linear function of dose, and hence may underestimate probability at low dose (Crump, 1979).
5. The model is excessively conservative, because it does not postulate a threshold or accommodate time to tumor data.

Multistage. The multistage model (Armitage and Doll, 1961; Crump et al., 1976) represents a generalization of the one-hit model and assumes that the carcinogenic process is composed of an unknown number of stages that are needed for cancer expression. Inherent in this model is the additional assumption that the effect of the carcinogenic agent in question is additive to a carcinogenic effect produced by external stimuli at the same stages. Such an assumption generally leads one to expect a linear dose–response curve at low exposure levels.

This assumes that carcinogenesis occurs in a single cell as a point of origin and, according to the multistage model, is the result of several stages that can include somatic mutation. The transitional events individually are assumed to depend linearly on dose rate. This then leads in general to a model in which the probability of tumor approximates a low-order polynomial in dose rate. In the low-dose region, which would relate to environmental levels, one finds that the responses are well approximated by a linear function of dose rate. The characteristic in which the low dose probability is proportional to the kth power of dose, where k is the number of stages, was considered by Armitage and Doll (1961) to be quite inconsistent with observation. They derived a multistage model, which by assuming that the effect of the agent at some stages was additive to an effect induced by external stimuli at those stages led to a lower power than k for D. Crump et al. (1976) discussed this model and, by assuming additivity at all stages, obtained as an expression for the required probability

$$P(D) = 1 - \exp\left\{-\sigma \sum_{i=o}^{\gamma} \alpha_i D^i\right\} \alpha_i \geq 0$$

where $\alpha = -\mu \neq \sigma$. Hartley and Sielken (1977) combined this model with time to response, obtaining a more general result. For $\alpha_1 > 0$ these models also imply low dose linearity because

$$\lim P'(D) = \alpha_1 \exp(-\alpha_0) \quad \text{as } D \to 0$$

Armitage and Doll [56] cited data relating lung cancer mortality rate to previous smoking habits as indicating a linear dose–response curve, but errors in reporting the amount smoked would lead to such a curve even if the true curve were convex. This supports the view that the apparent low-dose linearity in many epidemiologic studies is an artifact of errors in the reporting of dose. Crump et al. (1976) stress the crucial nature of the additivity assumption, pointing out that it can make orders-of-magnitude differences in the estimated risk associated with the low-dose exposure.

Crump (1979) describes a procedure for low-dose extrapolation in the presence of background that although based on the generalized model, reduces (if UCLs are used) to extrapolation using low-dose linearity. This is because the use of upper confidence limits on χ on the model is equivalent to admitting the possibility of a positive value of χ which at lose doses dominates the expression. Once UCLs on the VSD or risk at a given dose are used, there may be little practical difference, therefore, between use of the one-hit model and the generalization given by the Crump et al. equation.

Hartley and Sielken (1977) have developed a procedure based on maximum likelihood for the Armitage–Doll model. Their program is very general and allows for the inclusion of the effect of the time to a tumor.

In practice, these two approaches result in fitting a polynomial model to the dose–response curve such that (where t is time):

$$\frac{p(D,t)}{1 - P(D,t)} = gDh(t)$$

where $P(D,t)$ is the probability of the observance of a tumor in an animal by time t at a dosage D,

$$p(D,t) = \frac{DP(D,t)}{Dt}$$

where $g(D)$ is a function of dose such that

$$g(\text{dose}) = (a_1 + b_1 \text{ dose})(a_2 + b_2 \text{ dose})\ldots(a_n + b_n \text{ dose})$$
$$= c_0 + c_1 \text{ dose} + c_2 \text{ dose}^2 + \ldots + c_n \text{ dose}^n$$

where $a_i, b_i, c_i \chi 0$ are parameters that vary from chemical to chemical and $h(t)$ is a function of time. The probability of a tumor by time t and dosage D is

$$P(D,t) = 1 - \exp[-g(D)H(t)]$$

where

$$H(t) = \int_o^t h(t)\, D_t$$

This function generally fits well in the experimental data range but has limited applicability to the estimation of potential risk at low doses. The imitations arise, first, because the model cannot reflect changes in kinetics, metabolism, and mechanisms at low doses and, second, because low-dose estimates are highly sensitive to a change of even a few observed tumors at the lowest experimental dose.

A logical statistical approach to account for the random variation in tumor frequencies is to express the results in terms of best estimates and measures of uncertainty.

Important biologic mechanisms of activation and detoxification are not usually specifically considered. However, a steady-state kinetic model that incorporates the process of deactivation as well as other pharmacokinetic considerations has been offered by Cornfield (1977). He noted that whenever the detoxification response is irreversible, low exposure levels are predicted to be harmless. However, the presence of a reversible response suggests linearity at low-dose exposures. He additionally predicted that if multiple protective responses are sequentially operational, the dose–response relationship will look like a hockey stick "with the striking part flat or nearly flat and the handle rising steeply once the protective mechanisms are saturated." Despite its seemingly greater biologic veracity, the Food Safety Council (1978) challenged the multistage model general assumption of low-dose linearity on the basis of (1) the general absence of support for lose-wise additivity seen in many studies in which additivity has been evaluated and (2) studies that showed the effects of one carcinogenic agent offset or prevented the carcinogenic effects of another.

Crump (1979) has noted that biostatistical models such as the multistage model assume that the quantity of carcinogen finding its way to the critical sites is proportional to the total body exposure, which is clearly not the case across the entire dose range covered by the model.

Criticism of these models are summarized here:

1. These models do not consider the variation in susceptibility of the members of the population when deriving their dose-response relationships.
2. Low-dose linearity is not consistently found in experimental systems.
3. Low-dose linearity is assumed to occur by a mechanism of additivity to background levels; however, there is a lack of data supporting the additivity hypothesis.
4. They do not sufficiently recognize pharmacokinetic considerations including rates of absorption, tissue distribution, detoxification processes, repair, and excretion. (This would apply to the Mantel–Bryan model as well.)

Multihit. This model is also called the *K-hit* or *gamma multihit model*. It is a generalization of the one-hit model.

If k hits of a receptor are required to induce cancer, the probability of a tumor as a function of exposure to a dose (D) is given by

$$P(D) = 1 - \sum_{t=0}^{k-1} \frac{(\lambda D)^{l} e^{-\gamma D}}{i!} \approx \frac{(\gamma D)^{k}}{k!}$$

For small values of D, the k-hit model may be approximated by

$$P(D) = \gamma D^k$$

or

$$\log P(D) = \log \gamma + k \log D$$

Thus K represents the slope of log P(D) versus log D. By the same reasoning, if at least k hits are required for a response, then

$$P(D) = P(X \geq k) = \int_0^{\lambda D} \frac{u^{k-\tau} e^{-u} \, du}{(k-1)!}$$

Because this equation contains an additional parameter, k, it ordinarily provides a better description of dose–response data than the one-parameter curve. This can be generalized further by allowing k to be any positive number, not necessarily an integer. In this case the above formula can be described as that dose–response curve that assumes a gamma distribution of tolerances with shape parameter k. We note

$$\lim_{D \to 0} [P(D)/D^k] = \text{constant}$$

Thus, in the low-dose region, the equation is linear for $k = 1$, concave for $k < 1$, and convex for $k > 1$. At higher doses the gamma and the lognormal distributions are hard to distinguish, so that the model provides a blend of the probit model at high-dose levels and the logit at low ones.

Procedures for estimating the parameters of the k-hit model by nonlinear maximum likelihood estimation have been developed by Rai and Van Ryzin (1979). This method has the advantage of permitting the data to determine the number of hits needed to describe the results without introducing more than two parameters. If only one dose level gives responses greater than zero and less than 100%, unique values of the two parameters can no longer be estimated. The background effect in this model is taken care of using Abbott's correction.

The multihit model is discussed in some detail in the Food Safety Council report (1980). One derivation of this model follows from the assumption that k hits or molecular interactions are necessary to induce the formation of a tumor, and the distribution of these molecular events over time follows a Poisson process. In practice the model appears to fit some data sets reasonably well and to give low-dose predictions that are similar to the other models. There are cases, however, in which the predicted values are inconsistent with the predictions of other models by many orders of magnitude. For instance, the VSD as predicted by the multihit model appears to be too high for nitrolotriacetic acid and far too low for vinyl chloride (Food Safety Council, 1980).

Pharmacokinetic models. Pharmacokinetic models often have been used to predict the concentration of the parent compound and metabolites in the blood and at reactive sites, if identifiable. Cornfield (1977), Gehring and Blau (1977), and Anderson et al. (1980) have extended this concept to include rates for macromolecular events (e.g., DNA damage and repair) involved in the carcinogenic process. The addition of statistical distributions for the rate parameters and a stochastic component representing the probabilistic nature of molecular events and selection processes may represent a useful conceptual framework for describing the tumorigenic mechanism of many chemicals. Pharmacokinetic data are presently useful only in specific parts of the risk-assessment process. A more complete understanding of the mechanism of chemically induced carcinogenesis would allow a more complete utilization of pharmacokinetic data. Pharmacokinetic comparisons between animals and humans are presently most useful for making species conversions and for understanding qualitative and quantitative species differences. The modeling of blood concentrations and metabolite concentrations identifies the existence of saturated pathways and adds to an understanding of the mechanism of toxicity in many cases.

Taking advantage of the similarity of the probit and pharmacokinetic models in the 5% to 95% range, Cornfield (1977) developed an approximate method of estimating its parameters, particularly the value of T, the saturation dose. Risks at dosages below T are crucially dependent on K^*, the relative speed of the reverse, deactivation reaction, and this cannot be well estimated from responses at dosages above T, so that low-dose assessment using this model may be more dependent on further pharmacokinetic experimentation than on further statistical developments.

This model considers an agent subjected to simultaneous activation and deactivation reactions, both reversible, with the probability of a response being proportional (linearly related) to the amount of active complex. Denoting total amount of substrate in the system by S and deactivating agent by T and the ratios of the rate constants governing the back and forward reactions by K for the activation step and K^* for the deactivation step, the model is, for $D > T$

$$P(D) = \frac{D - S[p(D)] - y}{D - S[P(D)] - y + K}$$

where

$$y = K[P(D)]T/\{K[P(D)] + K^*[1 - P(D)]\}$$

and for $D < T$

$$P(D) \cong \frac{D}{S + K\left(1 + \dfrac{T}{K^*}\right)}$$

These equations follow from standard steady-state mass action equations. Thus, at low dose levels, $D < T$, the dose–response curve is nearly linear, but for deactivating reactions in which the rate of the back reaction is small compared to that of the forward reaction, K^* is quite small and the slope is near zero. In fact, in the limiting case in which $K^* = 0$ the dose–response curve has a threshold at $D = T$, but because the model is steady state and does not depend on the time course of the reaction, it cannot be considered to have established the existence of a threshold. For $K^* > 0$, the dose–response curve is shaped like a hockey stick with the striking part nearly flat and rising sharply once the administered dose exceeds the dose, T, which saturated the system. Because of the great sensitivity of the slope at low doses to the value of K^*/K, and insensitivity at high doses, responses at dose levels above $D = T$ probably cannot be used to predict those below T. This can be considered a limitation of the model, but it can equally well be considered a limitation of high-dose experimentation in the absence of detailed pharmacokinetic knowledge of metabolic pathways. The model can be generalized to cover a chain of simultaneous activating and deactivating reactions intervening between the introduction of D and the formation of activated complex, but this does not appear to change its qualitative characteristics. The kinetic constants, S, T, K, and K^* are presumably subject to animal-to-animal variation. This variation is not formally incorporated in the model, so that the possibility of negative estimates of one or more of these constants cannot be excluded.

Weibull. Another generalization of the one-hit model is the Weibull model:

$$P(D) = 1 - \exp(\alpha - \beta D^m),$$

where m and ϑ are parameters. Note that

$$\lim [P(D)/D^m =] = \text{constant}.$$

as the dose approaches zero. Thus, in the low-dose region, this last equation is linear for $m = 1$, concave for $m < 1$, and convex for $m > 1$. With a typical set of data, the Weibull model tends to give an estimated risk at a low dose that lies between the estimates for the gamma multihit and the Armitage–Doll models. The Weibull distribution for time to tumors has been suggested by human cancers (Cook et al., 1969; Lee and O'Neill, 1971):

$$I = bD^m(t - w)^k$$

where I is the incidence rate of tumors at time t, b is a constant depending on experimental conditions, D is dosage, w the minimum time to the occurrence of an observable tumor, and m and k are parameters to be estimated. Also, Day (1967), Peto et al. (1972), and Peto and Lee (1973) have considered the Weibull distribution for time to tumor occurrence. Theoretic models of carcinigenesis also predict the Weibull distribution (Pike, 1966). Theoretic arguments and some experimental data suggest a Weibull distribution by which tumor incidence is a polynomial in dose multiplied by a function of age. Hartley and Sielken (1977) adopted the form

$$H(t) = \sum_{i=1} \xi_i t^i$$

where $s_i \chi^0$. They noted that this function regarded as a weighted average of Weibull hazard rates with positive weight coefficients, s_j. The conventional statistical procedure of weighted least-squares provides one method of fitting the Weibull model to a set of data. With a background response measured by the parameter p, the model, using Abbott's correction is:

$$P = p + (1 - p)(1 - \exp(-\beta D^m))$$
$$= 1 - \exp(-(\alpha + \beta D^m)),$$

where $\alpha = \beta D^m$.

With a nonlinear weighted least-squares regression program, one can estimate the three parameters (m, α, β) directly. With only a linear weighted least-squares regression program, one can use trial and error on m to find the values of the three parameters that produce a minimum error sum of squares.

A nonlinear maximum likelihood method to obtain estimates of the parameters in the Weibull model also can be used. The use of the Weibull distribution for time or tumor leads to an extreme value distribution relating tumor response to dosage (Chand and Hoel, 1974). Hoel (1972) gives techniques for cases in which adjustments must be made for competing causes of death.

Logit. This model, like the probit model, leads to an S-shaped dose–response curve, symmetric about the 50% response point. Its equation (Berkson, 1944) is:

$$P(D) = 1/[1 + \exp\{-(\alpha + \beta \log D)\}]$$

It approaches zero response as D decreases more slowly than the probit curve, because

$$\lim 1[P(D)/D^\beta] = K$$

as dose approaches zero where K is a constant.

The practical implication of this characteristic is that the logit model leads to lower VSD than the probit model, one 25th as much in calculations reported by Cornfield et al. (1978), even if both models are equally descriptive of the data in the observable range.

Albert and Altshuler (1973) have developed a related model for predicting tumor incidence and life shortening based on the work of Blum (1959) on skin tumor response and on Druckrey (1967) for a variety of chemical carcinogens in rodents. They had investigated cancer in mice exposed to radium. The basic relationship used was $Dt^{11} = c$, where Di is dosage, t is the median time to occurrence of tumors, n is a parameter greater than α, and c is a constant depending on the given experimental conditions. It is of interest to determine the time it takes for a small proportion of the population to develop tumors. With this formulation, as the dosage is increased, the time to tumor occurrence is shortened. Albert and Altshuler (1973) used the log-normal distribution to represent time to tumor occurrence, assuming the standard deviation to be independent of dosage.

The log-normal distribution of tumor times corresponds closely to the probit transformation as employed in the Mantel–Bryan procedure.

Log-probit. The log-probit model assumes that the individual tolerances follow a log-normal distribution. Specific steps in the complex chain of events that lead to carcinogenesis are likely to have lognormal distributions. For example, it is reasonable to assume that the distribution of a population of kinetic rate constants for detoxification, metabolism, and elimination, in addition to the distribution of immunosuppression surveillance capacity and DNA repair capacity, can be adequately approximated by normal or log-normal distributions.

Tolerance-distribution models have been found to adequately model many types of biological dose–response data, but it is an overly simplistic expectation to represent the entire carcinogenic process by one tolerance distribution. A tolerance-distribution model may give a good description of the observed data, but from a mechanistic point of view there is no reason to expect extrapolation to be valid. The probit model extrapolation, however, has fit well in some instances (Gehring et al., 1977).

The log-probit model has been used extensively in the bioassay of dichotomous responses (see Finney, 1952). A distinguishing feature of this model is that it assumes that each animal has its own threshold dose below which no response occurs and above which a tumor is produced by exposure to a chemical. An animal population has a range of thresholds encompassing the individual thresholds. The log-probit model assumes that the distribution of log dose thresholds is normal. This model states that there are relatively few extremely sensitive or extremely resistant animals in a population. For the log-probit model, the probability of a tumor induced by an exposure to a dose D of a chemical is given by

$$P(D) = \Phi(\alpha + \beta \log_{10} D)$$

where Φ denotes the standard cumulative Gaussian (normal) distribution. Chand and Hoel (1974) showed that the log-probit dose–response relationship is obtained when the time-to-tumor distribution is log normal under certain conditions.

Nonlinear Dose Response. This model (Yee, 1996) initially was developed for predicting short-term, low-dose effects of gases.

- The best-fit model uses weighted measures in conjunction with probit method.
- In acute exposure animal studies, tolerance among members of a population tends to follow a lognormal distribution for any single endpoint as long as the operative mechanisms are identical across the range of interest.
- L_n is log-normally distributed with the population mean μ and variance σ^2.

It is convenient to linearize the relation between proportion P responding and the cumulative toxic exposure required to induce this level of response. The probit Y is written:

$$Y = K_1 + k_2 \log L_n, \quad K_1 = \mu/\sigma$$
$$Y = k_1 + k_2 \log C^n T \quad k_2 = 1/\sigma$$

It is often more convenient to express the probit relationship in the following form:
$$Y = b_0 + b_1 \log C + b_2 \log T$$
where b_0, b_1, and b_2 are experimentally derived regression coefficients
$$b_0 = k_1 \quad b_2 = k_2 \quad b_1 = nk_2 \text{ or } n = b_1/b_2$$

This model is robust in the sense that its predictive power is not unduly influenced by the inclusion of data that have a marked variance from the mean predictive value. It should be noted, however, that the addition or acquisition of data in the range of interest—particularly of human data—should serve to reduce the variability about the predictive mean. That is, confidence intervals should become smaller.

Miscellaneous. There are a large number of other proposed models for low-dose extrapolation, through these others have not gained any large following. Two examples of these are the extreme value and no-effect-level models.

Chand and Hoel (1974) showed that if the time-to-tumor distribution is a Weibull distribution, the dose–response model follows an extreme value model under certain conditions, with

$$P(D) = 1 - \exp[-\exp(I + \vartheta \log D)]$$

Park and Snee (1983) made the observation that many biologic responses vary linearly with the logarithm of dose, and that practical thresholds exists, and therefore the responses can be represented by the following model:

Response $= B_1$ if dose D^*

Response $= B_1 + B_2 \log (\text{dose}/D^*)$ if dose χD^*

This model incorporates a parameter D^* that represents a threshold below which no dose-related response occurs. In this model, B_1 is the constant response level at doses less than D^*, and B_2 is the slope of the log–dose response curve at doses χD^*. It has been found empirically that many quantitative toxicologic endpoints can be described adequately by the no-effect-level model. This model, therefore, may be useful for establishing thresholds for endpoints related to the carcinogenic process in situations in which information other than the simple presence or absence of a tumor is available. Both the model and predicted threshold are of value if carcinogenicity is a secondary event.

Critique and Comparison of Models

None of the models presented here (or any others) can be "proved" on the basis of biologic arguments or available experimental data, but some are more attractive than others on these grounds. The multistage model appears to be the most general model according to the values of the parameters. Unfortunately, most of these models fit experimental data equally well for the observable response rates at experimental dosage levels but they give quite different estimated responses if extrapolated to low dosage levels. There are now numerous sets of data that have been used to compare two or more of the models against each other. The comparisons presented here are examples from the literature, using data as presented in Table 11.6.

Table 11.7 shows that each of three models—the Armitage–Doll model, the Weibull model, and the multihit model—has a reasonable goodness-of-fit p value (.71, .80, and .93, respectively) in the experimental range. For example, assuming the Weibull model to be correct, the probability of seeing experimental data whose fit is not as good as the data that obtained for this experiment is approximately .80, indicating a high degree of fit. However, in this case the one-hit model has a goodness-of-fit p value $< .001$, indicating that this model is a poor fit to the data. Also in Table 11.7 the p value for the improvement of fit for the Weibull model over the one-hit model is shown to be $< .001$. The Weibull model clearly provides a statistically significantly better fit to these data than does the one-hit model using conventional p values of .01 or .05. The goodness-of-fit p values for the one-hit, Weibull, and gamma multihit model are based on usual chi-square tests; that for the Armitage–Doll model is based on the simulation procedure described by Crump et al. (1976). Likewise, the p values for the improvement of fit for the Weibull and multihit models over the one-hit model are based on likelihood ratio procedures that are not generally available for the Armitage–Doll model.

Table 11.8 presents the estimates of VSD for 10^{-4} and 10^{-6} using each of the four models. These VSDs have been calculated for each model by taking $P(D_o) - P(O) = 10^{-4}$ or 10^{-6}, because $P(D_o) - P(O)$ represents the additional risk due to the added dose D_o. Looking again at substance 11, ethylenethiourea, note that the range is from 5.5×10^{-2} to 63.0 ppm at a risk level of 10^{-4} and from 5.5×10^{-4} to 33.5 ppm at a risk level of 10^{-6}. Note that in this case the one-hit model, because of the imposed low-dose linearity, yields a much smaller VSD than the other three better-fitting models, which allow for low-dose nonlinearity but do not impose it. The nonlinearity in the observed data for ethylenethiourea is exhibited in the VSDs in Table 11.8 as well as in the estimates of the I_is for the Armitage–Doll model ($I_1 = 0$) in Table 11.7 and the estimates of m (3.30) and k (8.23) for the Weibull and multihit models respectively.

Table 11.9 attempts to summarize the major characteristics of the eight models presented here in terms of their operating characteristics. The performance of each model in any one particular case is dependent on the nature of the observed dose–response curve. All fit true linear data well but respond differently to concave or convex response curves. The actual choice of model must depend on what information is available and on the professional judgement of the investigator. The authors believe that to attempt to use any purely mathematical model is wrong, that an understanding of the pharmacokinetics and mechanisms of toxicity across the dose range is an essential

Table 11.7 Results of fitting four different models to data on 13 substances

Substance (test)	One-hit model		Armitage–Doll model		Weibull model			Gamma multihit model		
	Estimated VSD	Goodness-of-fit (p value)	Estimated VSD	Goodness-of-fit (p value)	Estimated VSD	Goodness-of-fit (p value)	Improvement over one hit (p value)	Estimated VSD	Goodness-of-fit (p value)	Improvement over one hit (p value)
A	3.4×10^{-5}	.07	7.9×10^{-4}	.49	4.0×10^{-2}	.64	.01	.28	.54	.009
B	1.6×10^{-4}	.32	4.0×10^{-4}	.77	3.1×10^{-2}	.81	.04	3.7×10^{-2}	.89	.04
C	8.4×10^{-8}	<.001	4.2×10^{-3}	.13	4.3×10^{-3}	.22	<.001	1.3×10^{-2}	.65	<.001
D	2.8×10^{-8}	.16	6.4×10^{-4}	.47	1.7×10^{-2}	.22	.10	4.9×10^{-2}	.19	.12
E	5.7×10^{-6}	.07	2.2×10^{-5}	.36	1.2×10^{-3}	.44	.03	6.7×10^{-3}	.55	.02
F	3.2×10^{-5}	.04	1.9×10^{-2}	.57	1.9×10^{-2}	.63	.003	7.7×10^{-2}	.72	.003
G	5.5×10^{-4}	<.001	4.5	.71	6.0	.80	<.001	33.5	.93	<.001
H	2.1×10^{-4}	.99	2.2×10^{-4}	.94	2.6×10^{-4}	.96	.94	2.6×10^{-4}	.96	.95
I	2.0×10^{-5}	<.001	1.9×10^{-4}	.09	0.52	.48	<.001	0.80	.48	<.001
J	4.3×10^{-5}	.33	0.33	.72	0.53	.99	.04	1.1	7.99	.04
K	5.2×10^{-6}	.53	1.6×10^{-3}	.73	1.7×10^{-3}	.85	.12	3.8×10^{-3}	.87	.11
L	3.7×10^{-5}	.78	5.7×10^{03}	.64	1.1×10^{-3}	.62	.67	3.8×10^{-3}	.62	.64
M	2.0×10^{-2}	.03	2.1×10^{-9}	.03	2.1×10^{-9}	.56	.002	3.9×10^{10}	.32	.002

Note: VSD, virtually safe dose at 10^{-6}.

Table 11.6 Experimental carcinogenicity results for 13 substances

Test number and substance	Species	Tumor or lesion	Dose units	Dose–response data (dose / no. of responses / no. of animals)
A. Aflatoxin B$_1$	Rat	Liver tumor	ppb	0/(0/18); 1/(2/22); 5/(1/22); 15/(4/21); 50/(20/25); 100/(28/28)
B. Bischloromethyl ether	Rat	Respiratory tumor	# of 6-h exposures at 100 ppb	10/(1/41); 20/(3/46); 40/(4/18); 60/(4/18); 80/(15/34); 100/(12/20)
C. Botulinum toxin	Mouse	Death	ng	.027/(0/30); .030/(4/30); .034/(11/30); .037/(10/30); .040/(16/30); .045/(26/30); .050/(26/30)
D. Dichlorodiphenyl-trichloroethane	Mouse	Liver hepatoma	ppm	0/(0/30); 2/(4/30); 10/(11/30); 50/(10/30); 250/(16/30)
E. Dieldrin	Mouse	Liver tumor	ppm	0/(4/111); 1.25/(4/105); 2.50/(11/124); 5.00/(44/60)
F. Dimethylnitrosoamine	Rat	Liver tumor	ppm	0/(17/156); 2/(11/60); 5/(25/58); 10/(44/60); 20/(15/23)
G. Ethylenethiourea	Rat	Thyroid carcinoma	ppm	0/(0/29); 5/(0/18); 25/(4/62); 125/(2/5); 250/(15/23)
H. Hexachlorobenzene	Rat	14th rib anomaly	mg/kg	0/(2/72); 10/(2/75); 73/(1/73); 250/(16/69); 500/(62/70)
I. Nitrilotriacetic acid	Rat	Kidney tumor	% in diet	0/(0/80); 10/(4/79)
J. Sodium saccharin	Rat	Bladder tumors	% in diet	
K. 2,3,7,8-tetrachlorodibenzo-p-dioxin	Rat	Intestinal anomaly	mg/kg	
L. Rapeseed (span) oil	Rat	Cardiovascular lesion	% in diet	
M. Vinyl chloride	Rat	Liver angiosarcoma	ppm	

Table 11.8 Estimated virtual safe dose by four models for 13 substances

		At 10^{-4}				At 10^{-6}			
Test	Dose unit	One-hit	Armitage–Doll	Weibull	Multihit	One-hit	Armitage–Doll	Weibull	Multihit
A	ppb	3.4×10^{-3}	7.6×10^{-2}	.40	1.2	3.4×10^{-3}	7.9×10^{-4}	4.0×10^{-2}	.28
B	no. of 6-h exposures								
C	ng	1.6×10^{-2}	4.0×10^{-2}	0.47	0.48	1.6×10^{-4}	4.0×10^{-4}	3.1×10^{-2}	3.7×10^{-2}
		8.4×10^{-6}	9.1×10^{-3}	9.2×10^{-3}	1.7×10^{-2}	8.4×10^{-8}	4.2×10^{-3}	4.3×10^{-3}	1.3×10^{-2}
D	ppm	2.8×10^{-2}	6.4×10^{-2}	0.41	0.76	2.8×10^{-4}	6.4×10^{-4}	1.7×10^{-2}	4.9×10^{-2}
E	ppm	5.7×10^{-4}	2.2×10^{-3}	1.8×10^{-2}	5.1×10^{-2}	5.7×10^{-6}	2.2×10^{-5}	1.2×10^{-3}	6.7×10^{-3}
F	ppm	3.2×10^{-3}	0.19	.19	0.41	3.2×10^{-5}	1.9×10^{-2}	1.9×10^{-2}	7.7×10^{-2}
G	ppm	5.5×10^{-2}	20.8	24.4	63.0	5.5×10^{-4}	4.5	6.0	33.5
H	mg/kg	2.1×10^{-2}	2.2×10^{-2}	2.4×10^{-2}	2.4×10^{-2}	2.1×10^{-4}	2.2×10^{-4}	2.6×10^{-4}	2.6×10^{-4}
I	% in diet	1.9×10^{-3}	1.9×10^{-2}	0.85	1.0	2.0×10^{-2}	1.9×10^{-4}	0.52	0.80
J	% in diet	4.3×10^{-3}	1.1	1.4	2.0	4.3×10^{-5}	0.33	0.53	1.1
K	mg/kg	5.2×10^{-4}	1.6×10^{-2}	1.7×10^{-2}	2.5×10^{-2}	5.2×10^{-6}	1.6×10^{-3}	3.8×10^{-3}	
L	% in diet	3.7×10^{-3}	5.7×10^{-3}	3.2×10^{-2}	6.7×10^{-2}	3.7×10^{-5}	5.7×10^{-5}	1.1×10^{-3}	3.8×10^{-3}
M	ppm	2.0	2.0	7.4×10^{-5}	3.0×10^{-2}	2.0×10^{-2}	2.0×10^{-2}	2.1×10^{-9}	3.9×10^{-10}

Table 11.9 Characteristics and requirements for use of major low-dose extrapolation models

	Low-dose linearity	Extrapolates low dose levels	Estimates virtual safe dose	Mechanistic (M) or tolerance (T) distribution	Requires metabolic data	Accommodates threshold	Takes time to tumor into account	Estimate of potential risk of low doses
One-hit (linear)	X	X	X	M				Highest
Multistage (Armitage–Doll)	X	X	X	M				High
Weibull (Chand and Hoel)	X		X	T		X	X	High
Multihit		X	X	M				Medium
Logit (Albert and Altshuler)	X		X	T		X	X	Medium
Probit (Mantel–Bryan)	X		X	T				Medium
Log-probit (Gehring et al.)		X	X	M	X	X	X	Low
Pharmacokinetic (Cornfield)		X	X	M	X	X	X	Lowest

step in the risk assessment of carcinogens. Any mathematical model must utilize such data, and as there is now significant evidence that many of these actual response curves are multiphasic, only models that can accommodate such nonlinear response surfaces have a chance of being useful.

Benchmark Dose Approach

The entire process of risk assessment as discussed to this point is applicable not just to carcinogens, but also to the other classes of toxic agents that result in some form of irreversible harm. The only difference is that the concept of a threshold dose level below which no ill effects are evoked is accepted for most of these other classes (the exception being mutagens) (Olin et al., 1995).

In recent years, a new approach has been proposed by regulatory representatives for the assessment of risk of quantal endpoints in addition to carcinogenicity (Glowa, 1991). Initially the focus was on developmental toxicity (Auton, 1994; Barnes et al, 1995; National Research Council, 1994), but the proposals have now expanded to include reproductive and neurotoxicants (U.S. EPA, 1995). This approach has been labeled the *benchmark dose*. In a very real sense, this is not a modeling approach but rather primarily a return to the application of "safety factors" (Weil, 1972) to bridge any uncertainties occuring because a lack of data.

Currently, human exposure guidelines for developmental toxicants are based on the no-observed adverse effect level (NOAEL) derived from laboratory studies. A NOAEL is defined as the highest experimental dose that fails to induce a significant increase in risk in comparison with the unexposed controls. A reference dose or reference concentration then is obtained by dividing the NOAEL by a suitable uncertainty factor allowing for difference in susceptibility between animals and humans (Nair et al, 1995; Slab and Pieters, 1995). The resulting reference dose then is used as a guideline for human exposure (Jarabek et al, 1990). Guidelines on the magnitude of the uncertainty factor to be used in specific cases have been discussed by Barnes and Dourson (1988). Current U.S. EPA uncertainty factors are presented in Table 11.10.

The NOAEL, restricted in value to one of the experimental doses, fails to properly take sample size into account (smaller and less sensitive experiments

Table 11.10 U.S. Environmental Protection Agency guidelines for uncertainty factors

Guidelines	Factors
Average → Sensitive human	≤ 10x
Animal	
LOAEL → NOAEL	≤ 10x
Database inadequacies	≤ 10x
Subchronic → Chronic	≤ 10x
Modifying factors: Juveniles	0–10x

lead to higher NOAELs than larger studies) and largely ignores the shape of the dose–response curve. The risk associated with doses at or above the NOAEL is not made explicit. However, Gaylor (1992) has shown, for a series of 120 developmental toxicity experiments, that the observed risk exceeds 1% in about one fourth of the cases. Leisenring and Ryan (1992) also found, based on the statistical properties of the NOAELs, that the NOAEL may identify a dose level associated with unacceptably high risk with a reasonably high probability. Because of the limitations associated with the use of the NOAEL (Gaylor, 1983, 1989; Kimmel and Gaylor, 1988), the U.S. EPA (1991) is considering the use of the benchmark dose (BMD) method, proposed by Crump (1984), as the basis for deriving the RfD for developmental toxicity (Leroux et al., 1996; Barnes et al, 1995).

The BMD is generally defined as the lower confidence limit (Crump, 1984, 1995; Crump et al., 1995) of the effective dose, d_α, that induces an α-percent increase in risk (ED_α). Although the α-percent increase in risk may refer to the excessive risk $\pi(0) = \alpha$, or relative risk $[\pi(d_\alpha) - \pi(o)]/[1 - \pi(0)] = \alpha$, the latter takes into account the background risk in the absence of exposure and is more sensitive to high spontaneous risk. If the background risk is $\pi(0) = 0$, then the two measures of risk are equivalent. It can be shown that the relative risk also has additional mathematical properties that facilitate computation and interpretation. The ED_α may be defined as the solution to the equation

$$\frac{\pi(d_\alpha) - \pi(0)}{1 - \pi(0)} = \alpha$$

where $\pi(d)$ represents an appropriate dose–response model for a particular endpoint. Crump (1984) discussed the estimating of BMD based on a dose–response model for a single endpoint. Allen et al. (1994a,b) estimated the BMDs using several dose–response models fitted to data from a large database. They found that the BMDs at 5% level are similar to NOAEL in magnitude on the average. Ryan (1992) and Krewski and Zhu (1994, 1995) used joint dose–response models to estimate the BMDs. A summary of such models is presented here:

Benchmark response model:

$$P(d,s) - \left[1 - \text{esp}\left\{-\left(\alpha + \beta(d - d_0)^w\right)\right\}\right] \cdot \exp\{-s(\theta_1 + \theta_2(d - d0))\}$$

National Center for Toxicologic Research model

$$P(d,s) = 1 - \exp\left\{-\left[(\alpha \times \theta_1 s) + (\beta + \theta_2 s)(d - d_0)^w\right]\right\}$$

Log-logistic model:

$$P(d,s) = \alpha + \theta_1 s + [1 - \alpha - \theta_1 s]/[1 + \exp(\beta + \theta_2 s - Y\log(d - d_0))]$$

Under the Weibull models for either the incidence of prenatal death or the incidence of fetal malformation, the ED_α is given by

$$d_\alpha = \left(\frac{-\log(1-\alpha)}{b}\right)^{1/\gamma}$$

where the subscript $k(k-1,2)$ for the parameters (b_k, gg_k) is suppressed for simplicity of notation. Note that the d_α is obtained by evaluating Eq. (31) at $(\hat{b}, \hat{\gamma})$. The variance of $\hat{d}_\alpha$ can be approximated by

$$\text{Var}(\hat{d}_\alpha) = \gamma^{-2} d_\alpha^2 C_1^T \Omega_1 C_1$$

using the δ-method, with the unknown parameters involved replaced by $(\hat{b}, \hat{\gamma})$. Here, Ω_1 is the covariance matrix for the estimates $(\hat{b}, \hat{\gamma})^T$ and

$$C_1 = (b^{-1}, \gamma^{-1} \log\{-b^{-1} \log(1-\alpha)\})^T$$

The ED_α for overall toxicity, based on the trinomial model $\pi_3 = 1 - (1-\pi_1)(1-\pi_2)$ is obtained as the solution to the equation

$$b_1 d_\alpha^\gamma + b_{2\alpha}^\gamma = -\log(1-\alpha)$$

The variance of $\hat{d}_\alpha$ based on the δ-method is given by

$$\text{VAR}(\hat{d}_\alpha) = \left[b_{???} d_\alpha \, d^{\gamma_1^{-1}} + b_{???} d_{\alpha 2}^{\gamma^{-1}}\right]^{-2} C_2^T \Omega_2 C_2,$$

where Ω_2 is the covariance matrix of the estimates $(\hat{b}_1, \hat{\gamma}_1, \hat{b}_2, \hat{\gamma}_2)^T$ and

$$C_2 = (d_\alpha^\gamma, b_1 d_\partial^{\gamma_1} \log_\alpha, d_\alpha^{\gamma_2}, b_2 d_\alpha^{\gamma_2} \log d_\alpha)^T$$

Because the variance estimates based on the δ-method depend on the dose–response models and the estimates of the unknown parameters, alternative methods, such as those based on likelihood ratio (Chen and Kodell, 1989), for obtaining confidence limits of ED_α may be used.

The ED_α for overall toxicity derived from the multivariate model $\pi 3 = 1 - (1-\pi_1)(1-\pi_2)$ is a more sensitive indicator of developmental toxicity than those for fetal malformation and prenatal death, in that the former is always below the minimum of the latter two (Ryan, 1992, Krewski and Zhu, 1994). In the absence of a strong dose–response relationship for one of the latter two endpoints, the ED_α for overall toxicity approximates their minimum. The estimates of the ED_α for overall toxicity-based multivariate dose–response models for the prenatal death rate *rim* and fetal malformation rate *y/s* are generally expected to be more efficient than estimates based on the univariate models for the combined rate $(y+r)/m$ (Ryan, 1992). In general, risk assessment that is based on multivariate dose–response models is preferred on the ground that it can account simultaneously for each individual source of risk.

The generalized score tests for trend and dose–response modeling of multiple outcomes from developmental toxicity experiments have been discussed by others (Kavlock et al., 1995). Conditional on the number of implants per litter, joint analyses of several outcomes are numerically more stable and statistically more efficient than separate analysis of a single outcome. The extramultinomial variation induced by the litter effects may be characterized using a parametric covariance function, such as the extended Dirichlet multinomial covariance. Alternatively, the Rao–Scott transformation, based on the concept of generalized design effects, may be used to allow for the approximation of the multinomial mean and covariance functions to the transformed data. Simple dose–response models, for example the Weibull model, in conjunction with a power transformation for the dose can be used to describe the dose–response relationship in developmental toxicity data.

The method of generalized estimating equations has been employed for model fitting (Fan and Chang, 1996). These equations are not only flexible in distributional assumptions, but also computationally simpler than the maximum likelihood estimation based, for example, on the Dirichlet multinomial distribution. The generalized estimating equation estimates of the model parameter are nearly as efficient as the maximum likelihood estimates, although estimates of the dispersion parameters that are based on the quadratic estimating equations are less efficient.

Generalized score functions after local orthogonalization can be used to construct a rich class of statistics for testing increasing trends in developmental toxicity data. These generalized score functions unify many of the specific statistics previously proposed in the literature. Further investigation on the behavior of these generalized score tests under various conditions would be useful.

Joint dose–response models can be applied directly to estimate the BMDs in risk assessment for developmental toxicity. The BMD, based on a multivariate dose–response model for multiple endpoints, has the advantage that it simultaneously takes into account different sources of risk. For example, the BMD for overall toxicity is a more sensitive measure of risk in that it is less than or equal to the minimum of the BMDs for fetal malformation or prenatal death (Starr, 1995a,b).

Both public and professional perception of the entire process leading to risk assessments of carcinogens is not good. The wide acceptance and large sales of Efron's *The Apocalyptics: Cancer and The Big Lie* (1984), which presents a broad-based critique on the entire process surrounding our understanding of environmental carcinogenesis, is an all too telling indicator of the public's increase loss of faith. The reversals of regulatory actions on benzene and formaldehyde, in part because the faulty nature of the risk assessments presented to support these actions, have reinforced public doubts.

Such doubts are not limited to the laity. Gori (1982), formerly a deputy director of the National Cancer Institute, has presented an overview and general critique of the entire process from a regulatory perspective. Hickey (1984) addressed the specific case of low-level radiation effects (where we have the most human data) from a statistician's point of view, pointing out that existing epidemiology data does not match the EPA's risk assessment. And certainly there is no consensus within toxicology, as the contents of this chapter should make clear. The consensus within the toxicology community is clearly that a more mechanistic and pharmacokinetics-based modeling process is call for. Park and Snee (1983) present an excellent outline of such an approach.

IMPACT OF MODELING ON RISK ASSESSMENT

As we have seen, the field of risk assessment, as it is practiced in toxicology, and the area of modeling of dose–response relationships are immutably bound. Both seemed to be fixed in place for some years during the 1970s and 1980s, but since the early 1990s they have become very active.

The purpose of these activities is a shared one, though there remain several divergent perspectives on approach. The desire all around is to be as accurate and precise with estimates of risk as possible and also clearly understand and minimize the variability (confidence limits) around such estimates.

These goals can be served first and foremost by gathering and using the best available data in the areas of exposure measurement and biologic response. New technologies allow better exposure monitoring, now frequently including either direct measurement of the molecules of interest in both target and surrogate/model species or measurement of a biomarker that is well correlated with such exposures. And progress continues on utilizing more objective and precise measurements of response in the exposed species. Careful consideration of the best biologic model in which to study the response remains an area of insufficient focus at present. It is clear, however, that the most accurate predictive model for responses in humans are humans of the same subpopulation as is of concern.

Those models that make the fewest assumptions and most clearly characterize error (that is, have clearly defined confidence limits associated with each predictive point, curve, or surface) are both scientifically and societally best. The substitution of conservative assumptions (under the label of "safety factors") for the best possible data and models is neither scientifically or societally justified, nor will it necessarily insure the safety of those individuals with whom we are concerned.

REFERENCES

Albert, R. E., and Altshuler, B. 1973. Considerations relating to the formulation of limits for unavoidable population exposures to environmental carcinogens. In *Radionuclide carcinogenesis*, ed. J. E. Ballou et al., pp. 233–253. AEC Symposium Series, CONF-72050. Springfield, VA: NTIS.

Albert, R. E., Burns, F. J., and Altshuler, B. 1979. Reinterpretation of the linear non-threshold dose-response model in terms of the initiation–promotion mouse skin tumorigenesis. In *New concepts in safety evaluation*, ed. M. A. Mehlman, R. E. Shapiro, and H. Blumenthal, pp. 88–95. New York: Hemisphere Publishing.

Allen, B. C., Kavlock, R. J., Kimmell, C. A., and Faustman, E. M. 1994a. Dose-response assessment for developmental toxicity: II. Comparison of generic benchmark dose estimates with NOAELs. *Fundam. Appl. Toxicol.* 23:487–495.

Allen, B. C., Kavlock, R. J., Kimmell, C. A., and Faustman, E. M. 1994b. Dose-response assessment for developmental toxicity: III. Statistical models. *Fundam. Appl. Toxicol.* 23:496–509.

Anderson, M. W., Hoel, D. G., and Kaplan, N. L. 1980. A general scheme for the incorporation of pharmacokinetics in low-dose risk estimation for chemical carcinogenesis: Example—vinyl chloride. *Toxicol. Appl. Pharmacol.* 55:154–161.

Arley, N. 1961. Theoretical analysis of carcinogenesis, in *Proceedings of the Fourth Berkeley Symposium on Mathematical Statistics and Probability*, ed. J. Neyman, pp. 1–18. Berkeley: University of California Press.

Armitage, P., and Doll, R. 1961. *Stochastic models for carcinogenesis from the Berkeley Symposium on Mathematical Statistics and Probability*, pp. 19–38. Berkeley: University of California Press.

Association of Food and Drug Officials of the U.S. 1959. *Appraisal of the safety of chemicals in foods, drugs and cosmetics*. Washington, DC: Author.

Auton, T. R. 1994. Calculation of benchmark doses from teratology data. *Regul. Toxicol. Pharmacol.* 19:152–167.

Barnes, D. G., Daston, G. P., Evans, T. S., Jarabek, A. M., Kavlock, R. J., and Kimmel, C. A. 1995. Park C. Spitzer benchmark dose workshop: criteria for use of a benchmark dose to estimate a reference dose. *Regul. Toxicol. Pharmacol.* 21:296–306.

Barnes, D. G., Dourson, M. 1988. Reference dose (RfD): Description and use in health risk assessments. *Regul. Toxicol. Pharm.* 8:471–486.

Berkson, J. 1944. Application of the logistic function to bio-assay. *J. Am. Stat. Assoc.* 39:357–365.

Blum, H. F. 1959. *Carcinogenesis by ultraviolet light*. Princeton, NJ: Princeton University Press.

Borzelleca, J. F. 1984. Extrapolation of animal data to man, in *Concepts in Toxicology*, vol. I, ed. A. S. Tegeris, pp. 294–304. New York: Karger.

Calabrese, E. J. 1983. *Principles of animal extrapolation*. New York: John Wiley.

Carlborg, F. W. 1979a. Cancer, mathematical models and aflatoxin. *Food Cosmet. Toxicol.* 17:159–166.

Carlborg, F. W. 1979b. Comments on aspects of the EPA's water quality criteria: EPA Methodology Hearings. In *EPA methodology document*. Cincinnati, OH: EPA.

Chand, N., and Hoel, D. G. 1974. A comparison of models for determining safe levels of environmental agents. In *Reliability and biometry statistical analysis of lifelength*, ed. F. Proschan and R. J. Serfling. Philadelphia: SIAM.

Chen, J. J., and Kodell, R. L. 1989. Quantitative risk assessment for teratological effects. *J. Am. Stat. Assoc.* 84:966–971.

Cook, P. J., Doll, R., and Fellingham, S. A. 1969. A mathematical model for the age distribution of cancer in man. *Inst. J. Cancer* 4:93–112.

Cornfield, J. 1977. Carcinogenic risk assessment. *Science* 198:693–699.

Cornfield, J., Carlborg, F. W., and Van Ryzin, J. 1978. Setting tolerance on the basis of mathematical treatment of dose-response data extrapolated to low doses. In *Proceedings of the First International Toxicology Congress*, pp. 143–164. New York: Academic Press.

Crump, K. 1995. Calculation of benchmark doses from continuous data. *Risk Analysis* 15:79–85.

Crump, K., Allen, B., Faustman, E., Donison, M., Kimmel, C., and Zenich, H. 1995. The use of the benchmark dose approach in health risk assessment. Risk Assessment Forum, EPA/630/R-94/007, February.

Crump, K. S., Hoel, D. G., Langley, C. H., and Peto, R. 1976. Fundamental carcinogenic processes and their implications for low dose risk assessment. *Cancer Res.* 36:2973.

Crump, K. S. 1984. A new method for determining allowable daily intakes. *Fundam. Appl. Toxicol.* 4:854–871.

Crump, K. W. 1979. Dose response problems in carcinogenesis. *Biometrics* 35:157–167.

Day, T. D. 1967. Carcinogenic action of cigarette smoke condensate on mouse skin. *Br. J. Cancer* 21:56–81

Deichmann, W. B. 1975. Cummings Memorial Lecture—1975. The market basket: Food for thought. *Am. Ind. Hyg. Assoc. J.* 36:411.

Dinman, B. D. 1972. "Non-concept" of "Non-threshold" chemicals in the environment. *Science* 175:495-497.

Dixon, R. L. 1976. Problems in extrapolating toxicity data from laboratory animals to man. *Envir. Health Perspect.* 13:43-50.

Dixon, R. L., and Nadolney, C. H. 1985. Assessing risk of reproductive dysfunction associated with chemical exposure. In *Reproductive toxicology*, ed. R. L. Dixon. New York: Raven Press.

Druckrey, H. 1967. Quantitative aspects in chemical carcinogenesis. In *Potential carcinogenic hazards from drugs*, UICC Monograph Series, vol. 7, ed. R. Truhaut, p. 60. Berlin: Springer-Verlag.

Efron, E. 1984: *The apocalyptics: Cancer and the Big Lie*. New York: Simon and Schuster.

Fan, A. M., and Chang, L. W. 1996. *Toxicology and risk assessment*. New York: Marcel Dekker.

FDA Advisory Committee on Protocols for Safety Evaluation. 1971. Panel on carcinogenesis report on cancer testing in the safety evaluation of food additives and pesticides. *Toxicol. Appl. Pharmacol.* 20:419-438.

Finney, D. J. 1952. *Statistical methods in biological assay*. New York: Hafner.

Food Safety Council. 1980. Quantitative risk assessment. *Food Cosmetics Toxicology.* 18:711-734.

Friedman, L. 1973. Problems of evaluating the health significance of the chemicals present in foods. In *Pharmacology and the future of man*, vol. 2, pp. 30-41. Basel: Karger.

Gad, S. C. 1998. *Statistics and experimental design for toxicologists*, 3rd ed. Boca Raton, FL: CRC Press.

Gad, S. C., and Chengelis, C. P. 1988. *Animal models in toxicology*. New York: Marcel Dekker.

Gad, S. C., and Chengelis, C. P. 1997. *Acute toxicology testing*, 2nd ed. San Diego, CA: Academic Press.

Gaylor, D. W. 1983. The use of safety factors for controlling risk. *J. Toxicol. Environ. Health*, 11:329-336.

Gaylor, D. W. 1989. Quantitative risk analysis for quantal reproductive and developmental effects. *Environ. Health Perspect.*, 79:243-246.

Gaylor, D. W. 1992. Incidence of developmental defects at the no observed adverse effects (NOAEL). *Regul. Toxicol. Pharmacol.* 15:151-160.

Gehring, P. J., and Blau, G. E. 1977. Mechanisms of carcinogenicity: Dose response. *J. Environ. Pathol. Toxicol.* 1:163-179.

Gehring, P. J., Watanabe, P. G., and Young, J. D. 1977. The relevance of dose-dependent pharmacokinetics in the assessment of carcinogenic hazards of chemicals. In *Origins of Human Cancer, Book A*, ed. H. Hiatt, J. D. Watson, and J. A. Weinstein, pp 187-203. Bar Harbor, ME Cold Spring Harbor Laboratory.

Glowa, J. 1991. Dose-effect approaches to risk assessment. *Neurosci. Biobehav. Rev.* 15:153-158.

Gori, G. B. 1982. Regulation of cancer-causing substances: Utopia or reality. *Chem. Eng. News* (September 6):25-32.

Gross, M. A., Fitzhugh, O. G., and Mantel, N. 1970. Evaluation of safety for food additives: An illustration involving the influence of methylsalicylate on rat reproduction. *Biometrics* 26:181-194.

Guess, H. A., and Hoel, D. G. 1977. The effect of dose on cancer latency period *J. Environ. Pathol. Toxicol.* 1:279-286.

Guess, H. A., Crump, K. S., and Peto, R. 1977. Uncertainty estimates for low-dose-rate extrapolations of animal carcinogenicity data. *Cancer Res.* 37:3475-3483.

Guzelian, P. S., Henby, C. J., and Olin, S. S. 1992. *Similarities and differences between children and adults: Implications for risk assessment*. Washington, DC: ILSI Press.

Haimes, Y. Y. 1998. *Risk modeling, assessment, and management*. New York: John Wiley & Sons.

Hallenbeck, W. H. 1993. *Quantitative risk assessment for environmental and occupational health*, 2nd ed. Boca Raton, FL: Lewis Publishers.

Hammond, E. C., Garfinkel, L., and Lew, E. A. 1978. Longevity, selective mortality, and competitive risks in relation to chemical carcinogenesis. *Environ. Res.* 16:153-173.

Hartley, H. O., and Sielken, R. L. 1977. Estimation of "safe doses" in carcinogenic experiments. *Biometric* 33:1-30.
Hickey, R. J. 1984. Low-level radiation effects: Extrapolation as "science." *Chem. Eng. News* (January 16:34-36).
Hoel, D. G. 1972. A representation of mortality data by competing risks. *Biometrics* 28:475-488.
Hoel, D. G., Gaylor, D. W., Kirschstein, R. L., Saffiotti, V., and Schneiderman, M. A. 1975. Estimation of risks of irreversible delayed toxicity. *J. Toxicol. Environ. Health* 1:133.
Jarabek, A. M., Menache, M. G., Overton, J. H. Jr., Dourson, M. L., and Miller, F. J. 1990. The U.S. Environmental Protection Agency's inhalation RfD methodology: Risk assessment for air toxics. *Toxicol. Ind. Health* 6:279-301.
Jusko, W. J. 1972. Pharmacodynamic principles in chemical teratology: Dose-effect relationships. *J. Pharm. Exp. Ther.* 183:469-480.
Kavlock, R. J., Allen, B. C., Faustman, E. M., and Mimmel, C. A. 1995. Dose-response assessments for developmental toxicity: IV. Benchmark doses for fetal weight changes. *Fundam. Appl. Toxicol.* 26:211-222.
Kimmel, C. A., Ross, D. C., and Francis, E. S., eds. 1990. Proceedings of the workshop on the qualitative and quantitative comparability of human and animal developmental neurotoxicity. *Neurotoxicol. Teratol.* 12:173-292.
Kimmel, C. A., and Gaylor, D. W. 1988. Issues in qualitative and quantitative risk analysis for developmental toxicity. *Risk Analysis* 8:15-20.
Klaassen, C. D., and Doull, J. 1980. Evaluation of safety: Toxicology evaluation. In *Casarett and Doull's toxicology*, ed. J. Doull, C. D. Klaassen, and M. O. Amdur, pp. 26. New York: Macmillan.
Krewski, D., and Zhu, Y. 1995. A simple data transformation for estimating benchmark doses in developmental toxicity experiments. *Risk Analysis* 15:29-39.
Lee, P. N., and O'Neill, J. A. 1971. The effect of both time and dose applied on tumor incidence rate in benzopyrene skin painting experiments. *Br. J. Cancer* 25:759-770.
Leisenring, W., and Ryan, L. 1992. Statistical properties of the NOAEL. *Regul. Toxicol. Pharmacol.* 15:161-171.
Leroux, B. G., Leisenring, W. M., Moolgavkar, S. H., and Faustman, E. M. 1996. A biologically based dose-response model for development. *Risk Analysis* 16:449-458.
Lijinsky, W., Rueber, M. D., and Riggs, C. W. 1981. Dose response studies of carcinogenesis in rats by nitrosodiethylamine. *Cancer Res.* 41:4997-5003.
Littlefield, N. A., Farmer, J. H., and Gaylor, D. W. 1980. Effects of dose and time in a long-dose carcinogenic study. *J. Environ. Pathol. Toxicol.* 3:17-34.
Mantel, N. 1963. Part IV: The concept of threshold in carcinogenesis. *Clin. Pharmacol. Ther.* 4:104-109.
Mantel, N., Bohidar, N. R., Brown, C. C., Cimenera, J. L., and Tukey, J. W. 1975. An improved Mantel-Bryan procedure for "safety" testing of carcinogens. *Cancer Res.* 35:865-872.
Mantel, N., and Bryan, W. R. 1961. Safety testing of carcinogenic agents. *J. Natl. Cancer Inst.* 27:455-470.
Mantel, N., and Scheniderman, M. A. 1975. Estimating "safe" levels, a hazardous undertaking. *Cancer Res.* 35:1379-1386.
Nair, R. S., Stevens, M. S., Martens, M. A., Ekuta, J. 1995. Comparisons of BMD with NOAEL and LOAEL values derived from subchronic toxicity studies. *Arch. Toxicol. Suppl.* 17:44-54.
National Research Council 1994. *Science and judgment in risk assessment*. Washington, DC: National Academy Press.
Olin, G., Farland, W., Park, C., Rhomberg, L., Schenplein, R., Starr, T., and Wilson, J. 1995. *Low-dose extrapolation of cancer risks*. Washington, DC: ILSI Press.
Park, C. N., and Snee, R. D. 1983. Quantitative risk assessment: State-of-the-art for carcinogenesis. *American Statistician.* 37:427-441.
Perera, F. 1997. Environment and cancer: Who are susceptible. *Science* 278:1068-1073.
Peto, R. 1978. The carcinogenic effects of chronic exposure to very low levels of toxic substances. *Environ. Health Perspect.* 22:155-159.

Peto, R., and Lee, P. N. 1973. Weibull distributions for continuous carcinogenesis experiments. *Biometrics* 29:457–470.

Peto, R., Lee, P. N., and Paige, W. S. 1972. Statistical analysis of the bioassay of continuous carcinogens. *R. J. Cancer* 26:258–261.

Pike, M. C. 1966. A method of analysis of a certain class of experiments in carcinogenesis, *Biometrics* 22:142–161.

Rai, K., and Van Ryzin, J. 1985. A dose–response model for teratological experiments involving quantal responses. *Biometrics* 41:1–9.

Rai, K., and Van Ryzin, J. 1979. Risk assessment of toxic environmental substances based on a generalized multihit model. In *Energy and Health*, pp. 99–177. Philadelphia: SIAM Press.

Rall, D. P. 1977. Species differences in carcinogenicity testing. In *Origins of human cancer*, ed. H. H. Hiatt, J. D. Watson, and J. A. Winsten, pp. 1283–1290. Cold Spring Harbor, NY: Cold Spring Harbor Laboratories.

Rall, D. P. 1979. Relevance of animal experiments to humans. *Environ. Health Perspect.* 32:297–300.

Roberts, C. N. 1989. *Risk assessment: The common ground*. Suffolk, UK: Life Science Research.

Ryan, L. 1992. Quantitative risk assessment for developmental toxicity. *Biometrics* 48:163–174.

Schmidt-Nelsen, K. 1984. *Scaling: Why is animal size so important*. New York: Cambridge University Press.

Schneiderman, M. A., Mantel, N., and Brown, C. C. 1975. *Ann. N. Y. Acad. Sci.* 246:237–248.

Slab, W., and Pieters, M. N. 1995. Probabilistic approach to assess human RfDs and human health risks from toxicological animal studies. In *Proceedings for the Annual Meeting of the Society for Risk Analysis and the Japan Section of SRA*, Abstract D8.04-A;60.

Smith, R. L. 1974. The problem of species variations. *Ann. Nutr. Alim.* 28:335.

Spector, W. S. 1956. *Handbook of biological data*. Philadelphia: W. B. Saunders.

Starr, T. B. 1995a. *Concerns with the benchmark dose concept*. Presented at the Toxicology Summer Forum, Aspen, CO, July 14.

Starr, T. B. 1995b. The benchmark dose concept: Questionable utility for risk assessment? In *Proceedings of the Annual Meeting of the Society for Risk Analysis and the Japan Section of SRA*, abstract H2.03:86-7.

Tomatis, L. 1979. The predictive value of rodent carcinogenicity tests in the evaluation of human risks. *Ann. Rev. Pharmacol. Toxicol.* 19:511–530.

U.S. Environmental Protection Agency. 1995. *Proposed guidelines for neurotoxicity risk assessment*. Fed. Reg. 60:52032–52056.

U.S. Environmental Protection Agency. 1976. *Fed. Reg.* 41:21402, 42:10412.

U.S. Environmental Protection Agency. 1984a. Proposed guidelines for mutagenicity risk assessment. *Fed. Reg.* 49:46314–46321.

U.S. Environmental Protection Agency. 1984b. Proposed guidelines for exposure assessment. *Fed. Reg.* 49:46304–46312.

U.S. Environmental Protection Agency. 1991. Guidelines for developmental toxicity risk assessment. *Fed. Regist.* 56:63797–63826.

Weil, C. S. 1972. Statistics vs safety factors and scientific judgment in the evaluation of safety for man. *Toxicol. Appl. Pharmacol.* 21:454–463.

Weil, C. S. 1984. Some questions and opinions: Issues in toxicology and risk assessment *Am. Ind. Hyg. Assoc. J.* 45:663–670.

Wilson, J. S., and Holland, L. M. 1982. The effect of application frequency on epidermal carcinogenesis assays. *Toxicology*, 24:45–53.

Yanysheva, N. Y., and Antomonov, Y. G. 1976. Predicting the risk of tumor-occurrence under the effect of small doses of carcinogens. *Environ. Health Perspect.* 13:95–99.

Yee, E. 1996. *A non-linear dose–response model with an application to the reconstruction of the human mortality response surface from acute inhalation toxicity with sarin*, SM 1476, DRES. Ottawa, Canada: CRAD.

CHAPTER
TWELVE

OVERVIEW OF ENVIRONMENTAL DECISION-SUPPORT SOFTWARE

T. M. Sullivan and P. D. Moskowitz

Brookhaven National Laboratory, Upton, New York

M. Gitten

Environmental Project Control, Maynard, Massachusetts

One important use of toxicologic data is to estimate human health effects caused by exposure. The toxicologic data are used as the basis for setting regulatory limits on exposure of workers and the public to various chemical and radiological compounds. These limits form the basis for making decisions on the characterization, monitoring, and remediation of environmental contamination. This chapter discusses the development of decision-support software (DSS) tools developed to support analysis of decisions concerning environmental management.

DSS packages are computer-based programs that facilitate the use of data, models, and structured decision processes in decision making. The optimal DSS should attempt to integrate, analyze, and present environmental information to remediation project managers to select cost-effective clean-up strategies. The optimal system should have a balance between the sophistication needed to address the wide range of complicated sites and site conditions that can be encountered and ease of use (e.g., it should not require data that typically are not known, it should have robust error checking of problem definition through input). This description of decision support defines the characteristics of DSS, but not the components. As such, the definition is vague and a wide range of

---

This work was performed under the auspices of the U.S. Department of Energy under contract no. DE-AC02-76CH00016.

software can be considered as DSS. The particular questions that are answered by any piece of environmental DSS fall into the following categories:

- Data analysis, including visualization of site-characterization data, contamination data, integration of data from different sources, and data-worth analysis (value of additional data toward making a better decision)
- Cost/benefit analysis
- Risk (dose) analysis
- Remedial action analysis, including optimization of design and comparison between different alternatives
- Regulatory compliance analysis

A DSS code can evaluate one or several of these categories. For example, DSS exists for optimal design of landfill cover systems. This software has a specific application and does not address other remedial alternatives. On the other extreme, DSS exists that can simulate several remedial action alternatives for multiple contaminants and provide a risk assessment and cost/benefit analysis of each. The variety of waste-management problems and environmental conditions is so vast that currently no DSS system covers all aspects relevant to environmental remediation problems. As such, no DSS system applies to every situation. Care must be taken by the analyst to match the capabilities of the DSS with the problem requiring a decision.

Many software packages that address specific components necessary to evaluate remedial problems are available. For example, there are software packages to evaluate groundwater flow, contaminant transport, cover design, cost/benefit analysis, and so forth. A common approach in the development of DSS is to combine existing software for the various aspects of the remediation problem and place it in a single shell that integrates the output from one module into the input of the next module. For example, for data-worth analysis, a module for geostatistical analysis might be combined with cost/benefit analysis. This indicates that the structure of the DSS should be modular and permit incorporation of new or improved modules in the system as necessary. This also implies that the DSS should be a "living" code that receives maintenance (i.e., upgrades) over time to keep the modules current.

This chapter provides a review of existing DSS and discusses the strengths and limitations of some DSS packages. General limitations of DSS also are discussed.

The methods used to identify existing DSS packages are presented in the next section. A listing of DSS packages, their function, and their developers are listed in the following section. For clarity of exposition, the DSS packages are grouped by their functional objectives and presented in the section after that. Subsequent sections discuss issues important to the implementation and use of DSS packages and summarize the chapter and present conclusions.

IDENTIFICATION OF DSS

The sheer amount of data collected to define the nature and extent of environmental contamination problems make software tools essential to effectively manage and analyze the data and scenarios involved with remediation of contaminated sites. To identify DSS a variety of sources were used to collect information. The scope of the review included software under development by government agencies and private industry. Software developed outside the United States and Canada was not considered in this study. Preliminary data collection was performed using Internet and literature searches. This identified software packages as well as contacts to obtain more detailed information on DSS packages.

The results of this search identified thousands of software code packages that can be used to assist in the analysis of environmental problems. Most of these codes, however, address only a single issue that is important to environmental remediation. For example, hundreds of groundwater flow codes are available. These codes have varying levels of sophistication, ranging from simple analytical solutions for a single fluid in a one-dimensional homogeneous media to three-dimensional numerical simulation of multiphase flow in the presence of a heat source in a fractured porous media. Although these codes that address a single issue may be used to analyze certain aspects of the problem, they are not considered DSS because they do not integrate their analysis into a decision-making framework. These types of codes may be used as separate modules in DSS.

Based on the available literature and conversations with environmental software developers, an analysis was made of the different software packages as to their ability to act as a decision-support tool. Packages that simulated only a single component of the remedial problem, did not contain expert system-type guidance in addressing decision endpoints, or were not sufficiently sophisticated to be of use in actual remedial situations were discarded from further consideration. The next section lists the software categorized as a potential DSS.

DSS TOOLS

Table 12.1 is an alphabetical listing and brief description of software determined to meet the criteria for DSS. This listing is based on the available information and the literature provided by the code developers. As stated previously, hundreds of software packages were identified in this review. Therefore, the list contains only software that addresses multiple issues in environmental decision making. It is not meant to be exhaustive or to imply that other code packages do not exist. Hundreds of code packages exist that perform single functions of decision making, such as risk assessment or cost analysis. This list in Table 12.1 represents the codes identified as having decision support characteristics.

Table 12.1 Summary of decision-support characteristics

	Description	Comments	Sponsor
API-DSS	Decision-support system for analyzing risks associated with hazardous contaminants; multi-media assessment	Limited to chemicals common in petroleum industry	American Petroleum Institute
Benefits Analyzer	Multiattribute analysis to weight benefits of different alternatives	Uses "soft" data for defining selection	DOE
BIOSVE	Helps to assess optimum design for bioremediation, soil vapor extraction, and vacuum-enhanced recovery	Remedial action design tool	Scientific Software Group
CES	Chooses appropriate landfill cover design based on costs	Limited applicability	EPA
Coleman Data Fusion	Integrates geophysical data from different sources to define subsurface features	Site character-ization tool	DOE
CURE	Cost estimation for remedial alternatives considering uncertainties	Project management	DOE
EnviroPro Designer	Analysis of plant operation and maintenance to minimize pollution and environmental impact	Focuses on operations and maintenance issues	Intelligen
EPRI-DSS (MYGRT and ROAM)	Risk assessment; remedy selection; cost/benefit analysis through grouping a series of codes into a single platform	Under development	EPRI
FLEX	Determines liner	Limited suitability applicability	EPA
GAES 2.0	Expert system to recommend appropriate geophysical measurements for a waste site	Optimum selection of geophysical measurement techniques	EPA
GANDT	Defines optimum monitoring network to define plume location	Sampling plan for aqueous phase	DOE
GMS	Visualization of site data; geostatistical analysis of contaminant data; useful interfaces for flow and transport analysis	Not optimized for decision support	DOD, EPA, DOE
HyperVentilate	Determines the feasibility of vapor extraction groundwater cleanup	Best for preliminary design	EPA
Lynx-GMS	Geostatistical analysis to define extent of contamination	Soil contamination characterization	Lynx

Table 12.1 *Continued*

	Description	Comments	Sponsor
MAPER	Site characterization by fusion of different data sources	Subsurface characterization	DOE
MARS	Remedy selection for light non-aqueous phase liquids	Plume characterization	Vendor Scientific Software
MODLP	Well-placement optimization	Pump and treat technology	DOE
OASIS	Expert system to choose between various ground-water fate and transport models	Simple models embedded Output in terms of concentration	EPA
OPTMAS	Geostatistical techniques to estimate the extent of soil contamination and design sampling plans	Plume characterization and sampling for soils	DOE
PHOENIX	Budgeting and planning for decontamination and decommissioning work	Program management for decontamination and decommissioning	DOE
PLANET	Optimizes pump layout for remediation efforts	Pump and treat	DOE
PLUME	Geostatistical techniques to estimate the extent of soil contamination and define sampling plans	Plume characterization and sampling for soils	DOE
Petroleum Release Decision Framework	Framework for decision-support tools	Tools for visualization and data management	American Petroleum Institute
PRECIS	Probabilistic risk evaluation for multiple pathways	Risk assessment	DOE
PROBE	Prioritizes waste reduction and clean-up projects based on cost effectiveness	Multiattribute analysis	DOD
PROTOCOL	Optimizes field sampling design for hazardous waste sites	Sampling plan	EPA
RAAS	Remedy selection and risk assessment	Simulates a wide range of remedial alternatives	DOE
Racer/Envest–Equis–CTGS–Auto Cad–Arc View–GMS	Coupled set of codes under a single platform	Unclear as to how this system works as a unit	Delta Research
RAS	Selects appropriate remedial actions for groundwater	Adding bioremediation, solid vapor extraction, and surfactant enhanced recovery	DOD

152 TOXICOLOGY IN RISK ASSESSMENT

Table 12.1 *Continued*

	Description	Comments	Sponsor
SADA	Geostatistical analysis to support estimation of nature and extent of soil contamination	Plume characterization and sampling for soils	DOE
SDS 2.0/CLUSTER	Develops cost-effective field-sampling plan		DOD
SEDSS	Probabilistic health-based risk analysis; system guides the user through each step of the compliance demonstration process	Determines if regulatory compliance objectives are met	EPA, DOE National Research Council
SELECT	Risk assessment for exposure to contaminants in the air and water	Volatile organic compounds in air and water; adding radionuclides and heavy metals	Lawrence Livemore National Laboratory
SitePlanner	Data visualization and simple volume estimation	Plume characterization	DOE
SmartSampling	Economic risk–based decision analysis for defining sampling needs for soil contamination	Plume characterization and sampling for soils	DOE, EPA
TOOL	Air sparging decision-support tool	Limited applicability	DOE
TCF	Decision-support tool to help ensure that compliance objectives are met	Geared towards facility management	Private: Automated Compliance Systems

Note: DOD, Department of Defense; DOE, Department of Energy; EPA, Environmental Protection Agency.

ORGANIZATION OF DSS BY FUNCTION

The preceding section presented an undifferentiated list of DSS (Table 12.1). As seen from the list, the objectives of the different software packages are quite varied. Some software has been developed to assess a single remediation issue; other software has more general applicability. The role of this section is to categorize the software based on its primary objectives. Some programs consider multiple objectives and are listed as such. The categories are as follows:

- Site characterization: defines the hydrogeology of the site and provides data-visualization tools to examine the data
- Plume characterization: defines the location and extent of contamination
- Data-worth analysis: defines the benefit of collecting additional data, the risks associated with not collecting more data, and optimum location for additional data collection
- Remedy selection: defines potential remedial alternatives
- Remedial design optimization: analyzes and optimizes remedial designs
- Risk assessment: defines risk (dose) associated with different remedial alternatives
- Cost/benefit analysis: defines the costs associated with different remedial alternatives

The first three categories refer to the collection, management, and interpretation of data. A clear distinction is drawn between hydrogeologic data and contaminant concentration data in the first two categories. The third category, data-worth analysis, has components of economic analysis and risk analysis. Because they are applied to data collection efforts, however, they are placed in their own unique category. The last four categories refer to the selection of different remedial alternatives and the consequences of that selection.

Site Characterization

Coleman Data Fusion System: integration of multiple sources of geophysical data
GMS: Data management and visualization
SitePlanner: Data management and visualization
GAES 2.0: Selection of geophysical measurement techniques
MAPER: Integration of multiple sources of geophysical data
PRDF: Data management and visualization
SELECT: Data management and visualization

Besides GMS and SitePlanner, there are many data-management and visualization tools that exist and can be used in environmental problems. These include MapIt, ModelCad, ARC/INFO, ArcCad, and ArcView, to list a few. These other packages were not included in this review because their objective is more geared towards data management. This does not imply they are not useful tools. Some of them have been used extensively in the environmental remediation field.

Plume Characterization

GANDT: Probabilistic flow and transport analysis
GMS: Geostatistical analysis
Lynx-GMS: Geostatistical analysis
MYGRT: Integral-transform methods for quasianalytical solutions of flow and transport
OPTMAS: Geostatistical analysis used for definition of soil contamination
PLUME: Geostatistical analysis
SADA: Geostatistical analysis
SmartSampling: Geostatistical analysis

Because of the spatially sparse data typically encountered in conducting environmental remediation studies, most plume-characterization programs use geostatistical techniques to optimize the amount of information that can be inferred from the data. One DSS package, GANDT, uses a probabilistic flow and transport analysis to guide data collection. It is more relevant for groundwater-contamination problems.

Data Worth

GANDT: Flow and transport estimate of data worth for well placement
MYGRT: Multiple sensitivity analysis to evaluate data worth
MODLP: Optimizes well emplacements
OPTMAS: Geostatistically based method to optimize analytical sampling for soil contamination
PLANET: Optimizes well emplacements
PLUME: Geostatistical based estimate of data worth for soil sampling
SADA: Geostatistical based estimate of data worth for soil sampling
SmartSampling: Geostatistical based estimate of data worth for soil sampling
SEDSS: Probabilistic estimates of data worth based on likelihood of data collection helping to meet performance objective

Two categories of data-worth analysis were found in this study. The first type includes programs that address well placement. These are based on water-flow analysis. The second type examines questions pertaining to whether the collection of additional data will guarantee compliance with regulatory objectives or provide better characterization of the plume. Most of these are based on geostatistical techniques.

Remedy Selection

MARS: Assists in remedy selection for light non-aqueous phase liquids
RAAS (ReOpt): Over 100 different remedial alternatives in the database
RAS: Remedial alternative selection
EPRI-DSS (ROAM): Remedial option assessment methodology

These packages use information about the site and the contamination problem to recommend potential remedial options.

Remedial Action Design Optimization

BIOSVE: Optimizes biodegradation, soil vapor extraction, and vacuum-enhanced recovery
CES: Optimizes landfill design
FLEX: Optimizes selection of geomembrane liner materials
HYPERVENTILATE: Optimizes soil vapor extraction applications.
OASIS: Optimizes bioremediation
TOOL: Optimizes air sparging systems

Generally these packages focus on specific remedial alternatives and attempt to optimize design. They are not able to compare between remedial alternatives.

Risk Assessment

API-DSS: Probabilistic risk assessment for air and groundwater
EPRI-DSS (MYGRT): Groundwater pathway risk assessment
HRS: Screening models to rank hazardous wastes
PRECIS: Probabilistic risk assessment from ingestion, inhalation, direct exposure, and groundwater pathways.
RAAS (MEPAS): Inhalation, surface water, groundwater, direct exposure, and ingestion pathways
SEDSS: Probabilistic risk assessment of the groundwater pathway
SELECT: Air- and water-quality risk assessment.

In addition to the software packages listed here, many computer codes calculate risk (dose) from environmental contamination. For example, RESRAD calculates the dose resulting from soil or building contamination. All of the codes listed here have other functions that provide additional information to support decisions. Codes that estimate only risk were not included in this analysis.

Remedial Alternatives Cost/Benefit

Benefit Analyzer: Multiattribute analysis for ranking remedial alternatives while incorporating "soft" data
CES: Analysis for various landfill designs
CURE: Probabilistic analysis of costs for remediation activities; based on RACER
DQO/DEFT: Develops a data sampling plan to meet data-quality objectives
OECERT: Analysis for remediation of unexploded ordinances
PROBE: Ranks hazardous waste risk reductions through various mitigation processes
RACER/ENVEST–Equis–CTGS–AutoCad, ArcView–GMS: Cost-estimating program for remedial alternatives; was reviewed by the Department of Energy's cost estimation group and ranked as one of the better cost estimation programs; does not have information for radioactive or mixed wastes and would need to be expanded for these contaminants
SELECT: Allows financial analysis of different environmental remedial options

Evaluation of Decision-support Software

A screening evaluation of the strengths and weaknesses of 19 software packages was performed. The selection of these codes from Table 12.1 was based on three criteria: (1) the code's ability to address a wide range of site applications, (2) the recognition of the code throughout the United States, and (3) if the code has been used on field-scale applications. The review focused on providing information to environmental managers concerning the ability of the software to address their site-specific problems. The review listed the code developer or software vendor, point of contact, and operating platform of each package. It then rated the DSS based on the ability to address:

- DSS function (site characterization, plume characterization, risk assessment, remedy selection, remedial design optimization, and cost/benefit analysis)
- Types of contaminants modeled (organic, inorganic, radioactive, mixed waste, etc.)
- Phase of the contaminant modeled (liquid, gas, or nonaqueous)
- Site environmental characteristics addressed (unsaturated flow, fracture flow, etc.)
- Class of regulatory problems addressed: (1) active hazardous waste sites (e.g., Resource Conservation and Recovery Act), (2) abandoned or unpermitted waste sites (e.g., Comprehensive Environmental Recovery and Comprehensive Liability Act), (3) low-level radioactive waste, and (4) uranium mill tailings waste
- Other technical criteria including complexity of the software and ease of using the software, visualization of model results, application to site-specific problems, and technical comments

Each software package was rated in each category with a *Consumer Reports*-style rating of high, medium, or low. The software packages reviewed included BIOSVE, CURE, MARS, RAAS, RACER, SELECT, API-DSS, GANDT, GMS, MAPER, MARS, OPTMAS, PLANET, PLUME, PRECIS, RAAS, SADA, SEDSS, SELECT, SitePlanner, and SmartSampling. The evaluation is reported by Sullivan et al. (1997).

ISSUES WITH DECISION-SUPPORT SOFTWARE

As part of this review, issues with the development of DSS have come to light. This section lists some of these issues and discusses their importance to the future development of DSS.

Development Costs

Anecdotal information suggests that the development costs for some larger programs run in the millions of dollars. The large development costs necessitate funding through government agencies, as few businesses are willing to make that large of an investment. Because businesses (e.g., environmental firms) are the intended end users of the software, there is a technology-transfer step needed before widespread application of many DSS models. This often leads to a large gap between what has been developed and what is actually used on environmental problems.

Acceptance

For the most part, DSS is in its infancy and is not a mature area of code development. Many codes listed as DSS in the previous section are under development and either have not been released for general use or have been released within the last few years. The newness of the DSS has prevented widespread application in the field. It will take time to gain regulatory acceptance of new software. Software programs that have received regulatory acceptance generally have long track records and have received substantial technical review. For example, many packages use MODFLOW, which is the most commonly used groundwater flow code in the United States. Software based on concepts new to environmental remediation problems, such as geostatistical analysis of the contamination data, requires longer to gain acceptance.

More work is needed on the demonstration of the utility of these types of software in the decision process. Anecdotal information indicates that large cost savings can be accomplished by using this type of software. For example, SmartSampling was used for a problem involving soil contaminated with lead at Sandia National Laboratory, and their analysis showed that fewer than 100 of the 300 samples taken were necessary. In general, however, the cost savings are not documented, and it is not clear whether other approaches could be taken to lead to similar cost savings.

Connection Between Data Collection and Remedy Selection / Risk Assessment

The review of DSS has indicated two major groups: software that supports data collection and that which supports remedy selection or risk assessment. There is apparently little connection between the two. Data-collection activities do not directly influence remedy selection or risk-assessment activities, and vice versa. Better communication between these groups is needed. The SEDSS program attempts to bridge this gap between data collection and risk assessment. It is under development, however, and it remains to be seen how successful it will be. Data-collection activities are independent of remedy selection activities in all DSS.

Maintenance and Training

Many DSS packages involve multiple disciplines and probably cannot be used without extensive training. Training is a key to proper implementation of the software and to gaining acceptance of these tools. In addition, the DSS should be viewed as living code that will require upgrading as new technologies, improved process models, and new data become available. The databases supported by these codes also will require maintenance to keep up with changes.

Data Management and Portability

Many DSS packages manage large amounts of data. These data include applicable regulations, site-characterization data (well data, contaminant data, hydrogeologic data, etc.), site maps, Environmental Protection Agency–approved sampling protocols, results of and assumptions used in risk assessments, and costing data. It is important that these data can be maintained and are compatible with other computer platforms and software systems.

In addition, it would be extremely useful if the code user is permitted to overwrite default assumptions or insert additional information into the database to tailor the code to the specific application at hand.

Handling "Soft" Data

Most existing DSS handles quantitative aspects of decision support (e.g., analysis of data, estimation of costs, probabilities of exceedence of performance objectives, data worth) but does not account for "soft" data (e.g., regulatory acceptance, programmatic objectives, public perception, etc.). The Benefits Analyzer from Sandia approaches this problem using a multiattribute analysis. However, it is not clear how it integrates qualitative and quantitative results into the decision process. Treatment of "soft" and sparse data often is performed using fuzzy set theory that qualitatively ranks the attributes and estimates the probability of success or failure. Fuzzy set theory has been used extensively in civil-engineering problems such as structural and earthquake analysis.

Availability and User Support

DSS packages are available on many platforms, such as UNIX, Mac, DOS, and the Internet. The utility of these code packages depends on the equipment that the user has. In general, UNIX-based programs are more difficult to operate than personal computer (Mac or DOS)-based programs, and fewer people have access to UNIX-based machines. Availability over the Internet eliminates many machine incompatibility problems.

The eventual distribution for many government-sponsored code packages has not been decided. If distributed from software clearing houses, the ability to maintain and upgrade the software is diminished. If distributed over the Internet, support must be provided to maintain the code and upgrade it as necessary. In any event, if any of these codes are to see widespread use, user support is necessary. This will come in the form of providing advice on how to operate the code as well as more general advice on how to simulate the problem best.

Gaps in DSS

In general, DSS often acts as modular platforms that integrate a variety of software applications under a single shell. As such, incorporating any model into the framework to address various aspects of the remedial process is conceptually possible. In practice, although software is available to simulate many remedial processes that occur, very often it is not integrated into DSS. For example, multiphase flow simulations needed to examine large spills of nonaqueous phase liquids are not used in DSS software. Other complex cases that require sophisticated modeling involve flow and transport in fractured sites.

The software that addresses risk assessment does not perform detailed modeling of remedial alternatives and how that affects the source. The models that conduct detailed modeling of remediation alternatives do not perform risk assessments.

The software that addresses risk assessment does not consider ecologic risks, nor is there guidance on balancing ecologic and human health risks.

There may be gaps in modeling of specific remedial alternatives. The emphasis of this study was on DSS and not on detailed modeling of remediation efforts.

One Code Fits All

Because of the scope and complexity of the set of remediation problems it is impractical, if not impossible, to have a code of general applicability that would be useful for all potential situations. In addition, codes that work well under one set of conditions may not work well under other situations. Applicability of any model is site- and problem-specific.

Level of Complexity

There exists a trade-off between simple models that are easy to use and more complex models that more accurately reflect the situation. Conceptually, the use of more accurate models (which usually involves more detailed models) can lead to better resolution of the contamination problem with less uncertainty than with simpler models. This can translate into lower remediation costs. On the other hand, simpler models are easier to use and defend and gain regulatory acceptance more easily. The appropriate level of complexity for a given problem is site- and problem-specific.

CONCLUSIONS

Environmental DSS, defined as computer software that facilitates the use of data, models, and structured decision processes in decision making, has been identified through literature searches, Internet searches, and personal communications. DSS sponsored by the government and private industries in the United States was the focus of this study. Over 40 different code packages were identified. Preliminary evaluation based on available literature was used to evaluate and categorize each DSS package based on its capabilities and functions. The major categories of functions have been given.

No single code package attempts to address all areas. Several, however, address more than one area. In general, software packages that address multiple issues tend to address the data-collection problem or remedy selection and application. Only one code attempts to integrate the data-collection problem with risk assessment.

A screening level review of 19 of the DSS packages identified in this report has been completed (Sullivan et al., 1997). The review rates the software in a *Consumer Reports* style, with a ranking of high, medium, or low capability in the areas of DSS functionality, types of contaminants modeled, environmental characteristics modeled, regulatory class of problem addressed, and other technical categories (e.g., ease of use, visualization tools, field applications).

Many issues related to the continued use and development of DSS are discussed and include the following:

- Costs: In general, the more elaborate codes are expensive to develop with development costs ranging up to several million dollars.
- Maintenance: For all DSS, after the initial development maintenance must be performed. This includes upgrading databases as regulations and recommended data change, upgrading process models, training, and user support. Depending on the database associated with the code and the user base, this may be a substantial effort.

- Acceptance: DSS packages are new and need to gain regulatory acceptance. Training of regulators in the theory behind the DSS models as well as the application of the DSS is needed. In addition, because these are new code packages, it is likely that benchmarking and comparison to field data will be needed. Situations in which application of DSS software has led to reduced costs (through improved sampling efficiency or better remedy selection) need to be documented in a defensible manner.
- Gaps: For the most part, the current DSS packages are quantitative and not geared towards incorporation of "soft" data into the decision process. Guidance on the use of soft data has not been supplied.

ACKNOWLEDGMENTS

The authors thank Paul Beam and Skip Chamberlain of the Department of Energy's Office of Environmental Management for their guidance and critical review of this work.

REFERENCE

Sullivan, T. M., Gitten, M., and Moskowitz, P. D. 1997. *Evaluation of selected environmental decision support software*, BNL-64613. Upton, NY: Brookhaven National Laboratory.

CHAPTER
THIRTEEN

APPLICATION OF RISK-ASSESSMENT TECHNIQUES TO MILITARY DEPLOYMENTS: OPERATION DESERT STORM, OPERATION JOINT ENDEAVOR, OPERATION DESERT FOCUS

Jack M. Heller

U.S. Army Center for Health Promotion and Preventive Medicine, Aberdeen Proving Ground, Maryland

The U.S. Army uses risk-assessment methodologies to assist its decision-making process in many critical areas, particularly to protect human health. Several examples are presented that show how the military uses and adapts this technique to its everyday operations, both in the continental United States and abroad (Fig. 13.1).

Deployed military forces frequently are exposed to environmental contaminants and diseases that may put them at risk of adverse acute or chronic health effects (Fig. 13.2). The U.S. Army Center for Health Promotion and Preventive Medicine (CHPPM) often is tasked to measure those exposures and assess the

- Conus
  - Restoration
  - Game Consumption
  - Permitting
- Deployments (Past and Present)
  - Operation Desert Storm (Southwest Asia)
  - Operation Vigilant Warrior (Southwest Asia)
  - Operation Joint Endeavor (Bosnia)
  - Operation Desert Focus (Southwest Asia)

Figure 13.1 Risk assessment in the military.

164 TOXICOLOGY IN RISK ASSESSMENT

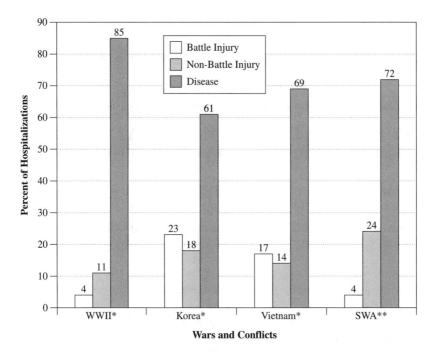

Figure 13.2 Percentage of Army hospitalizations during combat due to injury and disease since World War II. *Neel, Spurgeon. Medical Support of the U.S. Army in Vietnam 1965 to 1970. Department of the Army, U.S. GPO, Washington, DC, 1973. **Unpublished data.

potential for adverse health effects. The CHPPM's first major effort at measuring the environmental exposures of a deployed force, and attempting to determine the health consequences of that exposure, occurred during Operation Desert Storm (ODS) as a result of the concern over troop exposures to oil-fire smoke. The objectives of the health-risk assessment were (1) to identify the contaminants produced by the oil fires, (2) to determine the concentrations of contaminants at troop receptor points, and (3) to determine the health risks (cancer and noncancer) from exposure to the various contaminants. The two biggest challenges of that effort were collecting adequate exposure data (i.e., sampling) and evaluating the data for potential health risks (i.e., risk assessment). To assess the environment, and subsequent risk to troops caused by the oil fires, approximately 5000 environmental (air and soil) and industrial hygiene (air) samples were collected (Tables 13.1, 13.2, and 13.3) at 10 major troop locations throughout Kuwait and Saudi Arabia (Fig. 13.3). Sampling was conducted for 52 specific analytes using U.S. Environmental Protection Agency (EPA)–approved methods (Table 13.4) and was carried out from early May through early December 1991 (Fig. 13.4). The exposure data then were used to support a classic EPA "Superfund" health-risk assessment that evaluated all relevant

Table 13.1 Ambient air samples collected

Analyte	Number collected
Poly aromatic hydrocarbons	437
Volatiles	803
Acid gas	487
NO_X	86
SO_X	90
Ozone	92
Mercury	191
Metals	803
Total suspended particulate	224
Particulate matter < 10 μm	591
Radiologic (gross alpha, beta, and gamma)	215
Total	4019

Table 13.2 Soil samples collected

Analyte	Number collected
Metals	150
Poly aromatic hydrocarbons	80
Total	230

Table 13.3 Industrial hygiene samples collected

Analyte	Number collected
Poly aromatic hydrocarbons	437
Dust	28
Coal tar pitch volatiles	208
Volatiles	803
Acids	27
SO_X/NO_X	40
Total	785

environmental media and pathways. This included inhalation of metals and chemicals associated with particles, gases, and vapors; dermal absorption from contact with soil or sand; and incidental ingestion of soil or sand. Although the exposure had occurred and was continuing to occur, this approach was considered adequate to determine the potential for adverse health effects (cancer and noncancer) in the troop population. The toxicity assessment used the standard EPA values of slope factor for determining cancer risk and reference dose/concentration for determining noncancer risk. The risk-characterization step also used standard EPA methodology (Fig. 13.5) and cancer risk/noncancer risk standards. The methodology predicts outcomes that are population-based

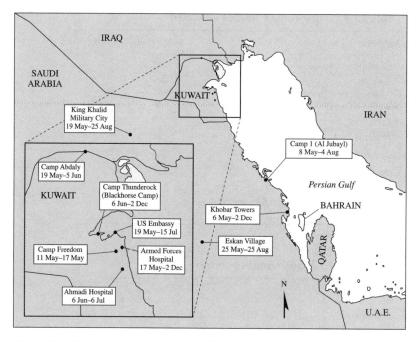

Figure 13.3 U.S. Army environmental sampling locations in 1991.

for both cancer and noncancer endpoints. EPA methodology at Superfund sites considers excess cancer risks greater than 1E-4 (one cancer in a population of 10,000) and noncancer hazard indices (the ratio of the chemical intake to the reference dose is greater than 1) greater than 1 to be problematic.

Results of the health-risk assessment indicated a small potential for adverse health effects to occur in the troop population as a result of exposure to petrochemical emissions from the oil fires. Total excess cancer risks were in the 7E-7 to 2E-6 range, and noncancer hazard indexes ranged from 0.6 to 5.0 throughout the theater of operation (Tables 13.5 and 13.6). The majority of the risks resulted from exposures to benzene and heavy metals. This risk assessment addressed total or absolute risk to the deployed force because the sample data could not distinguish between contaminants coming from the oil fires and those emanating from industrial or natural background sources (i.e., incremental risk). Another way of assessing the risk to troops was to compare the results from the industrial hygiene sampling (i.e., personal sampling) with American Conference of Government Industrial Hygienists threshold limit values. Table 13.7 compares the maximum results from the industrial hygiene sampling with threshold limit values and shows the detected contaminant level to be acceptable. However, following the conflict in the Persian Gulf troops began experiencing health problems upon their return to the United States. This situation prompted the Congress to pass two laws, PL102-190 and PL102-585, that required the Department of Defense (DOD) to set up a registry of all ODS veterans. The

Table 13.4 Sampled pollutants of concern

Volatile organic compounds		
Benzene	Toluene	m-Xylene
o-Xylene	p-Xylene	Propylbenzene
Ethylbenzene	Heptane	

Polycyclic aromatic hydrocarbons		
Acenaphthene	Acenaphthylene	Anthracene
Benzo(a)anthracene	Benzo(a)pyrene	Benzo(b)fluoranthene
Benzo(e)pyrene	Benzo(g,h,i)perylene	Benzo(k)fluoranthene
Binhenyl	Chrysene	Carbazole
Dibenzo(ah)anthracene	Dibenzofuran	2,6-dimethylnapthalene
Fluoranthene	Fluorene	Ideno(1,2,3-cd)pyrene
1-methylnapthalene	2-methylnapthalene	Naphthalene
Phenanthrene	Pyrene	

Acid gases		
Acetic	Formic	Hydrochloric
Nitric	Sulfuric	

Criteria pollutant gases		
Nitrogen dioxide/nitrogen oxide	Ozone	Sulfur dioxide

Particulates, metals, inorganics		
Particulate matter $< 10\ \mu m$	Total suspended particulate	Aluminum
Arsenic	Beryllium	Calcium
Cadmium	Chromium(3)	Chromium(6)
Iron	Mercury	Magnesium
Sodium	Nickel	Lead
Vanadium	Zinc	Sulfates
Nitrates	Chlorides	

registry was to be used to determine the oil-fire smoke exposure of all ODS veterans and also to conduct scientific research into other potential Gulf War exposures.

- Oil-well fire smoke/petrochemicals
- Chemical/biologic warfare agents
- Pesticides
- Vaccines
- Depleted uranium
- Pyriodostigmine bromide
- Particulate matter

The U.S. Army was given the DOD lead for Persian Gulf health issues, and the CHPPM was tasked with the responsibility of determining troop oil-fire exposure

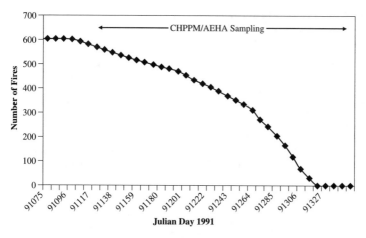

Figure 13.4 Chronology of extinguishment of oil fires.

and potential health risk. To accomplish this mandate the CHPPM selected geographic information system (GIS) technology. The GIS is capable of analyzing and displaying large quantities of spatially and temporally referenced environmental exposure, health outcome, demographic, and troop location data (Fig. 13.6). GIS accomplishes the following:

- Mapping environmental exposures
- Environmental health-risk assessment
- Assessing space and time relationships
- Integrating medical outcomes with potential exposures
- Assessing health risks during ODS, Bosnia, and future deployments

Because the CHPPM's environmental sample data only covered a limited geographic area and time period, modeled exposure data was required. Modeled

> - Carcinogenic Risk = Intake $\times$ Slope Factor
> $$(1E\text{-}4 - 1E\text{-}6)$$
> - Non-Carcinogenic Risk =
> $$\text{Hazard Quotient} = \frac{\text{Intake}}{\text{RfD}}$$

Figure 13.5 Risk-characterization formulas.

Table 13.5 Cancer risk levels for the eight monitoring sites

Site	Cancer risk
Khobar Towers, Al Jubayl, Saudi Arabia	2E-6
Camp 1, Al Jubayl, Saudi Arabia	1E-6
Eskan Village, Riyadh, Saudi Arabia	1E-6
King Khalid Military City, Saudi Arabia	7E-7
Camp Freedom Military Hospital, Kuwait	1E-6
Camp Thunderock, Doha, Kuwait	2E-6
United States Embassy, Kuwait City, Kuwait	2E-6
Al Ahmadi Hospital, Ahmadi, Kuwait	1E-6

Table 13.6 Noncarcinogenic risk levels for the eight monitoring sites

Sites	Hazard index
Khobar Towers, Al Jubayl, Saudi Arabia	2
Camp 1, Al Jubayl, Saudi Arabia	2
Eskan Village, Riyadh, Saudi Arabia	1
King Khalid Military City, Saudi Arabia	0.6
Camp Freedom Military Hospital, Kuwait	2
Camp Thunderock, Doha, Kuwait	2
United States Embassy, Kuwait City, Kuwait	4
Al Ahmadi Hospital, Ahmadi, Kuwait	5

Table 13.7 Maximum sample results

Location	Analysis	Results	Threshold limit value
Kuwait	Benzene	0.19	32
Kuwait	Toluene	0.75	377
Kuwait	Xylene	3.21	434
Kuwait	NO_2	6.70	5.6
Kuwait	SO_2	1.90	5.2
Kuwait	Nitric acid	0.12	5.2
Kuwait	Sulfuric acid	0.05	1.0
Saudi Arabia	Total particles	2.30	10
Saudi Arabia	Respirable particles	2.00	Compound-specific
Saudi Arabia	Coal tar	0.21	0.2

exposure data, if combined with field samples, expands the time period, locations, exposed populations, and contaminants that can be assessed. To accomplish the modeling effort the CHPPM enlisted the aid of the National Oceanic and Atmospheric Administration (NOAA) Air Resources Laboratory.

The CHPPM used the output from the NOAA Hybrid Single-Particle Lagrangian Integrated Trajectories (HY-SPLIT) Model, in conjunction with

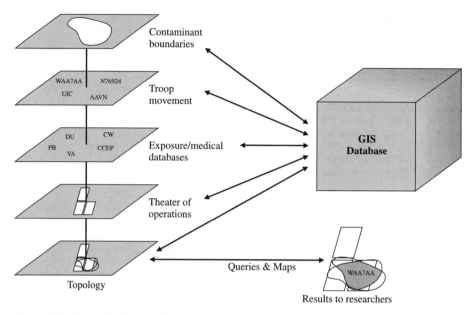

Figure 13.6 Geographic information systems concepts.

their Advanced Very High Resolution Radiometer (AVHRR) satellite images, to determine where the oil-fire plume impacted troops on a daily basis and at what level (Figs. 13.7–13.10). The GIS can combine the daily troop and plume location data to produce any number of informative data displays (Figs. 13.11 and 13.12). Daily troop unit locations were obtained from the U.S. Armed Services Center for Research of Unit Records, Troop Movement Database. The center has examined over 5 million records (e.g., unit logs, situation reports) since 1993 in order to place troop units geographically (by latitude and longitude) on a daily basis. To enhance the information in the Troop Movement Database the center has enlisted the aid of battalion and division intelligence and operations officers. These personnel were able to provide additional information that has improved the location data for individual troop units (Figs. 13.13 and 13.14). With all the effort and information that has been incorporated in the Troop Movement Database, there are still some problems with the data. For example, not all units have complete location data; some units have no location data; some units have multiple locations on a single day, making exposure assessment difficult; individuals may not always have been with their units; and there are service differences that complicate the data. The individual personnel in each troop unit were determined from the Defense Manpower Data Center's

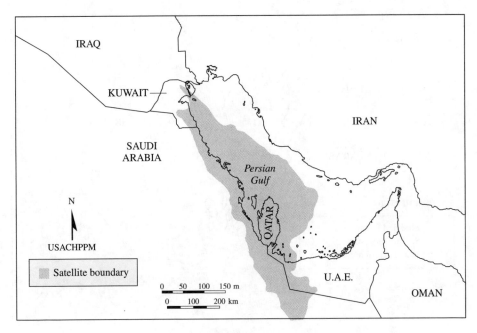

Figure 13.7 "Super plume" boundary satellite data for oil well fires on May 20, 1991.

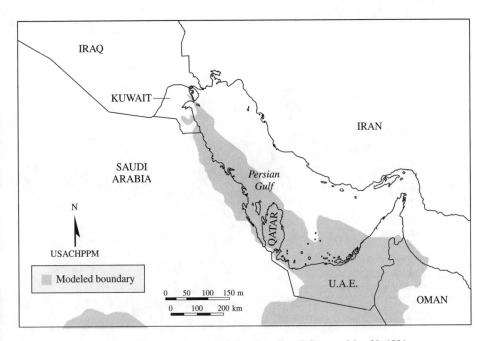

Figure 13.8 "Super plume" boundary modeled data for oil well fires on May 20, 1991.

172 TOXICOLOGY IN RISK ASSESSMENT

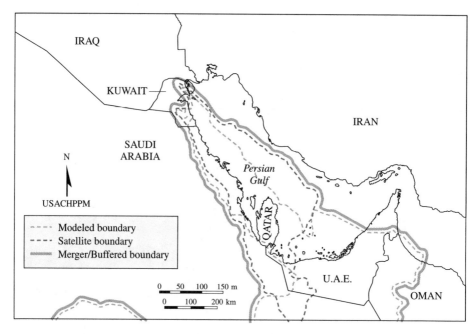

Figure 13.9 "Super plume" boundary merged satellite and modeled data for oil well fires on May 20, 1991.

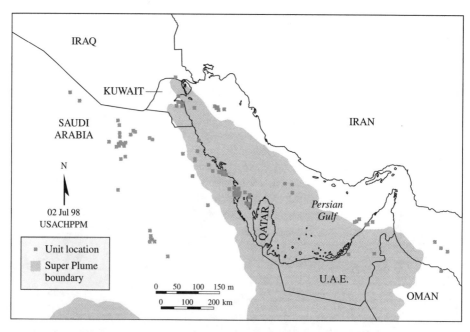

Figure 13.10 "Super plume" boundary merged satellite and modeled data for oil well fires on May 20, 1991, with troop unit locations included.

RISK ASSESSMENT IN MILITARY DEPLOYMENTS **173**

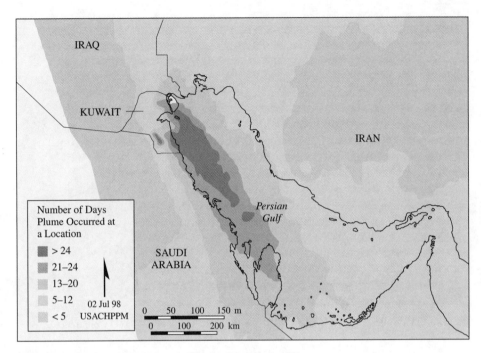

Figure 13.11 Smoke-plume frequency distribution, March 1991.

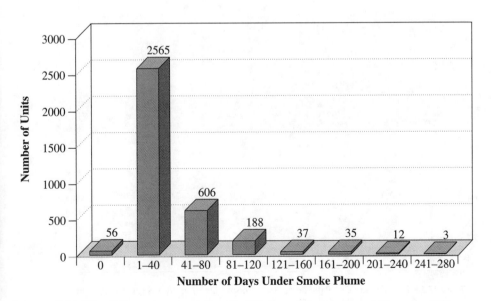

Figure 13.12 Oil well fire exposure groupings for U.S. force, February through December 1991.

174 TOXICOLOGY IN RISK ASSESSMENT

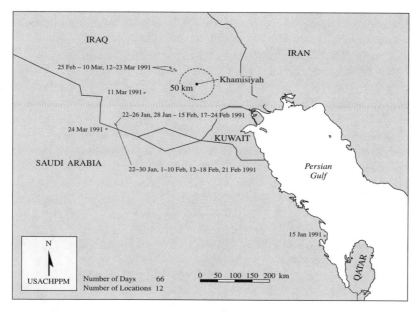

Figure 13.13 Locations of 3rd Brigade/101st Airborne Division before S3/G3 Conference.

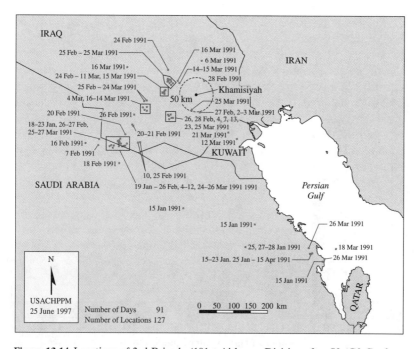

Figure 13.14 Locations of 3rd Brigade/101st Airborne Division after S3/G3 Conference.

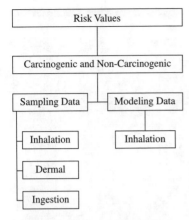

Figure 13.15 Algorithm of military risk assessment.

Persian Gulf Registry. Once the individuals that make up a unit are identified, the GIS can calculate an individual service member's exposure and resultant health risk using standard EPA exposure and toxicity factors (i.e., body weight, breathing rate, skin surface area, reference dose/concentration, and cancer slope factor [Figs. 13.15 and 13.16]). For this health-risk assessment some of the exposure factors were modified to account for the deployment situation and the military population. The risk levels shown in Figure 13.16 are for troop units, because of individual privacy requirements. However, the individuals in each unit can be identified by social security number from the Defense Manpower Data Center Persian Gulf Registry, and the individual risks can be calculated based on their number of days in theater and their exposure.

The potential exposures and contributing causes of ODS veterans' health problems are numerous (see list, p. 167). Unfortunately the data available to assess these exposures are very limited. Therefore, the CHPPM GIS is being used to assist in the evaluation of other suspected environmental exposures and the medical outcomes potentially associated with those exposures:

- Deployment
    Out patient
    In patient
- Post Deployment
    Registries
        VA Gulf War Health Examination Registry
        DOD Comprehensive Clinical Evaluation Program
    Hospitalization

Much of this work is being carried out using troop proximity to a particular event, such as a chemical agent alarm or detection or a Scud missile impact, as a surrogate for exposure (Fig. 13.17). Other exposures, for example to chemical weapons, are being modeled from reports of events that occurred during the war and with the aid of simulations (Fig. 13.18). Troops who were potentially

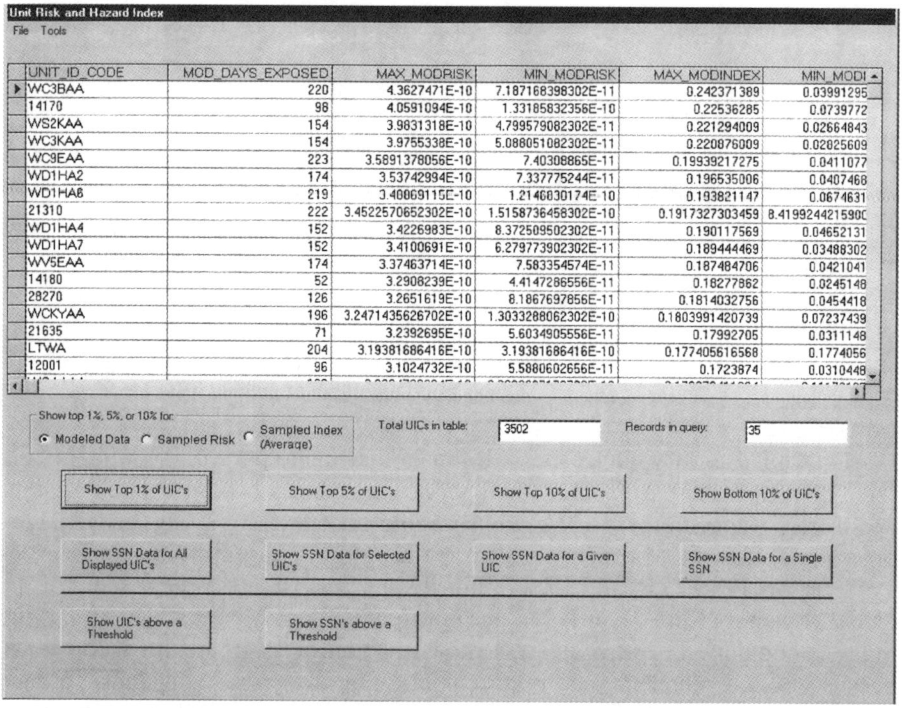

176 TOXICOLOGY IN RISK ASSESSMENT

Figure 13.16 Unit risk and hazard indices.

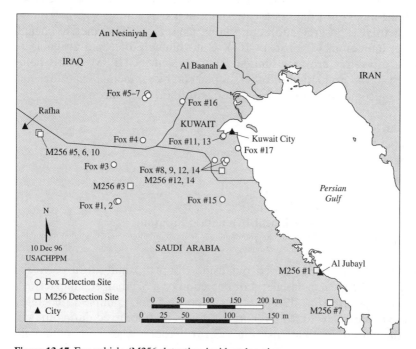

Figure 13.17 Fox vehicle/M256 detection incident locations.

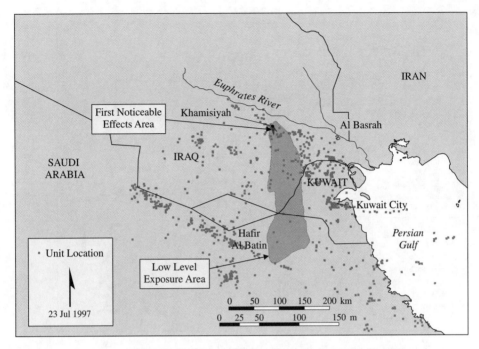

Figure 13.18 Modeled exposure for Khamsiyah pit demolition, day 1, March 10, 1991.

exposed are having their medical outcomes, such as hospitalizations and participation in DOD and Veterans Administration health registries, compared with unexposed troops or troops who did not deploy to the Persian Gulf region. This methodology is being used to try and determine if an exposure occurred. The situation with ODS veterans' health problems and the lack of adequate record keeping with respect to environmental exposures, troop locations, medical records, pesticide usage, and so forth has led the DOD to institute numerous changes.

Prior to the deployment to Bosnia, the DOD initiated the development of a directive and an instruction for joint medical surveillance for deployments. These documents have since been finalized and issued. Included in DOD Directive 6490.2, Joint Medical Surveillance, August 30, 1997, and DOD Instruction 6490.3, Implementation and Application of Joint Medical Surveillance for Deployments, August 7, 1997, are the responsibilities for determining environmental exposures, ascertaining potential health threats associated with the exposures, and reporting results back to field commanders and medical personnel. The CHPPM, in collaboration with other DOD activities, has assumed a large role in this area, with environmental sampling and risk assessment activities currently being conducted in Bosnia for Operation Joint Endeavor and

178 TOXICOLOGY IN RISK ASSESSMENT

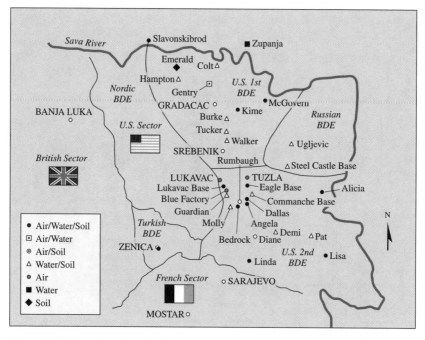

Figure 13.19 Operation Joint Endeavor environmental monitoring efforts.

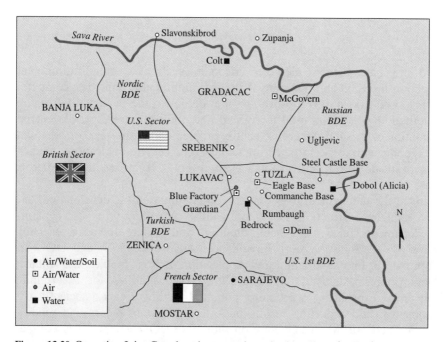

Figure 13.20 Operation Joint Guard environmental monitoring efforts (to date).

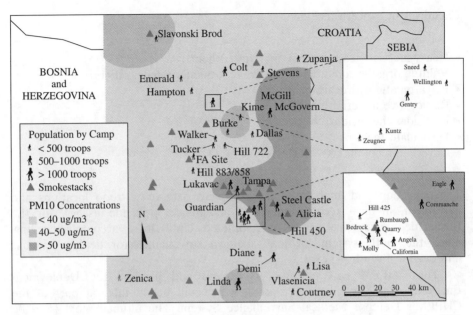

Figure 13.21 Particulate matter concentrations with smokestacks, June 1996 through August 1996.

Operation Joint Guard as follows:

- Assess acute and chronic health risks from environmental contaminants
- Provide upfront intelligence for environmental health
- Consider environmental exposures in predeployment planning
- Assess preliminary environmental baseline conditions prior to full deployment
- Provide timely environmental health-risk assessment to deployed force leadership
- Enhance medical surveillance

The CHPPM mission is to assess acute and chronic exposures for a wide variety of environmental contaminants and report the potential for adverse health effects back to the field (Figs. 13.19–13.21). The contamination sources of concern in this case include:

- Power plants
- Industrial facilities
- Agricultural operations
- Mining
- Military operations

Chemicals of concern include:

- Heavy metals—lead, arsenic, mercury, others
- Volatile organic compounds—benzene, toluene, xylene, others
- Polyaromatic hydrocarbons
- Radioactive materials
- Pesticides/herbicides
- Particulate matter
- Criteria air pollutants—SO_2, NO_2, CO, O_3

The collection and analysis of the complete data (e.g., troop locations and movement, medical records, medical surveillance, pesticide usage), for the Bosnia deployment has yet to be completed. Until this is accomplished, how much the DOD system for joint medical surveillance for deployment has improved will not be known.

The CHPPM is continuing to expand and improve the Deployment Environmental Surveillance Program, which will be an integral part of the CHPPM's Defense Medical Surveillance System. The ultimate goal is to be capable of responding immediately to a military deployment anywhere in the world. This would include "operations other than war" such as the peacekeeping effort in Bosnia or disaster relief efforts such as hurricane Andrew. To meet this challenge the Deployment Environmental Surveillance Program is expanding to

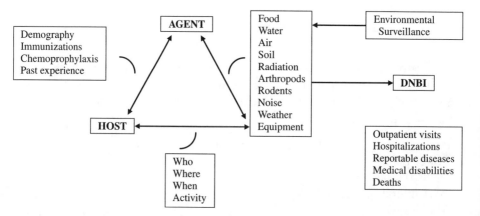

Figure 13.22 Comprehensive military medical/public health surveillance.

map larger areas of the world and determine the environmental and health threats that exist in regions on a spatial and temporal basis. GIS capability is increasing with respect to the diversity of dispersion models; it is capable of using environmental data and interfacing with the NOAA real-time meteorologic prediction network. The ultimate aim of this system is protecting the health of U.S. forces worldwide and reducing the incidence of disease and non-battle injury (Fig. 13.22).

CHAPTER
FOURTEEN

APPLICATION OF RISK-ASSESSMENT TECHNIQUES TO MILITARY SCENARIOS: MULTIPATHWAY EXPOSURE ASSESSMENT FOR CHEMICAL AGENT INCINERATORS

Hsieng-Ye Chang

U.S. Army Center for Health Promotion and Preventive Medicine, Aberdeen Proving Grounds, Maryland

Health-risk assessments (HRAs) are used for risk-management decisions for activities under both the Comprehensive Environmental Response, Compensation, and Liability Act (Superfund) and the Resource Conservation and Recovery Act (RCRA). In the permit process for boilers or industrial furnaces burning hazardous waste, HRAs are used by the respective regulatory agencies to determine if air emissions from operation of the incineration facility would result in increased health risks to human and ecologic health. An operating permit may be approved or denied depending on the degree of departure of the estimated health risks from the regulatory health benchmarks. Under the U.S. Environmental Protection Agency (EPA)'s (1993b) draft combustion strategy, facility owners seeking to renew an expiring permit and those wanting to operate a new facility both are required to submit a health risk evaluation as part of the RCRA part B permit application. Chemical-agent incinerators are considered hazardous-waste incinerators, and therefore the operator is required to submit a permit application to the regulating authority.

In general, HRAs are performed twice for each chemical-agent incineration facility. Because the proposed facilities have not yet been constructed, facility-specific emissions data are not available. Therefore, in order to complete the HRA for the part B permit application, air emissions are estimated from similar facilities, namely, the Johnston Atoll Chemical Agent Disposal System located in the Pacific Ocean. As data from the Tooele Chemical Agent Disposal Facility, Utah, become available, they will be incorporated for future HRAs. Once the facility has obtained the necessary operating permit, a trial burn is performed, after which actual facility emissions data are available. An HRA is conducted at that time using facility-specific emissions data.

Although some facilities were required to perform HRAs prior to the draft combustion strategy, those HRAs were not as extensive those required of HRAs today. Prior to the EPA's call for more stringent permit conditions in 1993, HRAs consisted only of an evaluation of exposure from inhalation of air emissions. Stricter requirements for combustion facilities were promulgated by the public's ever-increasing concern with health impacts from combustion emissions. As a consequence, HRAs were expanded to include indirect exposures in addition to direct exposures to air emissions.

Indirect exposure generally refers to any exposure that does not involve direct contact with substances in the primary media of substance release. Therefore, for incinerator HRAs, any exposure involving direct contact with air is considered a direct exposure because air is the primary media in which stack emissions come in contact with once substances are released. Air is also the primary mode of transport. Once deposited, a substance can accumulate in the medium in which it has been deposited (surface soil or water), or it can be transported to or taken up by another media. For example, surface-soil erosion is a physical means by which a substance can be transported to a surface body of water. Similarly, a substance may be taken up by a plant via root uptake. These mechanisms are referred to as *fate* and *transport processes* and depend on a substance's as well as the environment's physical and chemical properties. Indirect exposure pathways are also commonly referred to as *multipathway* or *foodchain* pathways.

The earliest known EPA guidance for performing indirect exposures to combustion emissions dates back to as early as 1990 (U.S. EPA, 1990, 1993a). Because indirect exposures were not required at that time, however, this guidance was not widely used, although the HRA for the Waste Technologies Industries incinerator, Ohio, generally implemented this methodology (U.S. EPA, 1996a). In April 1994, the EPA's Office of Solid Waste and Emergency Response released a guidance for performing a screening-level multipathway HRA (U.S. EPA, 1994a). The screening approach reduces the extensiveness of site-specific data collection required by previous EPA methodologies by focusing on individuals whose activities represent high-end trends of the population.

The U.S. Army Center for Health Promotion and Preventive Medicine (USACHPPM) was tasked to evaluate potential health risks from air emissions for several of the proposed chemical-agent disposal facilities (CDFs). These HRAs are performed by quantifying both cancer and noncancer health effects from exposure to various media. At the time the EPA screening methodology was released, the USACHPPM was developing an HRA work plan for the proposed chemical agent incineration facility at the Anniston Army Depot (ANAD), Alabama. The ANAD CDF was among the first of several proposed CDFs requiring an operating permit. Being the first agency to implement the new guidance, USACHPPM had the opportunity to work closely with regulatory agencies to discuss technical issues and problems encountered in using this guidance. The nature of the new guidance in combination with the paucity of fate and transport data, as well as the lack of toxicity information for many compounds, provided many challenges throughout the HRA process. In addition to the completed HRA for the ANAD CDF, the ACHPPM recently completed the HRA for the CDF at Pine Bluff Arsenal, Arkansas. Other HRAs are at the developmental stage. Although many technical issues were encountered, this chapter presents only some of the major issues that arose during the health-risk evaluation of air emissions from the proposed CDF.

EXPOSURE-ASSESSMENT ISSUES

One of the major issues that reflects the lack of toxicity data involves an acute exposure assessment. Wary of possible exposure to uncontrolled stack releases such as those occurring during an accident, the regulatory community requested the inclusion of an acute inhalation assessment. Although each incineration unit that processes chemical agents has added safety measures to ensure that no accidental release lasts longer than 15 minutes, the HRA conservatively models for maximum air concentrations from events up to 1 hour in duration. The evaluation looks at both an on-site worker and a resident. The resident may be an on-site or off-site individual, depending on whether or not a housing area exists on the installation. Even if an on-site housing area is present, air concentrations at an off-site fenceline location may be higher depending on the location of the housing area as well as local meteorologic conditions. For instance, the on-site housing area may not be directly downwind of the stack plume.

The issue of what toxicity data to use for the acute evaluation was the topic of discussion during several meetings of EPA and state regulatory personnel. To date, no methodology exists to satisfactorily quantify potential exposure from this pathway. Although short-term exposure limits have been used for various purposes, such as the American Industrial Hygiene Association's emergency response planning guidelines, data are limited. In addition, the regulatory community does not think that these guidelines are protective of human health. The methodology that eventually was applied for the acute analysis involves a comparison between a compound's modeled air concentration and its acute toxicity value. An acute hazard index then is obtained by summing the acute hazard quotients and comparing them to a regulatory target level of unity:

$$AHQ_i = Ca_i/ATV_i$$

where AHQ_i is the acute hazard quotient for substance i, Ca_i is the modeled 1-hour air concentration for substance i (in micrograms per cubic meter); and ATV_i is the acute toxicity value of substance i (in micrograms per cubic meter).

As mentioned previously, toxicity data for evaluating 1-hour exposures are limited. Therefore, upon the recommendation of the regulatory community, occupational exposure limits, namely threshold limit values (TLVs) published by the ACGIH (American Conference of Governmental and Industrial Hygenists), are used as the acute threshold concentrations. In addition, a safety factor of

100 is applied for the resident scenario to account for the sensitive subpopulation (children, the elderly, asthmatics).

Although TLVs may not be the best data to use for quantifying acute inhalation exposure, occupational exposure limits developed by various agencies constitute the most complete list of values than any other database. It should be noted, however, that TLVs are developed not for quantifying health risks, but rather to monitor chemical concentrations in the work environment to ensure the protection of workers. Unless otherwise stated, TLVs are developed for a normal 8-hour work day, 40 hours a week. Many areas of uncertainty are involved with the use of these values to estimate acute inhalation exposure, but they are not presented here.

In January 1995, the California EPA's Office of Environmental Health Hazard Assessment (OEHHA) released a draft document titled *Technical Support Document for the Determination of Acute Toxicity Exposure Levels for Airborne Toxicants*. This document specifically addresses 1-hour inhalation exposure to airborne substances. Values were derived based on literature studies, and the resulting acute threshold values are referred to as *relative exposure levels* (RELs). Although RELs are available only for a limited list of air pollutants, the document does provide a value for hydrochloric acid (HCl) that is not available in the American Conference of Governmental Industrial Hygienists (1996) TLV tables (a short-term exposure limit or a ceiling value is provided, but not a time-weighted average). Inclusion of the HCl REL of 60 $\mu g/m^3$ in the ANAD HRA resulted in exceedance of the regulatory benchmark level of unity.

Further inquiry into the OEHHA document indicated that the agency was updating its document. The OEHHA was investigating an alternate REL for HCl based on a recent study by Stevens et al. (1992). Although OEHHA had developed an REL based on this study, the value was still under peer review and therefore could not be released. The Stevens et al. study is based on results from ten 18- to 25-year-old asthmatics who were exposed to HCl concentrations between 0.8 to 1.8 ppm while wearing half-face masks. Based on data from this study, an ACHPPM toxicologist, using the methodology outlined in the OEHHA guidance, derived an REL of 2000 $\mu g/m^3$ for HCl.

To ensure that the study is valid and that the derived REL is protective of the sensitive subpopulation, peer review was solicited from both physicians and toxicologists from other organizations. The proposed REL was also reviewed by EPA's Office of Research and Development as well as National Center for Environmental Assessment (NCEA) toxicologists. The latter reviewers suggested incorporating a safety factor of 3 to account for the lack of support from other studies (U.S. EPA, 1996b). In general, the consensus was that the Stevens et al. study is reliable and that the derived REL is valid. Subsequently, an HCl REL of 2000 $\mu g/m^3$ with an uncertainty factor of 3 was applied to the acute exposure assessment.

In some instances, data may be superceded as new information becomes available. An example of such involves chronic toxicity values proposed for chemical agents (Department of the Army, 1996). In June 1996, the Army proposed interim values for the nerve agents GA (tabun, or ethyl n-dimethylphosphoramidocyanidate), GB (sarin, or isopropyl methylphosphonofluoridate), and GD (soman, or 1,2,2-trimethylphosphonofluoridate) and for sulphur mustard, HD (β-β'-dichloroethyl sulfide), and Lewisite. These values were endorsed by the Army Office of the Surgeon General in August 1996 and proposed for interim use. In the mean time, the proposed toxicity values are pending approval from the National Research Council's Committee on Toxicology.

Although the CDF HRAs did include chronic evaluations of chemical agents, media-based agent-control limits were substituted for toxicity values (Oak Ridge National Laboratories, 1992). Replacing the media-based standards with the interim health-based toxicity values resulted in levels exceeding of the regulatory target health levels (1E-05 for cancer risk) for the inhalation of HD/HT alone.

Until that point of the assessment, the risk-assessment methodology used to quantify chronic health effects from inhalation of air emissions from the CDF had not been questioned. The EPA screening methology uses the unit risk to estimate the probability of developing cancer from inhalation. Unit risks, however, are based on a continuous lifetime facility operation or 70 years. Although most commercial facilties operate for longer time periods, the proposed CDFs typically have much shorter operational lives ranging from 2 to 10 years.

Two possible solutions exist to better characterize health risk from inhalation of CDF air emissions. One is to use the cancer slope factor approach as outlined in the *Risk Assessment Guidance for Superfund* (U.S. EPA, 1989). This method uses actual facility lifetime to estimate cancer risk from inhalation as opposed to the simple air concentration comparison to the unit risk approach. The second approach is also provided in an EPA guidance (1991), which suggests that if the unit risk is used, the facility lifetime should be weighted to obtain a cancer risk that is reflective of the projected facility operational life. For example, because the ANAD facility is expected to operate for 6 years to include buffer time for agent campaign delays, the estimated cancer risk from inhalation of HD would be:

$$\text{Cancer Risk}_{inh} = 6/70 \cdot \text{unit risk} \cdot C_a$$

where C_a is the modeled chronic air concentration for HD (in micrograms per cubic meter). This approach was deemed acceptable by the regulatory community.

FATE AND TRANSPORT ISSUES

Other issues encountered concern fate and transport modeling parameters for substances such as dioxins/furans and mercury, which tend to drive health-risk estimates. Two specific fate and transport issues are presented in this section.

The first issue concerns the air-to-plant biotransfer factor (Bv) of dioxins/furans. This parameter is critical for determining the uptake of substances in the vapor phase to above-ground edible portions of plants. The impacted plant then could be consumed as forage by cows or as vegetables by humans. According to the EPA's screening methodology, dioxins/furans are expressed as 2,3,7,8-tetrachlorodibenzo-p-dioxin (TCDD) toxicity equivalents using congener-specific toxicity equivalence factors. The toxicity equivalence factors are dependent on each congener's toxicity with respect to 2,3,7,8-TCDD, which has been deemed as the most toxic of all dioxin/furan congeners. Although the EPA (1994) provides a chemical-specific Bv value for the 2,3,7,8-TCDD toxicity equivalent, new data suggested that this value could be refined. In a November 1994 memorandum, the EPA modified the Bv value from an initally proposed value of 2.70E + 05 to 4.55E + 05 (Units of [μg TCDD/g plant tissue]/[μg TCDD/g air]).

Subsequent health-risk evaluation indicated that the estimated cancer risk for the subsistence-farmer scenario was slightly above the regulatory target level. At the same time, the EPA was considering another experimental study for deriving the Bv value of the 2,3,7,8-TCDD toxicity equivalent. In a paper presented by Lorber (1995), the author used results from a study by Welsch-Pausch et al. (1995) to derive congener-specific Bv values. Lorber indicated that the Welsch-Pausch et al. study provided the best data to date because photodegradation was factored into the experiment (personal communication from M. Lorber, 5 March 1996). Based on additional information provided by Lorber, the ACHPPM developed a Bv value of 8.39E + 04 for the 2,3,7,8-TCDD toxicity equivalent.

The second issue involves mercury partition coefficient values. As part of the fate and transport modeling process, three parameters are particularly important for determining mercury concentration in a surface waterbody. They are as follows:

- K_{ds} = soil–water partition coefficient ([g Hg/g dry soil]/[g Hg/mL water], or more simply, mL/g)
- K_{dbs} = sediment–water partition coefficient (mL/g)
- K_{dsw} = suspended sediment–water partition coefficient (mL/g)

It should be noted that EPA region VI had released a draft guidance for conducting incinerator HRAs in December 1994 (U.S. EPA, 1994b). Although similar to the EPA April 1994 guidance (U.S. EPA, 1994a), the region VI document contains additional exposure pathways and different input parameters. Because the proposed Pine Bluff CDF will be located in region VI, the HRA methodology must follow the one outlined in the region VI guidance. This guidance suggests values of 150 mL/g for each of three partition coefficients for Hg. Very high Hg concentrations were estimated in fish tissue using the EPA default parameters.

The EPA's *Mercury Report to Congress* (1996c), however, suggests very different values for the three partition coefficients. Values of 53,700 mL/g, 157,000 mL/g, and 650,000 mL/g are presented in the document for K_{ds}, K_{dbs}, and K_{dsw}, respectively. The increase of the K_{ds} value resulted in a slightly higher estimated Hg concentration in fish tissue. This is evident because as the K_{ds} value increases, Hg contribution from soil erosion into the surface waterbody also increases. On the other hand, an increase of the K_{dbs} value from 150 to 160,000 mL/g resulted in a significant decrease of Hg concentration in the water column (as much as 99%). As the concentration in the water column decreases, more Hg ends up in the bed sediment, which was roughly 60% higher in Hg concentration. Mercury concentration in fish tissue is estimated using the bioaccumulation factor and not the the biota-to-sediment accumulation factor; therefore, an increase in K_{dbs} would result in lower Hg concentration in fish tissue. The K_{dsw} value, however, did not result in significant changes to the Hg concentration in fish tissue.

In order to ensure that these partition coefficients provided in the Mercury Report to Congress are valid, the ACHPPM consulted Glenn Rice from the NCEA. Upon his recommendation, and with the approval of the regulatory community, the new values were incorporated into the HRA. In addition to the suggested values for the three partition coefficients, the mercury report also suggests a higher Hg bioaccumulation factor of 335,000 L/kg. To be consistent in the use of new data, this value also was incorporated into the HRA.

CONTINUING ISSUES

Although the EPA has established a guidance for performing combustion facility HRAs, the state in which each proposed CDF is located has final RCRA authority over the HRA methodology. Therefore, it is unlikely that the HRAs for proposed CDFs can be compared, because of different requirements. Some of the modifactions include additional exposure pathways and exposure scenarios. Other changes from the current guidance include the use of input parameters other than recommended EPA default values or more stringent acceptable target levels. Thus, the resolution of issues for one CDF HRA does not necessarily mean that they are resolved for another CDF HRA.

DISCUSSION

It is evident from the examples provided here that an issue can best be resolved if a problem with a methodology or data is identified early. However, the intricacy of the HRAs for the proposed CDF makes it very difficult to know the problem until it is encountered. The best way to deal with the situation is to be resourceful and to keep current with changes. Being resourceful means knowing where to find answers and whom to contact for method validation. The high profile of matters concerning chemical agents, as well as the public's unpopular perception of incineration, make it even more critical to obtain third-party endorsement for new methodologies or data. However, not all situations can be resolved even if emissions are reduced. Under such circumstances, the best action is to present all results and assumptions and let the regulatory community decide the best course of action.

ACKNOWLEDGMENTS

The resolution of each issue could not have been possible without a joint effort from everyone working on the CDF HRAs. Special thanks to my mentors Bonnie Gaborek and Dennis Druck for sharing their many years of risk-assessment experience.

REFERENCES

American Conference of Governmental Industrial Hygienists. 1996. *Threshold limit values for chemical substances and physical agents and biological exposure indicies*. Cincinnati, OH: Author.

Department of the Army. 1996. *Interim chronic toxicological criteria for chemical warfare compounds*. Aberdeen Proving Ground, MD: Author.

Lorber, M. 1995. Development of an air-to-leaf vapor phase transfer factor for dioxins and furans. *Organohalogen Compounds* 24:179–186.

Stevens, B., Koenig, J., Rebolledo, V., Hanley, Q., and Covert, D. 1992. Respiratory effects from the inhalation of hydrogen chloride in young adult asthamatics. *J. Med.* 34:923–929.

California Environmental Protection Agency. 1995. *Technical support document for the determination of acute toxicity exposure levels for airborne toxicants*. Sacramento, CA: Office of Environmental Health Hazard Assessment.

Oak Ridge National Laboratories. 1992. *Estimated general population control limits for unitary agents in drinking water, milk, soil, and unprocessed food items*, Prepared for the U.S. Department of the Army by ORNL. Washington, DC.

U.S. Environmental Protection Agency. 1989. *Risk assessment guidance for superfund: Vol. I, human health evaluation manual (Part A)*. Interim Final. Washington, DC: Office of Emergency and Remedial Response.

U.S. Environmental Protection Agency. 1990. *Methodology for assessing health risk associated with indirect exposure to combustor emissions*, interim final. Washington, DC: Office of Research and Development.

U.S. Environmental Protection Agency. 1991. *Upper-bound quantitative cancer risk estimate for populations adjacent to sulfur mustard incineration facilities*. Washington, DC: Office of Research and Development.

U.S. Environmental Protection Agency. 1993a. *Addendum to the methodology for assessing health risks associated with indirect exposure to combustor emissions*, external review draft. Washington, DC: Office of Research and Development.

U.S. Environmental Protection Agency. 1993b. *Draft strategy for combustion of hazardous waste*. Washington, DC: Office of Solid Waste.

U.S. Environmental Protection Agency. 1994a. *Implementation guidance for conducting indirect exposure analysis at RCRA combustion units*. Washington, DC: Office of Solid Waste.

U.S. Environmental Protection Agency. 1994b. Revised draft guidance for performing screening level risk analyses at combustion facilities burning hazardous wastes: Attachment c; draft exposure assessment guidance for RCRA hazardous waste combustion facilities. Washington, DC: Author.

U.S. Environmental Protection Agency. 1996a. *Draft risk assessment for WTI, volume V: Human health risk assessment: Evaluation of potential risks from multipathway exposure to emissions*. Washington, DC: Office of Research and Development.

U.S. Environmental Protection Agency. 1996b. *Memorandum from Daniel Guth, National Center for Environmental Assessment-RTP, to Rosemary Workman*. Office of Solid Waste.

U.S. Environmental Protection Agency. 1996c. *Mercury report to Congress*, SAB review draft. Cincinnati, OH: National Center for Environmental Assessment, and Office of Research and Development.

Welsch-Pausch, K., McLachlan, M., and Umlauf, G. 1995. Determination of the principal pathways of polychlorinated dibenzo-p-dioxins and dibenzofurans to Lolium multiflorum (Welsh Ray Grass). *Environ. Sci. Technol.* 29:1090–1098.

CHAPTER
FIFTEEN

A DRINKING WATER ADVISORY: CONSUMER ACCEPTABILITY ADVICE AND HEALTH EFFECTS ANALYSIS ON METHYL TERTIARY-BUTYL ETHER

Charles O. Abernathy, Julie T. Du, Amal Mahfouz, Maria M. Gomez-Taylor, and Joyce M. Donohue

U.S. Environmental Protection Agency, Washington, DC

The purpose of this drinking water advisory is to provide information to state and local drinking water facilities and public health personnel on the potential health effects of methyl tertiary-butyl ether (MtBE). This advisory may be revised in the future based on findings that decrease uncertainties in quantifying risk for the drinking water route of exposure. A final health advisory (HA) will be issued when the database is judged to be adequate. The organoleptic effects (taste and odor) of MtBE affect the acceptability of water at concentrations that appear to provide an additional basis for assessment of quality and usability of water resources.

MtBE, an octane enhancer that has replaced lead in gasoline, causes more complete combustion of gasoline and reduces atmospheric carbon monoxide and ozone levels (Agency for Toxic Substances and Disease Registry, 1996; U.S. EPA, 1997). MtBE may constitute up to 15% (v/v) of the gasoline mixture, and its production was estimated at 6.2 billion kg in the United States in 1994 (National Science and Technology Council, 1996). About 30% of gasoline is reformulated to achieve cleaner combustion; 84% of reformulated gasoline contains MtBE as an oxygenate. Presently 32 areas in 13 states are participating in the reformulated gasoline program. Because it is a volatile chemical, MtBE is released to air from reformulated gasoline. In some instances, drinking water sources may be contaminated. Leaking underground storage tanks for gasoline products are frequently the cause of groundwater contamination. According to

---

The opinions expressed in this manuscript are those of the authors and do not necessarily reflect those of the U.S. Environmental Protection Agency.

the toxic chemical release inventory published in 1995, approximately 5% of the MtBE released from industrial sources enters surface water or publicly owned water-treatment plants (Agency for Toxic Substances and Disease Registry, 1996). Surface waters also can become contaminated as noncombusted MtBE in gasoline is released into air and precipitated by rain and snow.

MtBE is a small, highly water-soluble molecule. It does not bind strongly to most soils and can travel relatively rapidly to and through surface and underground water. Although there has been no comprehensive monitoring of MtBE in water, MtBE has been reported in groundwater and drinking water derived from groundwater. Based on U.S. Geological Survey data, it appears that wells most susceptible to contamination are shallow groundwater wells in urban areas (U.S. Environmental Protection Agency, 1997). Recreational watercraft and other nonpoint sources can lead to contamination of shallow aquifers and surface waters. The occurrence data for MtBE in drinking water are limited and do not permit a full characterization of the drinking water contamination problem.

MtBE may represent 5% to 10% of the volatile organic compounds that are emitted from gasoline-burning vehicles in those areas in which it is added to fuels as part of a clean fuel program (ARCO Chemical Company, 1995). There are no reliable data on MtBE levels in food, but food does not appear to be a significant source of exposure to MtBE. Limited data suggest that MtBE does not bioaccumulate in fish or food chains.

MtBE, an aliphatic ether, is a colorless liquid with a characteristic odor. It has a low molecular weight (88.15 g/mol), high volatility (vapor pressure 245 mm Hg at 25°C), and high water solubility (40 to 50 g/L).

TOXICOKINETICS

There are no data on MtBE absorption in humans after ingestion, but absorption is rapid after inhalation exposure (Cain et al., 1994; Prah et al., 1994; Johanson et al., 1994). In animals, absorption of MtBE administered by oral, intraperitoneal, or inhalation routes is rapid and extensive (Bio/dynamics, 1994; Savolainen et al., 1985; Bio-Research Laboratories, 1990a, b, c; Miller et al., 1997). Dermal absorption in rats is limited but increases at higher dose levels (Bio-Research Laboratories, 1990a). MtBE is moderately lipophilic with a log K_{ow} of 1.24, which facilitates its absorption across the lipid matrix of cell membranes.

The metabolism and elimination of MtBE and its metabolites proceeds quickly in animals. After absorption, it is demethylated to form tertiary-butyl alcohol (TBA) and formaldehyde by the O-demethylase of the microsomal cytochrome P450 system (Brady et al., 1990). In rodents, TBA is further metabolized to formaldehyde or conjugated with glucuronic acid to form glucuronide, which is excreted in urine (Cederbaum and Cohen, 1980). Other oxidative metabolites of TBA include 2-methyl-1,2-propanediol and alpha-hydroxy isobutyric acid (Bio-Research Laboratories, 1990a; Miller et al., 1997). Formaldehyde may be reduced to methanol or oxidized to formic acid and then carbon dioxide.

After absorption, MtBE is distributed to all major tissues. In blood, MtBE has a very short half-life of 10 to 30 minutes. A minor long-term exponential decay component in humans exposed to MtBE via inhalation suggests that some MtBE can deposit in the tissues (Prah et al., 1994; Johanson et al., 1994). Animal studies showed that 24 to 96 hours after single short-term exposures, the total residual levels in various tissues (brain, muscle, skin, fat, liver, and kidney) were low regardless of exposure route (Bio/dynamics, 1994; Savolainen et al., 1985; Bio-Research Laboratories, 1990a,b,c; Miller et al., 1997). Although toxicokinetic models are being developed for MtBE (Borghoff et al., 1996; Rao and Ginsberg, 1997), more data are needed prior to using these models for route-to-route dose extrapolation.

In the absence of an adequate toxicokinetic model, the U.S. Environmental Protection Agency (EPA) utilized the method selected by the interagency task force on MtBE (National Science and Technology Council, 1996, 1997) to convert inhalation exposure concentrations to dose values. The National Science and Technology Council (NSTC) (1996) conversion method assumes that for a given exposure concentration of MtBE, the adjusted external human equivalent dose would be the same regardless of the animal species used in the study. The method also assumes 100% absorption of MtBE as a default value in the absence of reliable inhalation absorption data. The equation used for the dose conversion by the NSTC (1997) is as follows:

$$\text{Human equivalent dose (HED)} = \frac{C(\text{ppm}) \times 10^{-6} \text{ ppm}^{-1} \times MM \times RR \times EC}{MV \times BW}$$

where:

C = atmospheric concentration
MM = molar mass expressed in milligrams (88,150 mg for MtBE)
MV = molar volume at 20°C (24.04 L)
RR = human respiration rate (20,000 L/day)
EC = exposure condition (# h/24 h × [# days/week])
BW = Average human body weight (70 kg)

The value of 10^{-6} ppm^{-1} in the equation is a unit-adjustment factor that expresses the amount of the contaminant that is present in each unit of inspired air.

If the concentration of MtBE is 1 ppm and the exposure condition is continuous (24 hours per day and 7 days per week), the EC is 1 and the HED is calculated as 1.05 mg/kg-d as follows:

$$\text{HED} = \frac{1\,\text{ppm} \times 10^{-6}\,\text{ppm}^{-1} \times 88.150\,\text{mg} \times 20{,}000\,\text{L/day}}{24.04\,\text{L} \times 70\,\text{kg}} = 1.05\,\text{mg/kg-d}$$

In cases in which exposures are conducted for 6 hours per day and 5 days per week, the EC is equal to $(6/24) \times (5/7)$ or 0.1786. Consequently, 1 ppm of MtBE is equivalent to 0.1875 mg/kg-d. The NSTC (1997) methodology for extrapolation of inhalation exposure doses to oral doses in studies with MtBE is presented in order to be consistent with the risk assessment values of those provided in the NSTC report (1997). This methodology generates significant uncertainties.

HEALTH-EFFECTS DATA

Human Studies

There are few data on the effects of MtBE in humans, and no data are available for the oral route of exposure. In two studies in which 37 and 43 human volunteers, respectively, were exposed to low levels of MtBE in air (1.39 or 1.7 ppm) for 1 hour (Cain et al., 1994; Prah et al., 1994), no significant increases in symptoms of eye, nasal, or pulmonary irritation were noted. There were also no significant effects on mood or in the results from several performance-based, neurobehavioral tests. In both studies, the women ranked the quality of the air containing MtBE lower than the control atmosphere. The results from studies of neurologic effects (headache, dizziness, disorientation, fatigue, emotional distress, etc.), gastrointestinal problems (nausea, diarrhea), and symptoms of respiratory irritation in individuals exposed to MtBE vapors through MtBE-containing fuels are inconclusive (Hakkola et al., 1996; Moolenaar et al., 1994; White et al., 1995).

Perfusion of MtBE through the bile duct and gallbladder once was used as a clinical treatment for gallstones. This procedure could permit some of the MtBE to enter the blood stream. Effects reported in patients treated by this procedure included sedation, perspiration, bradycardia (slow heart beat) and elevation of liver enzymes (Allen et al., 1985; Wyngaarden, 1986; ARCO Chemical Company, 1980). However, these signs may not be caused solely by MtBE exposure. Concurrent exposure to anesthesia and the infusion process itself also may have contributed to the observed symptoms.

Animal Studies

Acute and subchronic noncancer effects. Studies of the systemic effects of MtBE have been conducted in animals. From an acute standpoint, MtBE is not very toxic. The oral LD_{50} in rats is 3.9 g/kg; treated animals exhibit central nervous system depression, ataxia, and labored breathing (ARCO Chemical Company, 1980). In a 14-day study, rats were given MtBE, orally, in corn oil at 0,

537, 714, 1071, or 1428 mg/kg-d. At the highest dose, anesthesia was immediate, but recovery was complete within 2 hours. There was a dose-related decrease in body-weight gain, but it was significant only in females at the highest dose. Increases in relative kidney weights were noted in the males at the two highest doses and in females at 1428 mg/kg-d. No treatment-related lesions were noted at any dose (Robinson et al., 1990).

Rats were given MtBE in corn oil by gavage at doses of 0, 100, 300, 900, or 1200 mg/kg-d for 90 days. Anesthesia was evident at the highest dose, but full recovery occurred in 2 hours. There was a significant decrease in final body weight of females only at the highest dose. Diarrhea was seen in the treated animals but was considered to be the consequence of the bolus dosing regimen. In females, there were increases in relative kidney weights at 300, 900, and 1200 mg/kg-d; in males, increases were noted only at the two highest treatment levels. Reductions in blood urea nitrogen, serum calcium, and creatinine levels were observed in males, and a reduction in cholesterol in females was reported, but these were not clearly dose-dependent. Based on the alterations in kidney weights, a no-observed-adverse-effects level (NOAEL) and a lowest-observed-adverse-effects level (LOAEL) of 100 and 300 mg/kg-d, respectively, are identified by this study.

In another study, rats were given 0, 250, or 1000 mg/kg-d MtBE in olive oil via gavage for 4 days per week for 2 years. This dosing regimen resulted in 7-day time-weighted average daily doses of 0, 143, or 571 mg/kg-d. Survival appeared to be decreased in female rats after 16 weeks, but no statistics were reported. There was no reporting of hematologic, clinical chemistry, or urinalysis parameters or any indication as to whether or not these endpoints were evaluated. The authors did not observe any differences in food consumption or final body weights among the groups. In addition, they did not report any noncancer histopathologic changes (Belpoggi et al., 1995). Because of the limited scope, intermittent treatment schedule, and scant data reporting, evaluation of this study is difficult.

The NOAEL (100 mg/kg-d) from the subchronic study was used to calculate a human no-effect drinking water concentration of 3500 μg/L for kidney effects from MtBE. The increase in kidney weights at 300 mg/kg-d and higher was considered to be an adverse effect, because increases in organ weights may be markers for adverse organ effects (Weil, 1963). The calculation of the drinking water concentration is based on a 70-kg adult drinking 2 L of water per day and uses an uncertainty factor (UF) of 1,000. The UF reflects 10-fold UFs for the less-than-lifetime length of the study, for interspecies and intraspecies variability.

Kidney toxicity also was observed in both males and females in a 2-year inhalation study in F344 rats (Chun et al., 1992). In fact, the EPA derived a reference concentration of 3 mg/m^3 based on the kidney and liver effects of MtBE in this study (U.S. EPA, 1993). The subchronic and chronic inhalation data support the conclusion that, after MtBE exposure, kidney toxicity is of concern. The use of the subchronic study (Robinson et al., 1990) for risk assessment, however, has two significant uncertainties: the study duration and extrapolation of dose from a single daily bolus dose in corn oil to the small, intermittent doses from drinking water exposure.

Reproductive studies. Data were available on the reproductive effects of MtBE from two inhalation studies in rats. A two-generation reproduction study was conducted at Bushy Run Research Center using target concentrations of 0, 400, 3000, or 8000 ppm of MtBE for 6 hours per day, 5 days per week for 10 weeks before mating and during mating, gestation, and lactation days 5 to 21 (Bevan et al., 1997b; Biles et al., 1987). Statistically significant reductions in body weight and body-weight gains in male and female F_1 and F_2 pups were noted with the 3000-ppm and 8000-ppm exposures during the latter periods of lactation. At 3000 ppm, only transient body weight reductions were noted in F_1 males and females during their premating period. At 8000 ppm, pup survival was significantly reduced ($p < .01$) in the F_1 litters on lactation days 0 through 4 and in F_2 litters on postnatal day 4. Clinical signs of toxicity were noted in both generations at 3000 and 8000 ppm; these included hypoactivity and lack of startle reflex. Ataxia and blepharospasm (eyelid twitching) were observed at 8000 ppm. The NOAEL and LOAEL for both parental and pup toxicity were 400 and 3000 ppm, respectively (Bevan et al., 1997).

A one-generation study (Biles et al., 1987) in rats was carried out with two matings, using target concentrations of 0, 300, 1300, or 3400 ppm of MtBE vapor for 6 hours per day, 5 days per week, prior to and during mating. Exposure was continued during 5-day mating intervals. In males, exposure continued until the end of the second mating to produce the F_{1b} litters. In females, exposure continued during the gestation period and lactation days 5 to 21, but not during the first 4 days of the lactation period. A NOAEL and a LOAEL may be identified at 300 ppm and 1300 ppm, respectively, based on pup viability in the F_{1b} litters. However, this study has limited usefulness in the evaluation of reproductive toxicity because of some noted problems (e.g., the loss of one entire litter of 12 pups at birth in the middose group).

Developmental studies. Four inhalation studies were evaluated: one in rats (Conaway et al., 1985), two in mice (Conaway et al., 1985; Bevan et al., 1997a), and one in rabbits (Bevan et al., 1997a). Studies by Conaway et al. in the rat and mouse were performed at target concentrations of 0, 250, 1000, or 2500 ppm of MtBE for 6 hours per day on days 6 to 15 of gestation. Dams were sacrificed at gestation day 20 for rats and gestation day 18 for mice. The concentrations for the studies at Bushy Run Research Center (Bevan et al.) in mice and rabbits were 0, 1000, 4000, or 8000 ppm. Mice were exposed on days 6 to 15 of gestation, and rabbits were exposed on days 6 to 18 of gestation. Mice dams were sacrificed on gestation day 18 and rabbits on gestation day 28. In the Conaway et al. rat study, no effects were noted in rats at 2500 ppm. In the Bushy Run rabbit study, no developmental toxicity was noted at 8000 ppm, but maternal toxicity was noted at 4000 ppm and above.

For mice, maternal toxicity was observed at the two higher concentrations (4000 and 8000 ppm) in the study at Bushy Run. Also, fetal skeletal variations and reduction in fetal weight were noted at the higher doses (Bevan et al., 1997a). In the Conaway et al. (1985) mouse study, there was a dose-related increase in the incidence of skeletal malformations per litter, with incidence of 7.4% in the control group compared with 11.5%, 16% and 22.2% in the 250-, 1000-, and 2500-ppm groups, respectively. These malformations included cleft palate, scrambled and fused sternebra, and angulated ribs. Cleft palate occurred in two fetuses of one litter in the control group; one fetus in the 1000-ppm group; two fetuses, each in a different litter, in the 2500-ppm group; and none in the 250-ppm group. There were also 17%, 11%, and 17.3% resorptions in the 250-, 1000-, and 2500-ppm groups, respectively, compared with 9% in control. Based on the incidence of skeletal malformations in these two mice studies, an NOAEL for developmental effects in mice can be projected in the range of 250 ppm to 1000 ppm. The NOAEL of 400 ppm for parental toxicity in the rat two-generation reproductive study falls within the NOAEL range for developmental effects. The developmental NOAEL values are projected as equivalent to doses of 65.6 mg/kg-d to 262.5 mg/kg-d, respectively, using the NSTC convention. These NOAEL values can be used to calculate projected human no-effect drinking water concentrations of 2.3 to 9.2 mg/L. These conversions assume that a 70-kg adult consumes 2 L of water per day. An UF of 1000 was applied to the NOAEL. The UF includes 10-fold factors for inter- and intraspecies variability, and for acute exposure plus limitations associated with the conversion of the inhaled dose to an oral dose.

Neurotoxicity studies. Inhalation exposure of animals to high levels of MtBE is associated with depression of the central nervous system (CNS) in the period immediately after exposure (Daughtrey et al., 1997). Symptoms after a 6-hour exposure to an atmosphere containing 4000 or 8000 ppm MtBE included labored respiration, ataxia, decreased muscle tone, abnormal gait, impaired treadmill performance, and decreased hind-limb grip strength. These effects were not noted 6 and 24 hours after the cessation of exposure. At 800 ppm, no apparent effects were noted after a 6-hour exposure. Subchronic exposures to the same daily exposure conditions used for the acute study gave no indication that repetitive exposure exacerbated the acute CNS response. Although there was a significant decrease in the absolute, but not the relative, brain weight in the high-dose group after 13 weeks, there were no significant changes in brain or peripheral nervous system histopathology. These studies identified 800 ppm as an NOAEL and 4000 ppm as an LOAEL for acute effects of MtBE on the central nervous system. The 800-ppm NOAEL for acute neurotoxic effects is projected to be equivalent to a dose of 210 mg/kg-d based on the NSTC convention. Using this value, the projected human no-effect concentration for neurologic effects of MtBE from drinking water is 7.4 mg/L for a 70-kg adult drinking 2 L of water per day. The UF of 1000 included 10-fold factors for a frank toxic effect, interspecies variability, and intraspecies variability.

Mutagenicity studies. Several studies were available to assess the mutagenicity of MtBE. With one exception, MtBE did not exert genetic toxicity. Positive results were noted in a mouse lymphoma assay in the presence of microsomal enzymes (ARCO Chemical Company, 1980), probably because of the formaldehyde produced from in vitro metabolism (Stoneybrook Laboratories, 1993). The objective of the mutagenicity studies is to determine whether MtBE's carcinogenic activity is associated with positive genetic activity (McKee et al., 1997). MtBE was negative in sex-linked recessive lethal test in *Drosophila melanogaster* (Hazelton Laboratories America, 1989) and in the Ames assays using *Salmonella* spp., both with and without metabolic activation (ARCO Chemical Company; Life Science Research; 1989b). Chromosome aberrations (ABS) or sister chromatid exchange (SCE) induction tests in Chinese hamster ovary cells were negative with or without activation (ARCO Chemical Company). In addition, MtBE did not cause mutations in cultured Chinese hamster V79 cells (Life Science Research, 1989a) and was negative at the hprt locus in mouse lymphocytes (Ward et al., 1995). Moreover, there was no increase in unscheduled DNA synthesis in the hepatocytes of CD1 mice exposed to MtBE vapor at concentrations of up to 8000 ppm for 6 hours per day for 2 consecutive days (Bushy Run Research Center, 1994). It also did not cause DNA damage in the primary rat hepatocytes culture test (Life Science Research, 1989c), nor was it clastogenic in a rat in vivo cytogenetic assay (ARCO Chemical Company, 1980). Accordingly, the overall weight of evidence from the mutagenicity studies indicated that MtBE is not mutagenic.

Carcinogenic effects. There are three chronic cancer studies of MtBE in two rodent species (one inhalation study in mice and one in rats, and one gavage study in rats). High doses of MtBE were used in all of the carcinogenicity studies, and some may have exceeded the maximum tolerated dose (MTD).

Oral study When MtBE was administered orally to Sprague–Dawley rats (gavage in olive oil, at doses of 0, 250, or 1000 mg/kg-d, 4 days per week for 2 years), no significant differences in food/water consumption or body weight gain were observed. A dose-related increase was caused in the incidence of leukemia and lymphomas in the females (2/58 in the controls, 6/51 in the low-dosed group and 12/47 in the high-dosed group), and an increase in the testicular interstitial Leydig cell adenomas in high-dosed males (18.3% vs. 3.3% in the controls and/or low-dosed animals). Survival was decreased 15% and 20% in the low- and high-dosed females, respectively, after 9 to 12 months of treatment (Belpoggi et al., 1995). There are some limitations in data reporting, as quoted here (NSTC, 1997):

> The Belpoggi et al. study was published in the peer-reviewed literature. However, no detailed technical report of the bioassay is available. Lacking a detailed report about the bioassay, the NRC panel [1996] identified a number of issues and questions which reflects upon the risk assessment use of these data. The NRC noted that the morphological criteria used to classify histopathological findings for both the lymphoma-leukemia and interstitial cell tumor responses were not adequately described and that the study did not adequately address the impact on

tumor outcomes or differences in survival between controls and dosed groups. NRC went on to say that "because of the importance of this study for eventual use in risk assessment, the superficial reporting of the data and the nature of the observed lesions, the committee felt strongly that an independent in-depth review of the data, especially the pathology (microscopic slides) of the critical lesions is warranted (as was done with the inhalation studies) before the data are used for risk assessment." While the NRC raised questions about survival differences and the tumor outcome, it should be noted that Belpoggi et al. included statistical analyses that adjusted for intercurrent mortality. Several attempts by the Interagency Oxygenated Fuels Assessment Steering Committee to arrange for a pathology review of the Belpoggi et al. study have not been successful, hence, the underlying concerns raised by NRC review cannot yet be resolved.

Inhalation studies F344 rats were exposed to 0, 400, 3000, or 8000 ppm MtBE by inhalation (6 hours per day, 5 days per week for 2 years) (ARCO Chemical Company, 1980; Bird et al., 1997). Survival time was statistically and significantly reduced in the exposed male rats in a dose-related manner. The mean body weights of the 8000-ppm group (both sexes) were reduced (19% in the males at week 82 and 13% in the females). An increase in chronic, progressive nephropathy was observed in the exposed male and female rats. The combined incidence of renal tubular adenomas and carcinomas was increased significantly in the male rats exposed to the middose (controls, 1/35; low-dose, 0/32; middose, 8/31; high-dose, 3/20). The reduced survival rate of the high-dosed group may have decreased the sensitivity of the test to produce a dose-related increase in tumors (Table 15.1). A study by Prescott-Matthews et al. (1997) shows that MtBE caused a mild induction of α-2u-globulin nephropathy and enhanced renal cell proliferation in male F344 rats, suggesting that α-2u-globulin nephropathy may play a role in male rat kidney tumorigenesis.

The EPA (1991) published three criteria for establishing whether α-2u-globulin is responsible for the kidney tumor in male rats: (1) increased number and size of hyaline droplets in renal proximal tubule cells of treated rats, (2) accumulating protein in the hyaline droplets is α-2u-globulin, and (3) presence of additional aspects of the pathologic sequence of lesions associated with α-2-u-globulin nephropathy. The agency's policy states that if experimental data

Table 15.1 Renal tumor incidence of F344 male rats after inhalation exposure to methyl tertiary-butyl ether

Exposure concentration (ppm)	Human equivalent dose[a] (mg/kg-d)	Tumor incidence[b]	Survival-adjusted tumor incidence
0	0	1/50	1/35
400	75	0/50	0/32
3000	562.5	8/50	8/31
8000	1500	3/50	3/20

Source: Chun et al., 1992.
[a] See Toxicokinetics for NSTC's extrapolation of dose from inhalation exposure.
[b] Tumor type: Combined renal tubular adenomas and carcinomas.

do not meet the criteria in any one of the three categories, then α-2u-globulin alone is not considered responsible for the renal tumor formation and the renal tumor may be used for risk assessment. Based on the available data, the EPA concluded that the first criterion has been met but the second and third criteria have not.

The mechanism of action of MtBE kidney carcinogenesis in male rats is not well understood at the present time. In this case, the background of chronic progressive nephropathy (CPN) in both male and female rats and the apparent absence of one or more key α-2u-globulin pathologic factors complicate the evaluation. The absent factors may be masked by CPN, or the mild induction may be insufficient to elicit the full α-2u-globulin response. It is possible that other proteins related to α-2u-globulin also may be involved (Health Effect Institute, 1996).

An increased incidence of the interstitial testicular Leydig cell adenomas of the treated rats also was detected (Chun et al., 1992) (32 in the controls, 35 with the low dose, 41 with the middose, and 47 with the high dose). The increase in the incidence of Leydig cell adenomas of the male rats in this study (Chun et al.; Bird et al., 1997) was significantly different from the concurrent but not the historical controls. The concurrent control incidence was 64%, and the historical control values ranged from 64% to 98% in the same laboratory (Bird et al.). (Leydig cell adenomas occur at a high spontaneous rate in the F344 strain of rats.) This type of tumor, however, also was observed in Sprague–Dawley rats after oral exposure (Belpoggi et al., 1995). Because this rat strain does not have a high background incidence for this tumor, confidence in the conclusion that the appearance of the tumor in both studies is MtBE treatment–related is greater.

CD1 mice were exposed to 0, 400, 3000, or 8000 ppm MtBE by inhalation, 6 hours per day, 5 days per week, for 18 months (Bird et al., 1997; Burleigh-Flayer, 1992). Mortality rate was increased and the mean survival time was decreased in the high-dosed mice compared with controls. Body-weight gain also decreased in the 8000-ppm group compared with the controls (16% and 24% for males and females, respectively), indicating that the high dose exceeded the MTD. A significant increase was found in the incidence of hepatocellular carcinomas in male mice and of hepatocellular adenomas in female mice exposed to 8000 ppm of MtBE (Table 15.2). Because MtBE is generally negative in mutagenicity tests, neither the authors (Burleigh-Flayer et al., 1992) nor the National Research Council (1996) considered the liver tumors likely to be a direct DNA-acting phenomenon, and the National Research Council suggested the "non-genotoxic, hormonally-related mechanisms are the most plausible explanation for the development of mouse liver tumors."

The EPA calculated slope factors from the three cancer studies discussed previously (NTSC, 1997). The ability to calculate such estimates does not automatically imply great confidence in the data. Because of the inherent uncertainties in these values, they should be used cautiously. The slope factors are not likely to underestimate risk for the general population. The true risk is

Table 15.2 Hepatocellular tumors in female mice after inhalation exposure to methyl tertiary-butyl ether

Exposure concentration (ppm)	Human equivalent dose (mg/kg-d)	Tumor incidence		
		Adenoma	Carcinoma	Combined
0	0	2/50	0/50	2/50
400	75	1/50	1/50	2/50
800	562.5	2/50	0/50	2/50
8000	1500	10/50	1/50	11/50

Note: In the male mice, the combined hepatocellular tumor incidences for the control, low-, mid-, and high-dose groups were 12/47, 12/47, 12/46, and 16/37, respectively.
Source: Burleigh-Flayer et al., 1992.

likely to be lower and may be nearly zero. The first slope factor is based on the Belpoggi et al. (1995) study. Using the combined tumor incidence of lymphoma and leukemia in the female rats and a scaling factor of body weight raised to the $\frac{2}{3}$ power, a slope factor of 4×10^{-3} $(mg/kg\text{-}d)^{-1}$ can be calculated by the linearized, multistage model. (Based on the Proposed Guidelines for Carcinogen Risk Assessment [FR *61*, 17960, April 23, 1996], with the same tumor data, using a scaling factor of body weight raised to the $\frac{3}{4}$ power, an LED_{10} of 35.6 mg/kg-day and a slope factor of 2.8×10^{-3} $[mg/kg\text{-}d]^{-1}$ are obtained. The drinking water concentration is 12 $\mu g/L$ for a risk of one in a million using this slope factor.) The second is based on the Chun et al. (1992) data. Based on the combined renal tubular cell adenomas and carcinomas in the male F344 rats, using a scaling factor of body weight raised to the $\frac{2}{3}$ power, a slope factor of 6×10^{-4} per ppm can be calculated by the linearized, multistage model. The third is based on the Burleigh-Flayer et al. (1992) study. Based on the liver tumor incidence in the female CD1 mice, using a scaling factor of body weight raised to the $\frac{2}{3}$ power, a slope factor of 3×10^{-4} per ppm was calculated by the linearized, multistage model. Additional understanding of the mode of action of this response could alter substantially these estimates.

Carcinogenicity studies of MtBE metabolites. Formaldehyde and TBA, the metabolites of MtBE, have been evaluated for their carcinogenicity. The cancer data for the metabolites are relevant to the evaluation of the carcinogenicity of MtBE because it is rapidly converted to its metabolites.

TBA F344 rats were exposed to TBA via drinking water at concentrations of 0, 1.25, 2.5, or 5 mg/mL for 2 years. There was some evidence of carcinogenic activity in male rats based on increased incidences of renal tubular hyperplasia and renal tubular adenomas or carcinomas, and no evidence of carcinogenic activity in female rats. Increased nephropathy also was noted in all treated animals. Compared with controls, survival was less in the high-dosed animals, especially in the males (Cirrello et al., 1995; National Toxicology Program, 1995).

B6C3F1 mice were exposed to TBA in drinking water at concentrations of 0, 5, 10, or 20 mg/L for 130 weeks. There was equivocal evidence of carcinogenic activity in male mice (marginal increase in thyroid tumors), and some evidence in female mice (increased incidence of thyroid follicular cell hyperplasia and adenomas). The survival rate of males in the high-dose group was significantly lower than that of the control group. Thus, the National Toxicology Program (NTP) study (1995) shows no clear evidence of carcinogenicity in either species.

Formaldehyde Inhalation exposure of F344 rats to formaldehyde for 2 years at 0, 2, 5.6, or 14.3 ppm (6 hours per day, 5 days per week) induced squamous-cell carcinomas of the nasal cavity in both male and female F344 rats at the highest dose, but not in female B6C3F1 mice (same exposure conditions) (Kerns et al., 1983). Lifetime inhalation studies of formaldehyde in Sprague–Dawley rats at 14 ppm (Sellakumar et al., 1985) and Wistar rats at 10 ppm (Woutersen et al., 1989) also produced nasal tumors. Based on available data, the International Agency for Research on Cancer (1995) has stated that there is sufficient evidence of carcinogenicity of formaldehyde in animals by the inhalation route.

The evidence for carcinogenic activity, after exposure to formaldehyde via drinking water, is mixed. One study, in Sprague–Dawley rats using concentrations of 0, 10, 50, 100, 1000, or 1500 ppm, showed a dose-related increase in the incidence of leukemia and intestinal tumors (Soffritti et al., 1989). As in a chronic oral study (Belpoggi et al., 1995) of MtBE (conducted by the same laboratory), the reporting of the study is limited and the pathology also lacks independent review. Another 2-year drinking water study of formaldehyde using Wistar rats at doses ranging from 1.2 to 82 mg/kg-d showed no evidence of carcinogenicity (Til et al., 1989).

Organoleptic effects. In addition to its potential for causing adverse health effects, water containing MtBE may have unpleasant organoleptic (taste and odor) effects. Although taste and odor properties cannot be used to develop primary drinking water standards, they are of concern to most U.S. citizens. Unpleasant taste or odor can alert consumers that the water is contaminated with MtBE. Individuals do not respond equally to MtBE's taste and odor because of differences in individual sensitivity. The taste and odor responses reported in observed individuals for MtBE are in the 15- to 180-μg/L range for odor and the 39- to 135-μg/L range for taste (Prah et al., 1994; NTSC, 1997; Til et al., 1989, Young et al., 1996; Dale et al., 1997; American Petroleum Institute, 1993). These data must be viewed with caution, as the studies used relatively small numbers of subjects (3–19). The ranges, however, show the variability in individual response. In addition, the fact that the studies reported "similar" ranges for taste and odor suggests that the 15- to 180-μg/L range is probably a good estimate for the range over which different individuals in the population experience organoleptic effects.

HAZARD AND DOSE–RESPONSE CHARACTERIZATION

Hazard Characterization

The data on human responses to MtBE are scant. In controlled studies, there were no observable responses to short-term (1-hour) exposures to low concentrations of MtBE in air, although women felt the air quality was substandard (Cain et al., 1994; Prah et al., 1994). Other acute human studies are of limited value, because MtBE was part of a mixture of other chemicals, such as gasoline, medicines, or anesthesia (Hakkola et al., 1996; Moolenaar et al., 1994; White et al., 1995; Allen et al., 1995; Wyngaarden, 1986). Studies of gasoline/MtBE mixtures are inconclusive but suggest that MtBE-containing gasoline vapors may be irritating to eyes, the respiratory system, and the nervous system (Hakkola et al., Moolenaar et al., White et al.). There have been no long-term studies of human exposure to MtBE.

Animal studies identify the kidneys, brain, and developing fetus as potential targets of MtBE. Because the neurotoxicity data after inhalation exposures (Daughtrey et al., 1997) show transient CNS depression and decreased motor activity only at 8000 ppm, they provide little or no support to the hypothesis that low levels of MtBE in drinking water exert adverse effects on the human nervous system.

The collective evaluation of the reproductive and developmental studies of MtBE in animals indicate that inhalation exposure can result in maternal toxicity and adverse effects on the developing fetus (Bevan et al., 1997a,b; Conaway et al., 1995). The fetal toxicity in mouse developmental studies indicates that the mouse may be more sensitive to inhalation of MtBE vapors during gestation than the rat or rabbit. It seems likely, however, that MtBE is not a developmental or reproductive hazard at low concentrations.

Effects on the kidney were observed in rats after both oral and inhalation exposure. After short-term oral exposure, increases in kidney weights were noted (Robinson et al., 1990); in a longer-term inhalation study, histopathologic abnormalities were apparent (Chun et al., 1992). The oral data are confounded by the bolus dosing regimen and the 90-day duration of the study. The use of inhalation data to project effects from the oral exposures is generally not desirable but, with MtBE, there is a qualitative similarity in the observed effects. To use the inhalation data to calculate a human equivalent dose for risk assessment, however, introduces additional uncertainties.

In the animal carcinogenicity studies, there are two chronic inhalation studies available, one in rats showing increased incidence of renal and testicular tumors (Chun et al., 1992) and one in mice showing induction of liver tumors (Burleigh-Flayer et al., 1992). By the oral route, there is a gavage study in rats producing a dose-related increase in leukemia and lymphoma in females and an increase in testicular tumors in males (Belpoggi et al., 1995). In addition, formaldehyde, a metabolite of MtBE, is an animal carcinogen. After inhalation, it induces nasal tumors in rats (Burleigh-Flayer et al., 1992). In drinking water, one study showed a dose-related increase in leukemia (Saffritti et al., 1989); another study showed no evidence of carcinogenicity (Til et al., 1989).

The cancer studies of MtBE and its metabolites have limitations, such as route-of-exposure differences, high animal mortality rates, limited pathology reporting, and historical tumor incidence. In spite of the limitations, there are some consistent tumor findings for MtBE and its metabolites. This consistency contributes to the overall weight of evidence. A statistically significant increase in interstitial Leydig cell adenomas of the testes was detected in the exposed rats after both inhalation (Chun et al., 1992; Bird et al., 1997) and gavage (Belpoggi et al., 1995) exposures. In addition, the elevation of kidney tumors in male F344 rats treated with TBA (a metabolite of MtBE) via drinking water (Cirvello et al., 1995; National Toxicology Program; 1995) supports the increase of similar tumors in male rats after exposure to MtBE by inhalation (Chun et al., Bird et al.). The similarity in the findings of a dose-related increase in leukemia in rats (Sprague–Dawley, male and female combined) after exposure to formaldehyde (also a metabolite of MtBE) via drinking water and the increase of leukemia and lymphomas in female rats (same strain) after exposure to MtBE via gavage (Belpoggi et al., 1995) suggests a possible involvement of formaldehyde in the leukemogenic effect of MtBE. Issues remain unresolved related to these studies, however, as both provided limited reporting and no information on historical incidence of leukemia. (Unlike NTP carcinogenicity studies, the histopathology diagnoses from the inhalation studies of MtBE in rats and mice have not been subject to a full peer review. Also, there is a major difference between the oral and inhalation carcinogenicity studies of MtBE. Lengthy reports of the inhalation studies of MtBE in rats and mice were submitted to the EPA. These reports [Chun et al., Burleigh-Flayer et al., 1992] provide significantly more information than what is contained in the published peer-reviewed literature [Belpoggi et al., Bird et al.,]. For example, based on these reports, we can conclude that the inhalation studies were conducted in conformance with good laboratory practices; there is a lack of evidence to back up that the gavage study also was conducted in conformance with good laboratory practices.)

MtBE does not appear to react with DNA. In an array of in vitro and in vivo systems, the results have been negative overall. The possibility that the genesis of the rat kidney tumors involves the α-2u-globulin mechanism is being investigated, but, as yet, the evidence does not satisfy all the EPA criteria (U.S. EPA, 1991) for ascribing tumorigenicity to this mechanism. The nephropathy and toxicity associated with tumorigenicity in the rat kidney suggest that a number of factors, including the α-2u-globulin mechanism, may be at work. The observation of testicular tumors from MtBE and thyroid tumors from TBA suggest the need for examination of disruption of pituitary and thyroid hormone function, as such disruption is not uncommon with these tumors (Hill et al.,

1989; U.S. EPA, 1997), and it has been suggested that MtBE-induced mouse liver tumors also may be hormone-related. Although MtBE is not mutagenic, a nonlinear mode of action has not been established for MtBE. In the absence of sufficient data, it is prudent for the EPA to assume a linear dose–response relationship. Although there are no studies on the carcinogenicity of MtBE in humans, there are multiple animal studies (inhalation and gavage studies) showing carcinogenic activity and supporting animal carcinogenicity data on two of its the metabolites. The weight of evidence indicates that MtBE is an animal carcinogen and that the chemical poses a carcinogenic potential to humans (NTSC, 1997).

Characterization of Organoleptic Effects

There have been several studies of taste and odor response by humans. There is typically variation among individuals in organoleptic responses to a chemical, and this is the case for MtBE. The studies on MtBE have involved only a few individuals. Larger numbers of individuals could better characterize the full distribution of sensitivity of humans. Nevertheless, the existing studies were performed independently and show consistent distributions. This lends confidence to the conclusion that sensitive individuals respond to odor and taste at about 20 to 40 μg/L. In this advisory, the organoleptic values are rounded to one significant number, 20 and 40, to avoid the appearance of precision that use of two significant numbers would give. Because characterization of the full distribution of sensitivity is not provided by available data, the numbers should be regarded as approximate. For the same reason, a range is presented. The data are used only to estimate sensitive range and should not be mistaken as defining thresholds of human response, as they are not mean or median values for a large population.

Dose–Response Characterization

There are no chronic studies of MtBE exposure in humans; the pertinent data on potential adverse effects are from rodent studies. The available data do not provide sufficient information on the potential toxic effects from drinking water exposure, and they only present an uncertain view of the dose–response relationship. For quantitative assessment, the preferred data would be from studies of effects after oral exposure to MtBE in drinking water. For MtBE, the data are either from inhalation studies or from daily high bolus dose studies, using oil as a vehicle. Estimating drinking water dose equivalents based on inhalation studies or on bolus dosing studies would introduce significant uncertainties.

The results of the oral subchronic study, supported by inhalation exposure data, provide adequate support for the conclusion that MtBE may affect the kidney. At the present time, however, the EPA does not have high confidence in the use of this or any other study for quantitative purposes. Accordingly, this drinking water advisory does not recommend either a low-dose oral cancer risk number or a reference dose for MtBE. Instead, the drinking water advisory provides perspective by showing margins of exposure (MoEs) between observations of the range for concentrations having effects in animals and concentrations of MtBE in drinking water that generate a taste or odor response (20–40 μg/L). Because the use of drinking water is correlated to its potability, the organoleptic (taste and odor) effects of MtBE should be considered (Cain et al., 1994; Bio/dynamics, 1994; Young et al., 1996; Dale et al., 1997; American Petroleum Institute, 1993). Table 15.3 summarizes the MoE information. The values in Table 15.3 show the lower end of ranges of observation of effects in animals tested for cancer and noncancer responses and the appropriate MoEs, that is, the ratios of the effect levels to the sensitive range of human response to

Table 15.3 Estimation of margin of exposure for methyl tertiary-butyl ether (MtBE) on water concentration at 20–40 μg / L

			Margin of exposure	
Endpoint	Parameter	Concentration[d] (μg/L)	Compared with 40 μg/L	Compared with 20 μg/L
Noncancer[a]				
Kidney	NOAEL	3,500,000	90,000	180,000
Neurologic	NOAEL	7,400,000	185,000	370,000
Reproductive/ developmental	NOAEL	2,300,000 9,200,000	≥ 60,000	≥ 120,000
Cancer[b]				
Rat lymphoma and leukemia (gavage) in females	LED_{10}^c	805,000	20,000	40,000
Rat kidney tumor (inhalation) in males	LED_{10}^c	6,230,000	160,000	320,000
Mouse liver tumor (inhalation) in females	LED_{10}^c	11,025,000	280,000	550,000

Note: The margin of exposure is calculated by dividing the no-observed effects limit (NOAELs) for noncancer endpoints or the 95% lower bound on dose for a 10% extra risk (LED_{10}) for cancer effects by 40 μg/L, or 20 μg/L, which are the low ends of the taste and odor threshold, respectively.
[a] The data from Robinson et al. (1990) were used for the kidney effects. Data from Bevan et al. (1997) and Conaway et al. (1985) were used for the reproductive and developmental numbers, and the data of Daughtrey et al. (1997) were the basis for the neurotoxicity value.
[b] The data from Belpoggi gavage study and the Chun and Burleigh-Flayer inhalation studies were used in the calculation. Air concentration of MtBE in ppm was converted to mg/kg-d by the NSTC method: 1 ppm = 1.05 mg/kg-day (NSTC, 1996).
[c] The LED_{10} was calculated by applying the tumor incidence data to the multistage model. As indicated by the NSTC (1996), a lifetime adjustment factor of 2.37 (i.e., $[24/18]^3$) was applied to the mouse liver tumor data to account for the short duration of the study (18 months instead of 24 months). In addition, as done by NSTC, the rat kidney tumor incidence in the highest-exposure group was excluded from the risk analysis because this exposure group was terminated at 82 weeks (not 102 weeks) because of an extremely high mortality rate.
[d] The NOAEL and LED_{10} were initially calculated in mg/kg-d and then converted to μg/L, assuming a body weight of 70 kg and a water consumption rate of 2 L/d.

odor and taste (20 to 40 μg/L). The cancer LED_{10} values (95% lower bound of the dose for a 10% extra risk) are based on analyses of the Belpoggi et al. (1995), Chun et al. (1992), and Burleigh-Flayer et al. (1992) studies. The noncancer NOAEL values are from the studies of the kidney (Robinson et al., 1990), reproductive or developmental (Conaway et al., 1985; Bevan et al., 1997a) and neurotoxicity effects (Daughtrey et al., 1997) after inhalation exposure.

To avoid unpleasant taste and odor, the drinking water advisory recommends that a concentration in the range of 20 to 40 μg/L likely will protect sensitive members of a population. At 20 μg/L, the MoE is approximately 40,000 for cancer effects and over 100,000 for some noncancer effects. At 40 μg/L, the MoE is approximately 20,000 for cancer effects and 60,000 for noncancer effects. In the case of noncancer effects, the lower end of the developmental NOAEL range was used as the minimum effect level in the MoE calculation; the cancer value was calculated using the LED_{10}. (Based on the EPA's recently proposed guidelines for carcinogen risk assessment [U.S. EPA, 1996], the rationale supporting the use of the LED_{10} is that a 10% response is at or just below the limit of sensitivity for discerning a significant difference in most long-term rodent studies. The NOAEL in most study protocols is about the same as an LED_5 or LED_{10}—the lower 95% confidence limit on a dose associated with a 5% or 10% increased effect. The MoE value for cancer was obtained by dividing the concentration equivalent to the LED_{10} [23 mg/kg-d equivalent to 805,000 μg/L] by 20 μg/L to obtain a MoE of 40,200. The MoE for noncancer effects was obtained by dividing the concentration equivalent to the lower end of the NOAEL for the developmental toxicity range [65.6 mg/kg-day equivalent to 2,292,500 μg/L] by the environmental water concentration of 20 μg/L to obtain an MoE of 114,625. The calculations assume a 70-kg body weight and 2 L/d water consumption.) Comparison indicates that there are over four to five orders of magnitude between the 20- to 40-μg/L range and concentrations associated with observed ranges of effects in animals. Accordingly, there is little likelihood that a concentration of 20 to 40 μg MtBE in 1 L of drinking water would cause adverse effects in humans. It can be noted that at this range of concentrations, the MoEs are about 10 to 100 times greater than would be provided by an agency reference dose for noncancer effects. Additionally, they are in the range of margins of exposure typically provided by National Primary Drinking Water Standards under the Federal Safe Drinking Water Act.

ACKNOWLEDGMENTS

All of the members of the Drinking Water Health Assessment Team were involved in development of the drinking water advisory for MtBE. In addition to the authors of this report, the team includes Nick Baer, Nancy Chiu, Barbara Corcoran, Kris Khanna, and Mary Ko Manibusan. Jeanette Wiltse, Director of the Health And Ecological Criteria Division, also played a key role in development of the framework for the drinking water advisory.

REFERENCES

Allen, M. J., Borody, T. J., Bugliosi, T. F., May, G. R., LaRusso, N. F., and Thistle, J. L. 1985. Cholelitholysis using methyl tertiary-butyl ether. *Gastroenterology* 88:122–125.

American Petroleum Institute. 1993. *Odor threshold studies performed with gasoline and gasoline combined with MtBE, EtBE, and TAME*, API# 4592. Washington, DC: Author.

ARCO Chemical Company. 1980. *Methyl tertiary-butyl ether: Acute toxicological studies*. Unpublished study for ARCO Research and Development, Glenolden, PA.

ARCO Chemical Company. 1995. *Methyl t-Butyl Ether (MtBE): A status report of its presence and significance in US drinking water*. Presented to the Office of Water, U.S. Environmental Protection Agency.

Agency for Toxic Substance and Disease Registry. 1996. *Toxicological profile for methyl-tert-butyl ether*. Atlanta, GA: U.S. Department of Health and Human Services.

Belpoggi, F., Soffritti, M., and Maltoni, C. 1995. Methyl-tertiary-butyl ether (MtBE)—a gasoline additive—causes testicular and lymphohaematopoietic cancers in rats. *Toxicol. Indust. Health* 11:1–31.

Bevan, C., Tyl, R. W., Neeper-Bradley, T. L., Fischer, L. C., Panson, R. D., Kneiss, J. J., and Andrews, L. S. 1997a. Developmental toxicity evaluation of methyl tertiary-butyl ether (MTBE) by inhalation in mice and rabbits. *J. Appl. Toxicol.* 17:S21–S30.

Bevan, C., Neeper-Bradley, T. L., Tyl, R. W., Fischer, L. C., Panson, R. D., Kniess, J. J., and Andrews, L. S. 1997b. Two-generation reproductive study of methyl tertiary-butyl ether (MTBE) in rats. *J. Appl. Toxicol.* 17:S13–S20.

Biles, R. W., Schroeder, R. E., and Holdsworth, C. E. 1987. Methyl tert-butyl ether inhalation in rats: a single generation reproduction study. *Toxicol. Indust. Health* 34:519–534.

Bio-Research Laboratories. 1990a. *Mass balance of radioactivity and metabolism of methyl tert-butyl ether (MtBE) in male and female Fischer-344 rats after administration of ^{14}C MtBE by iv, oral, and dermal routes*, report #38843. Senneville, Quebec, Canada: Author.

Bio-Research Laboratories 1990b. *Pharmacokinetics of methyl tert-butyl ether (MtBE) and tert-butyl alcohol (TBA) in male and female Fischer-344 rats after single and repeat inhalation nose-only exposure to ^{14}C-MtBE* report #38844. Senneville, Quebec, Canada: Author.

Bio-Research Laboratories. 1990c. *Disposition of radioactivity of methyl tertiary-butyl ether (MtBE) in male and female Fischer-344 rats after nose-only inhalation exposure to ^{14}C MtBE*, report #38845. Senneville, Quebec, Canada: Author.

Bio/dynamics. 1994. *The metabolic fate of methyl tertiary-butyl ether (MtBE) following acute intraperitoneal injection*, Project No. 80089. Unpublished report submitted to American Petroleum Institute, Washington, DC.

Bird, M. G., Burleigh-Flayer, H. D., Chun, J. S., Douglas, J. F., Kneiss, J. J., and Andrews, L. S. 1997. Oncogenicity studies of inhaled methyl tertiary-butyl ether (MTBE) in CD-1 mice and F-344 rats. *J. Appl. Toxicol.* 17:S45–S56.

Borghoff, S. J., Murphy, J. E., and Medinsky, M. A. 1996. Development of a physiologically based pharmacokinetic model for methyl tertiary-butyl ether and tertiary-butanol in male Fischer-344 rats. *Fundam. Appl. Toxicol.* 30:264–275.

Brady, J. F., Xiao, F., Ning, W. J., and Yang, C. S. 1990. Metabolism of methyl tertiary-butyl ether by rat hepatic microsomes. *Arch. Toxicol.* 64:157–160.

Burleigh-Flayer, B. D., Chun, J. S., and Kintigh, W. J. 1992. *Methyl tertiary butyl ether: Vapor inhalation oncogenicity study in CD-1 mice*, report 91N0013A. Export, PA: Bushy Run Research Center.

Bushy Run Research Center. 1994. *Methyl tertiary-butyl ether: In vivo-in vitro hepatocyte unscheduled DNA systhesis assay in mice*, project ID 93N1316. Export, PA: Author.

Cain, W. S., Leaderer, B. P., Ginsberg, G. L., Andrews, L. S., Cometto-Muniz, J. E., Gent, J. F., Buck, M., Berglund, L. G., Mohsenin, V., Monhan, E., and Kjaergaard, S. 1994. *Human reactions to brief exposures to methyl tertiary-butyl ether*. Unpublished data from John B. Pierce Laboratory, New Haven, Connecticut.

Cederbaum, A. I., and Cohen, G. 1980. Oxidative demethylation of t-butyl alcohol by rat liver microsomes. *Biochem. Biophys. Res. Comm.* 97:730–736.

Chun, J. S., Burleigh-Flayer, H. D., and Kintigh, W. J. 1992. *Methyl tertiary ether*: *Vapor inhalation oncogenicity study in Fisher 344 rats*, report 91N0013B. Export, PA: Bushy Run Research Center.
Cirvello, J. D., Radovsky, A., Heath, J. E., Farnell, D. R., and Lindamood, C. 1995. Toxicity and carcinogenicity of t-butyl alcohol in rats and mice following chronic exposure in drinking water. *Toxico. Indust. Health* 11:151–165.
Conaway, C. C., Schroeder, R. E., and Snyder, N. K., 1985. Teratology evaluation of methyl tertiary-butyl ether in rats and mice. *J. Toxicol. Environ. Health* 166:797–809.
Dale, M. S., Moylan, M. S., Koch, B., and Davis, M. K. 1997. *MTBE: Taste and odor threshold determinations using the flavor profile method*. Presented at the Water Quality Technology Conference, Denver, CO.
Daughtrey, W. C., Gill, M. W., Pritts, I. M., Fielding Douglas, J., Kneiss, J. J., and Andrews, L. S. 1997. Neurotoxicological evaluation of methyl tertiarv-butyl ether in rats. *J. Appl. Toxicol.* 17:S57–S64.
Hakkola, M., Honkasalo, M. L., and Pulkkinen, P. 1996. Neuropsychological symptoms among tanker drivers exposed to gasoline. *Occup. Med.* 46:125–130.
Hazelton Laboratories America. 1989. *Mutagenicity test on methyl tertiary-butyl ether*. Drosophia melanogaster *sex-linked recessive lethal test*, study no. 1484-0-461. Kensington, MD: Author.
Health Effect Institute. 1996. *The potential health effects of oxygenates added to gasoline: A review of the current literature. A special report of the Institute's oxygenates evaluation committee.* Cambridge, MA: Health Effects Institute.
Hill, R. N., Erdreich, L. S., Paynter, O. E., Roberts, P. A., Rosenthal, S. L., and Wilkinson, C. F. Thyroid folicular cell carcinogenesis. *Fundam. Appl. Toxicol.* 12:629–697.
International Agency for Research on Cancer. 1995. Formaldehyde. In *IARC monographs on the evaluation of carcinogenic risks to humans: Wood dust and formaldehyde*, vol. 62, pp. 217–362. Lyon, France: Author.
Johanson, G., Nihlen A., and Lof, A. 1994. Toxicokinetics and acute effects of MtBE and MtBE in male volunteers. *Toxicol. Lett.* 82/83:713–718.
Kerns, K. D., Pavkov, K. L., Donofrio, D. J., Gralla, E. J., and Swenberg, J. A. 1983. Carcinogenicity of formaldehyde in rats and mice after long-term inhalation exposure. *Cancer Res.* 43:4382–4392.
Life Science Research. 1989a. *Gene mutation in Chinese hamster V79 cells, test substance*: *MTBE*, report no. 216002-M-03589. Rome: Author.
Life Science Research. 1989b. *Reverse mutation in* Salmonella typhimurium, *test substance*: *MtBE*, report no. 216001-M-03489. Rome: Author.
Life Science Research. 1989c. *Unscheduled DNA synthesis (UDS) in primary rat hepatocytes (autoradiographic method), test substance*: *MtBE*, report no. 216003-M-03689. Rome: Author.
McKee, R. H., Vergnes, J. S., Galvin, J. B., Douglas, J. F., Kneiss, J. J., and Andrews, L. S. 1997. Assessment of the in vivo mutagenic potential of methyl tertiary-butyl ether. *J. Appl. Toxicol.* 17:S31–S36.
Miller, M. J., Ferdinandi, E. S., Klan, M., Andrews, L. S., Douglas, J. F., and Kneiss, J. J. 1997. Pharmacokinetics and disposition of methyl t-butyl ether in Fischer-344 rats. *J. Appl. Toxicol.* 17:S3–S13.
Moolenaar, R. L., Hefflin, B. J., Ashley, D. L., Middaugh, J. P., and Etzel, R. A. 1994. Methyl tertiary butyl ether in human blood after exposure to oxygenated fuel in Fairbanks, Alaska. *Arch. Environ. Health* 49:402–409.
National Research Council. 1996. *Toxicological and performance aspects of oxygenated motor vehicle fuels*. Washington, DC: National Academy Press.
National Science and Technology Council. 1996. *Interagency assessment of potential health risks associated with oxygenated gasoline*. Washington, DC: National Science and Technology Council Committee on Environment and Natural Resources and Interagency Oxygenated Fuels Assessment Steering Committee.
National Science and Technology Council Committee on Environment and Natural Resources. 1997. *Interagency assessment of oxygenated fuels*. Washington, DC: Author.
National Toxicology Program. 1995. *Toxicology and carcinogenesis studies of t-butyl alcohol (CAS No.*

76-65-0) in F344/N rats and B6C3F1 mice (drinking water studies), Technical Report Series No. 436, NIH Publication No. 94-3167. Research Triangle Park, NC: National Institute of Health.

Prah, J. D., Goldstein, G. M., Devlin, R., Otto, D., Ashley, D., House, S., Cohen, K. L., and Gerrity, T. 1994. Sensory, symptomatic, inflammatory, and ocular responses to and the metabolism of methyl tertiary-butyl ether in a controlled human exposure experiment. *Inhalation Toxicology* 6:521–538.

Prescott-Mathews, J. S., Wolf, D. C., Wong, B. A., and Borghoff, S. J. 1997. Methyl tert-butyl ether causes $\alpha 2u$-globulin nephropathy and enhanced renal cell proliferation in male F344 rats. *Toxicol. Appl. Pharm.* 143:301–314.

Rao, H. V., and Ginsberg, G. L. 1997. A physiologically-based pharmacokinetic model assessment of methyl t-butyl ether in groundwater for a bathing and showering determination. *Risk Anal.* 17:583–598.

Robinson, M., Bruner, R. H., and Olson, G. R. 1990. Fourteen- and ninety-day oral toxicity studies of methyl tertiary-butyl ether in Sprague-Dawley rats. *J. Am. Coll. Toxicol.* 9:525–540.

Savolainen, H., Pfaffli P., and Elovaara, E. 1985. Biochemical effects of methyl tertiary-butyl ether in extended vapor exposure in rats. *Arch. Toxicol.* 57:285–288.

Sellakumar, A. R., Snyder, C. A., Solomon, J. J., and Albert, R. E. 1985. Carcinogenicity of formaldehyde and hydrogen chloride in rats. *Toxicol. Appl. Pharmacol.* 81:401–406.

Soffritti, M., Maltoni, C., Maffei, F., and Biagi, R. 1989. Formaldehyde: an experimental multipotential carcinogen. *Toxicol. Indust. Health* 5:699–730.

Stoneybrook Laboratories. 1993. *Actiuiated mouse lymphoma (L5178Y/TK/ + /) mutagenicity assay supplemented with formaldehyde dehydrogenase for methyl tertiary butyl ether*, status report 65579. Princeton, NJ: Author.

Til, H. P., Woutersen, R. A., Feron, V. J., Hollanders, V. M. H., and Falke, H. E. 1989. Two-year drinking-water study for formaldehyde in rats. *Food Chem. Toxicol.* 27:77–87.

U.S. Environmental Protection Agency. 1991. *Alpha 2μ-globulin assicuation with chemically induced renal toxicity and neoplasia in the male rat*: Risk assessment forum, EPA/625/3-91/019F. Washington, DC: United States Environmental Protection Agency.

U.S. Environmental Protection Agency. 1993. *Assessment of potential health risks of gasoline oxygenated with methyl tertiary-butyl ether (MtBE)*. EPA/600/R.93/206 (1993). Washington, DC: Office of Research and Development, US Environmental Protection Agency.

U.S. Environmental Protection Agency. 1996. Proposed guidelines for carcinogen risk assessment, EPA/600/P-92/003C. *Federal Register* 61:17960–18011.

U.S. Environmental Protection Agency. 1997a. *Assessment of thyroid follocular cell tumors*: Risk assessment forum, EPA/630/R-97/002. Washington, DC: Author.

U.S. Environmental Protection Agency. 1997b. *Drinking water advisory: Consumer acceptability advice and health effects analysis on methyl tertiary butyl ether (MtBE)*, EPA-822-F-97/009. Washington, DC: U.S. Environmental Protection Agency.

Ward, Jr., J. B., Daiker, D. H., Hastings, D. A., Ammenheuser, M. M., and Legator, M. S. 1995. Assessment of the mutagenicity of methyl-tertiary butyl ether at the HPRT gene in CD-1 mice [abstract]. *Toxicologist* 15:79.

Weil, C. S. 1963. Significance of organ-weight changes in food safety evaluation. In *Metabolic aspects of food safety*, ed. F. J. Roe, pp. 419–454. New York: Academic Press.

White, M. C., Johnson, C. A., Ashley, D. L., Buchta, T. M., and Pelletier, D. J. 1995. Exposure to methyl tertiary-butyl ether from oxygenated gasoline in Stamford, Connecticut. *Arch. Environ. Health* 50:183–189.

Woutersen, R. A., van Garderen-Hoetmer, A., Bruijntjes, J. P., Swart, A., and Feron, V. J. 1989. Nasal tumors in rats after severe injury to the nasal mucosa and prolonged exposure to 10 ppm formaldehyde. *J. Appl. Toxicol.* 9:39–46.

Wyngaarden, J. B. 1986. New nonsurgical treatment removes gallstones. *JAMA* 256:1692.

Young, W. F., Horth, H., Crane, R., Ogden, R., and Arnott, M. 1996. Taste and odor threshold concentrations of potable water contaminants. *Water Res.* 30:331–340.

CHAPTER
SIXTEEN

ARSENIC: MOVING TOWARD A REGULATION

Charles O. Abernathy, Irene S. Dooley, James Taft, and Jennifer Orme-Zavaleta

U.S. Environmental Protection Agency, Washington, DC, and Research Triangle Park, North Carolina

Although primarily perceived by many as a poison, arsenic has played important roles in medicine, agriculture and industry (Polson and Tattersall, 1969; Frost, 1970; Winship, 1970). Arsenic is constantly recycled among environmental compartments through such processes as burning of fossil fuels, volatilization, weathering of rocks, smelting of metals, and manufacturing (International Programme on Chemical Safety, 1981; Hindmarsh and McCurdy, 1986). Everybody is exposed to arsenic through food and water ingestion and environmental exposure (air and dermal); some may be occupationally exposed (International Programme on Chemical Safety, 1981; Webb et al., 1986).

Arsenic is a metalloid that exists in four valence states (-3, 0, $+3$, and $+5$). Because there is little or no human exposure to the -3 state and the 0 form is not absorbed in the gastrointestinal tract, they pose little or no risk. The inorganic forms (arsenate [$+5$] and arsenite [$+3$]) and their metabolites (monomethylarsonic acid and dimethylarsinic acid) are the most important species from the environmental standpoint. In the United States, food is the primary source of arsenic for most people. The average U.S. citizen ingests around 50 μg/d from his or her diet (Borum and Abernathy, 1994). Most of this ingested arsenic is from fish and shellfish, which primarily contain the organic derivatives, arsenobetaine and arsenocholine. These compounds are relatively stable and are excreted primarily as the parent molecules. Accordingly, they are believed to be relatively nontoxic (International Programme on Chemical Safety, 1981). About 10 to 15 μg of the arsenic in the diet, however, is inorganic and may be of public health concern. If arsenic levels in potable waters are 10 to 20 μg/L or above, drinking water contributes over one half of the inorganic arsenic exposure. In most areas, the concentrations of arsenic in the air are in the range between one and a few nanograms per cubic meter. Near power plants burning fossil fuel with high arsenic content or in the vicinity of smelters,

The opinions expressed in this manuscript are those of the authors and do not necessarily reflect the opinions and/or policies of the United States Environmental Protection Agency.

however, levels of 1 $\mu g/m^3$ may be reached. Although there has not been a lot of research of the dermal absorption of arsenic, the available data suggest that it is not a major source of exposure (Wester et al., 1993).

Exposure to arsenic can cause adverse effects after short- or long-term exposure. Acute effects include death, hepatic dysfunction, gastroenteritis, neurologic and hematologic effects, convulsions, and paralysis (International Programme on Chemical Safety, 1981; Fielder et al., 1986). Such effects are caused by exposure to large doses within a short period of time. However, these exposures generally do not simulate environmental situations, as most human exposures to arsenic are to small levels over an extended period of time. Accordingly, regulatory agencies, such as the U.S. Environmental Protection Agency (EPA), set drinking water standards that protect humans from such long-term, low-dose exposure. Generally, human data are scant, and animal toxicity data are usually used in formation of regulations. Arsenic is unusual in that there is a relatively large human data base (U.S. EPA, 1984, 1988). In addition, arsenic is the only element that the International Agency for Research on Cancer recognizes as a human carcinogen that lacks evidence supporting animal carcinogenicity (Wilbourne et al., 1986). Because exposure to arsenic in drinking water has been associated with the development of skin and internal cancers (Tseng, 1977; Tseng et al., 1968; Smith et al., 1992; Bates et al., 1992), one might anticipate that the risk assessment of arsenic would be relatively easy. This has not been the case, as there has been controversy over the use of skin-cancer data from Taiwan as the basis of a regulation, involving the following factors (Tseng, 1977; Tseng et al., 1968; Yang and Blackwell, 1961; Brown and Abernathy, 1997; Brown et al., 1997; Groschonig and Irgolic, 1997):

1. Prevalence study of humans (approximately 40,000)
2. Observed dose- and age-dependent responses
3. Midpoint (e.g., 170 μg As/L in low dose village) of exposure group was used as measure of arsenic exposure for entire village
   a. Arsenic concentration in low dose village wells ranged from 10 to 770 μg/L
   b. Limit of quantitation for Natelson method for arsenic is in 30 to 40 μg/L range
   c. Assumed water was only source of arsenic exposure. Absorption of arsenic from food (primarily) or inhalation/dermal exposure (potentially) could affect quantitation
4. Ecologic study
   a. No individual dosimetry
5. Other chemicals in water
   a. Metals and humic acids
6. Applicability of Taiwan data to U.S. population
   a. Dietary and nutritional influences
   b. Potential metabolic differences
7. Potential exposure to fungal toxins

The aim of this chapter is to review the regulatory history of arsenic and to discuss the process involved in reaching a decision on promulgating a new maximum contaminant level (MCL) for arsenic.

REGULATORY HISTORY AND BACKGROUND

In 1975, the EPA established the interim primary drinking water regulation for arsenic at 50 μg/L (U.S. EPA, 1975), based on a standard originally developed by the U.S. Public Health Service (1943) in the 1940s. Commenters had recommended an MCL of 100 μg/L based on there being no observed adverse health effects at this level. The EPA noted long-term chronic effects at 300 to 2750 μg/L, but no illness at 120 μg/L (U.S. EPA, 1976).

In 1980, the EPA set the surface-water quality criterion for discharges of arsenic at 0.022 μg/L (U.S. EPA, 1975). This Clean Water Act criterion was based on protecting human health from ingestion of contaminated water and aquatic organisms. The EPA's Risk Assessment Forum established an internal technical panel to review the quantification of arsenic cancer risk. This panel (U.S. EPA, 1988) verified 1×10^{-6} excess skin cancer risk from oral exposure to arsenic as 0.02 μg/L. In 1992, however, when the Clean Water Act criteria were recalculated using the updated cancer slope factor data, they gave a value of 0.018 μg/L for arsenic (U.S. EPA, 1992a).

In 1983, the National Academy of Sciences (NAS) Safe Drinking Water Committee endorsed the 50-μg/L interim standard as providing "a sufficient margin of safety" (U.S. EPA, 1985). Subsequently, the EPA requested public comment on whether the arsenic MCL should consider carcinogenicity, other health effects, and nutritional requirements, and whether MCLs are necessary for separate valence states (U.S. EPA, 1983). In 1985, the EPA proposed a maximum contaminant level goal (MCLG) of 50 μg/L based on the NAS conclusion that 50 μg/L balanced toxicity and potential essentiality. The EPA (1985) also requested comment on alternate maximum MCLGs of 100 μg/L based on noncarcinogenic effects and 0 μg/L based on carcinogenicity. The 1986 amendments to the Safe Drinking Water Act (PL 99-339) intervened by converting the 1975 interim standard to a National Primary Drinking Water Regulation, subject to revision by 1989.

After reviewing the EPA's arsenic health-effects studies, the EPA's Science Advisory Board (SAB) (1989) stated that (1) the essentiality of arsenic to human health is suggestive but not definitive; (2) hyperkeratosis may not be a precursor of skin cancer; (3) the Taiwan data (Tseng, 1977) are adequate to conclude that high doses of ingested arsenic can cause skin cancer; (4) the Taiwan study (Tseng, 1977) is inconclusive to determine cancer risk at levels ingested in the United States; and (5) arsenic (+3) levels below 200 to 250 μg/d may be detoxified. The SAB concluded that the dose–response relationship is nonlinear and reported that the 1988 Risk Assessment Forum report (U.S. EPA, 1988) did not apply nonlinearity in its risk assessment.

Review of the arsenic risk-assessment issues caused the agency to miss the 1989 deadline for proposing a revised National Primary Drinking Water Regulation, and a citizens' suit was filed against the EPA. A consent decree was entered by the court in June 1990 and was amended several times thereafter. (Since the 1996 amendments to the Safe Drinking Water Act included a new statutory deadline for the arsenic regulations, the existing litigation on arsenic was dismissed in November 1996.)

Arsenic has continued to be the subject of workshops and other information-gathering activities over the past several years (Table 16.1). The SAB reviewed the EPA's April 12, 1991, Arsenic Research Recommendations and recommended mechanism research projects (U.S. EPA, 1992b) that would substantially impact the risk assessment in 3 to 5 years. These were (1) investigation of chromosomes and the carcinogenic forms of arsenic, (2) study of human liver methylation, (3) research on arsenic species in urine at different exposures, and (4) comparisons of methylated arsenic excreted in the U.S., Taiwanese, Mexican, and Argentinian populations and to consider nutritional or genetic differences. If time were not a factor, however, the SAB ranked developing an animal model of arsenic-induced cancer as the highest priority.

In 1993, the SAB reviewed the EPA's draft Drinking Water Criteria Document on Inorganic Arsenic and concluded that current data support an association between high levels of arsenic and internal cancer in humans (U.S. EPA, 1993). The SAB recommended, however, against the use of the uncertainty factor of 3 that was used to derive the arsenic reference dose. They also recommended that the EPA account for the differences between U.S. and Taiwanese cancer risks.

The Office of Research and Development held an expert workshop to develop an epidemiology research strategy for arsenic in drinking water in March 1994 (U.S. EPA, 1994). The panel recommended that the EPA identify populations with exposure information suitable for analytic (versus ecologic) epidemiology studies of noncarcinogenic effects in the United States and develop biomarkers that are predictive of health risks rather than exposure. In addition, the panel encouraged researchers to pursue physiologically based pharmacokinetic models and metabolism studies for arsenic.

The American Water Works Association (AWWA) Research Foundation, AWWA Water Industry Technical Fund, and Association of California Water Agencies (1995) sponsored an Expert Workshop on Arsenic Research Needs held in Ellicott City, Maryland, May 31 through June 2, 1995. The final report from that meeting prioritized research in mechanisms, epidemiology, toxicology, and treatment.

On August 6, 1996, Congress passed the Safe Drinking Water Act Amendments of 1996 (PL 104-182), which included specific requirements for arsenic. In the 1996 amendments, Congress directed the EPA to devise a program of research that would support rule making by filling in critical gaps in

Table 16.1 Workshops and research recommendations to reduce uncertainties in risk assessment of arsenic

Date	Group	Result
1992	SAB	Recommended research for understanding mechanism for arsenic-induced carcinogenicity after reviewing Office of Research and Development recommendations
1993	SAB	Recognized internal cancer as an endpoint of arsenic exposure, recommended that the EPA consider differences in population sensitivity
1995	AWWARF, ACWA, AWWA	Expert Workshop on Arsenic Research Needs: prioritized research in mechanisms, epidemiology, toxicology, and treatment
1994	EPA	Developed epidemiology research strategy; made recommendations on noncarcinogenic effects in U.S. population, biomarkers, models, and metabolism
1997	EPA	National Research Council evaluation of risk assessment
1997	EPA	IRIS reassessment
1997	NCI, EPA	Conference on health effects, mechanisms, and NIEHS research needs

Note: ACWA, Association of California Water Agencies; AWWA, American Water Works Association; AWWARF, American Water Works Association Research Foundation; EPA, Environmental Protection Agency; IRIS, Integrated Risk Information System; NIEHS, National Institute for Environmental Health Science; SAB, Science Advisory Board.

the current understanding of the health risks associated with exposure to low levels of arsenic. The EPA was charged to conduct the research in consultation with the NAS, Federal agencies, and interested public and private entities. Furthermore, the agency was encouraged to enter into cooperative agreements for the research. Although Congress authorized funding of $2.5 million per year for 4 years, Congress appropriated $2 million to support this research over the first 2 years. Finally, the EPA is mandated by the 1996 amendments to propose a new national drinking-water regulation for arsenic by January 1, 2000, and to issue a final regulation no later than January 1, 2001.

Other sections of the 1996 amendments emphasize use of risk assessment, use of the best available peer-reviewed science for decision making, analysis of health benefits likely to occur, possible effects on sensitive populations, and costs of alternative options. The EPA must review and revise, as appropriate, each primary drinking water regulation every 6 years, to be at least as protective of health.

PLANS FOR DEVELOPING THE ARSENIC DRINKING WATER STANDARD

In view of the requirement for peer-reviewed science, the EPA recognizes that the results of the newly funded arsenic health-effects research program will not be fully available when the proposal is issued. Thus, the EPA will base the proposed regulation on information that is already available in the published peer-reviewed literature and on studies that are currently underway and that will be peer-evaluated in time. Because the 1996 amendments also require that the agency revisit drinking-water standards, as appropriate, there will be ample opportunity for the EPA to reevaluate the arsenic standard as the results of longer-term research become available. Figure 16.1 illustrates the process that the EPA will use to meet the statutory requirements for regulations and research. Having established a framework within which many of these activities can proceed in parallel, the agency believes that the statutory deadline is a challenging but realistic one.

Figure 16.2 is a schematic representation of how the agency will address scientific uncertainties about the health effects of arsenic identified in the research plan. In addition to the usual channels for funding both internal and external research, the EPA has entered into a joint solicitation agreement with the AWWA Research Foundation and the Association of California Water Agencies. A request for applications was issued, and the nearly $3 million of research funded by the parties began in the Fall of 1997. Other activities that are expected to contribute to improved characterization of the human-health risks associated with low-level exposure to arsenic include several programs of international research, evaluations of the existing data being conducted by the mode-of-action review panel and by the National Research Council, and revision

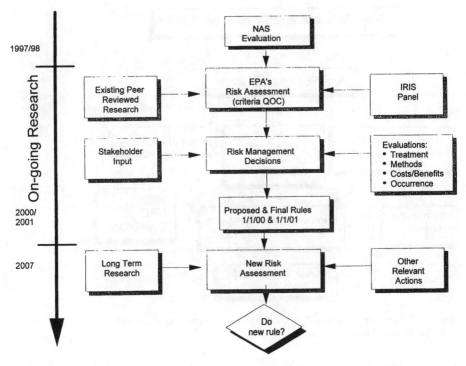

Figure 16.1 The Environmental Protection Agency's approach to meeting the statutory requirements for regulations and research.

of the methodology the EPA uses to establish MCLGs that will reflect the agency's draft cancer reassessment guidelines (U.S. EPA, 1996).

The four steps of risk assessment that are used to develop MCLGs for drinking water are as follow:

Hazard identification: data describing adverse effects of arsenic (illness, cancer, reproductive effects)
Dose–response relationship: quantify the relationship between the exposure (dose) and adverse health effects
Exposure analysis: number of people exposed, levels of arsenic exposure, duration of exposure, routes of exposure (water, food)
Risk characterization: likelihood of experiencing adverse effects

The agency's Office of Research and Development provides expertise and funding support in the areas of hazard identification, dose–response determination, and exposure analysis. Scientists from the Office of Science and Technology of the Office of Water analyze exposure and health data to

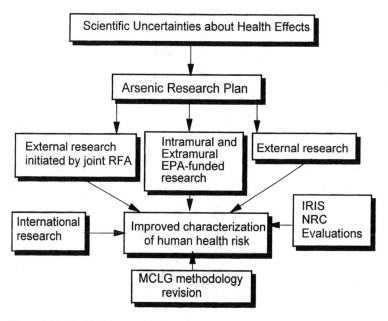

Figure 16.2 The Environmental Protection Agency's approach to addressing scientific uncertainties about the health effects of arsenic.

characterize the MCLG, or concentration, that allows an adequate margin of safety to avoid potential health threats from exposure to the contaminant.

Some of the agency's anticipated milestones for activities being undertaken in response to the arsenic mandate are summarized in Figure 16.3. Because the development, writing, and review of a new rule are time-consuming processes, information needs to be in place well in advance of the statutory deadline. Since 1997, the agency has held five stakeholder meetings to discuss the development of the regulation. There will be a 60-day comment period for the proposed rule and additional opportunities scheduled for input from the full range of stakeholders likely to be affected by the new regulation.

Figure 16.4 illustrates the risk-management components that will be considered by the EPA staff writing the proposed regulation. These factors include:

1. The availability of approved analytic methods for arsenic, including the number of private and public laboratories with the appropriate instrumentation, the number of laboratories proficient with the procedure, practical quantification levels, and cost of analyses
2. The performance efficacy of existing treatment technologies, including their technical and economic suitability for small systems, equipment requirements, maintenance needs, residuals, and other factors associated with each technology

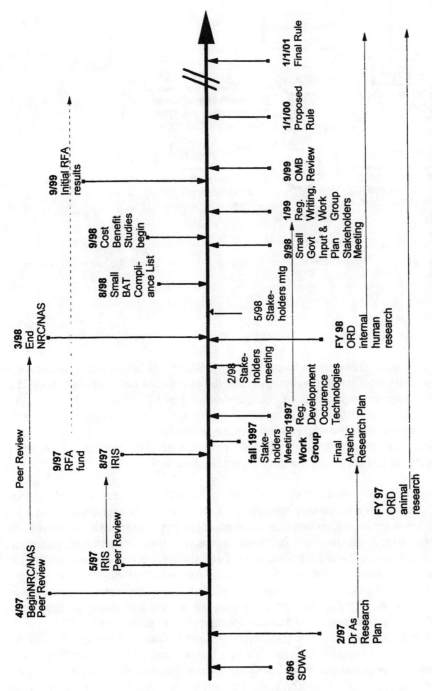

Figure 16.3 Schedule for completing arsenic-related activities in response to the Safe Drinking Water Act Amendments of 1996.

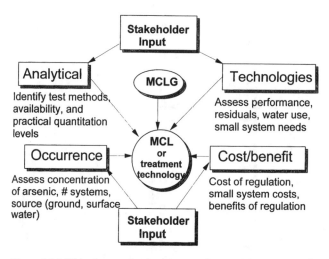

Figure 16.4 Risk characterization as one of several key factors inform the rulemaking process for arsenic.

3. The arsenic concentrations occurring in different drinking water systems, the number of contaminated sources, and the number of people being exposed to the range of concentrations being considered as MCL options
4. The costs of installing and maintaining treatment technologies and benefits associated with the decreased exposure to arsenic
5. Stakeholder input into all of these risk-management assessments, which is essential to developing an implementable standard

In addition, several other Congressional statutes and executive orders affect the regulatory development process. In writing proposed regulations, the EPA must consider the costs and benefits of regulatory alternatives and seek the views of tribes and state or local governments that may be significantly affected, in order to minimize the regulatory burdens and meet regulatory objectives. The EPA must develop compliance guidance for small groups and convene a small-business panel to provide advice during the development of proposed rules that would have a "significant economic impact on a substantial number of small entities" (section 609(b) of the Regulatory Flexibility Act).

The Executive Order for Environmental Justice requires the EPA to identify and address disproportionate health or environmental impacts on minority or low-income populations, providing them with an opportunity to input during the regulatory process. Children's health must be protected by considering disproportionate impacts on them.

REFERENCES

American Water Works Association Research Foundation, AWWA Water Industry Technical Fund, and Association of California Water Agencies. 1995. *Research needs report: Arsenic in drinking water report from International Expert Workshop.* Ellicott City, MD: Author.
Bates, M. N., Smith, A. H., and Hopenhayn-Rich, C. 1992. Arsenic ingestion and internal cancers: A review. *Am. J. Epidemiol.* 135:462–475.
Borum, D. R., and Abernathy, C. O. 1994. Human oral exposure to inorganic arsenic. In *Arsenic exposure and health,* eds. W. R. Chappell, C. O. Abernathy, and C. R. Cothern, pp. 119–128. Northwood, UK: Science and Technology Press.
Brown, K. G., and Abernathy, C. O. 1997. The Taiwan skin cancer risk analysis of inorganic arsenic ingestion: Effects of water consumption rates and food arsenic levels. In *Arsenic: Exposure and Health* (Eds. C. O. Abernathy. R. L. Calderon, and W. R. Chappell), pp. 260–271. Chapman and Hall, London.
Brown, K. G., Guo, H.-R., Kuo, T. L., and Greene, H. L. 1997. Skin cancer and inorganic arsenic: Uncertainty status of risk. *Risk Anal.* 17:37–42.
Fielder, R. J., Dale, E. A., and Williams, S. D. 1986. *Toxicity review, 16: Inorganic arsenic compounds.* London: HMSO Publications.
Frost, D. V. 1970. Arsenicals in biology: Retrospect and prospect. *Fed. Proc.* 26:194–208.
Groschonig, H., and Irgolic, K. J. 1997. The mercuric-bromide stain method and the Natelson method for the determination of arsenic: Implications for assessment of risks from exposure arsenic in Taiwan. In *Arsenic: Exposure and Health* (Eds. C. O. Abernathy. R. L. Calderon, and W. R. Chappell), pp. 17–32. London: Chapman and Hall.
Hindmarsh, J. T., and McCurdy, R. F. 1986. Clinical and environmental aspects of arsenic toxicity. *CRC Crit. Rev. Lab. Sci.* 23:315–347.
International Programme on Chemical Safety. 1981. *Environmental health criteria, 18: Arsenic.* Geneva: World Health Organization.
Polson, C. J., and Tattersall, R. N. 1969. *Clinical toxicology,* 2nd ed. Philadelphia: J. B. Lippincott.
Smith, A. H., Hopenhayn-Rich, C., Bates, M. N., Goeden, H. M., Hertz-Picciotto, I., Duggan, H. M., Wood, R., Kosnett, M. J., and Smith, M. T. 1992. Cancer risks from arsenic in drinking water. *Environ. Health. Perspect.* 97:259–267.
Tseng, W.-P. 1977. Effects and dose-response relationships of skin cancer and blackfoot disease with arsenic. *Environ. Health Perspect.* 19:109–119.
Tseng, W.-P., Chu, H. M., How, S. W., Fong, J. M., Lin, C. S., and Ye, S. 1968. Prevalence of skin cancer in an endemic area of chronic arsenicism in Taiwan. *J. Natl. Cancer Inst.* 40:453–463.
U.S. Environmental Protection Agency. 1975. Water programs: National interim primary drinking water regulations. *Fed. Reg.* 40:59566.
U.S. Environmental Protection Agency. 1976. *National interim primary drinking water regulations.* EPA-570/9-76-003. Washington, DC: Author.
U.S. Environmental Protection Agency. 1983. National revised primary drinking water regulations. Advance notice of proposed rulemaking. *Fed. Reg.* 48:45502.
U.S. Environmental Protection Agency. 1984. *Health assessment document for inorganic arsenic:* Final report, EPA-600/8-83-021F. Washington, DC: U.S. Environmental Protection Agency.
U.S. Environmental Protection Agency. 1985. National primary drinking water regulations: Synthetic organic chemicals, inorganic chemicals, and microorganisms. Proposed rule. *Fed. Reg.* 50:46936.
U.S. Environmental Protection Agency. 1988. *Special report on ingested inorganic arsenic: Skin cancer, nutritional essentiality,* Risk Assessment Forum, EPA/-625/3-87/013. Washington, DC: Author.
U.S. Environmental Protection Agency. 1989. *A critical examination of the evidence for a threshold for cancer risk in humans from inorganic arsenic,* SAB report. Washington, DC: Author.
U.S. Environmental Protection Agency. 1992a. Water quality standards: Establishment of numeric criteria for priority toxic pollutants. States' compliance. Final rule. *Fed. Reg.* 57:60848.

U.S. Environmental Protection Agency. 1992b. *An SAB report: Review of Arsenic Research Recommendations. Review by the Drinking Water Committee of the Office of Research and Development's Arsenic Research Recommendations,* EPA-SAB-DWC-92-018. Washington, DC: Author.

U.S. Environmental Protection Agency. 1993. *An SAB report: Review of the Draft Drinking Water Criteria Document on Inorganic Arsenic,* prepared by the Drinking Water Committee of the Science Advisory Board, EPA-SAB-DWC-34-005. Washington, DC: Author.

U.S. Environmental Protection Agency. 1994. *EPA Workshop on Developing an Epidemiology Research Strategy for Arsenic in Drinking Water.* Panel meeting report, Research Triangle Park, NC. Washington, DC: Author.

U.S. Environmental Protection Agency. 1996. Proposed guidelines for carcinogen risk assessment. *Fed. Reg.* 61:17960–18011.

U.S. Public Health Service. 1943. Public Health Service drinking water standards. *Public Health Reports* 58:69–111.

Webb, D. R., Sipes, I. G., and Carter, D. E. 1986. In vitro solubility and in vivo toxicity of gallium arsenide. *Toxicol. Appl. Pharmacol.* 76:96–104.

Wester, R. C., Maibach, H. I., Sedik, L., Melendres, J., and Wade, M. 1993. In vivo and in vitro percutaneous absorption and skin decontamination of arsenic from water and soil. *Fundam. Appl. Toxicol.* 20:336–340.

Wilbourne, J., Haroun, L., Heseltine, E., Kaldor, J., Partensky, D., and Vainio, V. 1986. Response of experimental animals to human carcinogens: An analysis abased upon the IARC Monographs programme. *Carcinogenesis* 7:1853–1863.

Winship, K. A. 1970. Toxicity of inorganic arsenic salts. *Adv. Drug React. Act. Poison Rev.* 3:129–160.

Yang, T.-H., and Blackwell, R. Q. 1961. Nutritional and environmental conditions in the endemic blackfoot area. *Formosan Sci.* 15:101–129.

CHAPTER
SEVENTEEN

THE EVOLUTION OF HEALTH-RISK ASSESSMENT: TRICHLOROETHYLENE AS A CASE STUDY

Elizabeth A. Maull

Institute for Environment, Safety and Occupational Health Risk Analysis, Brooks Air Force Base, Texas

Harvey J. Clewell

KS Crump Group, Inc., ICF Consulting, Ruston, Louisiana

Health-risk assessment, as it is applied to the environment, is a relatively new science. Risk assessment in the Federal government was defined in a 1983 as "the characterization of the potential adverse effects of human exposures to environmental hazards" (National Research Council, 1983). Another way to look at risk assessment is as the intersection of science (or toxicology) and policy or regulation. Those involved in risk assessment know that this intersection of policy with science is not always smooth.

Although risk assessment as applied to the environment has been well defined only since 1983, risk assessment in the regulatory community has existed for at least 40 years. The Delaney Clause of the Food Drug Cosmetic Act of 1958 focuses specifically on cancer-risk assessment. It states that for food additives there is no acceptable level of a carcinogen. The "no acceptable level" was based on results from nuclear testing, which suggested that there was no safe exposure level for ionizing radiation. The limited amount of research on chemicals available at that time supported the no-threshold approach for chemical carcinogens. The de minimus value for acceptable cancer risk had its beginning with the Food and Drug Administration (FDA), whose risk-based approach to carcinogen standard setting considered one additional cancer in the whole U.S. population (200 million at that time [1958]) as unacceptable (Rhomberg, 1997). The de minumus risk has been relaxed to one in one million excess cancer risk.

In hindsight, many members of the scientific community may question how we could have made the policy decisions that were made in the 1960s through the 1970s. In the context of what we then knew about cancer and our notions of the impact of environmental contamination on human health, perhaps the decisions were not inappropriate. From the period of the Second World War on, the United States experienced a 30-year period of industrial expansion with few or no regulatory controls. Rachel Carson's publication of *A Silent Spring* in 1962, along with the Love Canal incident in the 1970s, provided the genesis for the environmental movement. During this same decade, there was a perception that there was an increased cancer mortality rate within the United States (Higginson, 1993).

The end product of all this was a backlash on industrialization and the establishment of several agencies by then-President Richard Nixon to safeguard human health and the health of the environment. These agencies included the Environmental Protection Agency (EPA), the National Institute for Occupational Safety and Health, and Occupational Safety and Heath Administration. Although these were new agencies, many of the functions that were included within them were bits and pieces of previously existing regulatory groups that had been "downsized" during previous administrations (Albert, 1994). During this time, it was also thought that human cancers were caused by exposures to environmental contamination, primarily through industrial discharges (Higginson, 1993). One of President Nixon's largest initiatives during the 1970s was the war on cancer. By cleaning up the environment, by investing large amounts of research dollars into cancer-related projects, it was thought that we could reduce, if not eliminate, the threat from cancer (Albert, 1994).

Although many of the concerns and hopes of the 1960s and 1970s may have been unfounded, they did lead us as a nation down paths that were not only profitable from a scientific standpoint but also morally responsible. The practices of the 1950s through 1970s were likely to be unsustainable.

Trichloroethylene (TCE), a chemical used in the textile, dry cleaning, and food industries, had been in production in the United States since the 1920s. The scientific literature began to identify TCE as a potential cancer hazard in rodent bioassays in the 1970's. NIOSH published its Current Intelligence Bulletin on TCE in 1975, which presented preliminary results of a National Cancer Institute study in which elevated incidence in hepatocellular carcinomas was noted in B6C3F1 mice. At that time, it was estimated that there were more than 280,000 workers exposed to TCE in the United States. The NIOSH Current Intelligence Bulletin pointed out that there were no published reports of any association between TCE and cancer in humans.

Based on these early reports of carcinogenicity in the rodent bioassays, the FDA banned TCE from use in the food industry in 1977 (International Agency for Research on Cancer, 1979). TCE had been used as an extractant, especially in the decaffeination process for coffee. The FDA currently regulates TCE as an unintentional additive in foods (as an adhesive in the packaging) (Agency for Toxic Substances and Disease Registry, 1997).

By the late 1970s there were sufficient questions regarding how the FDA tackled risk assessment that the Congress of the United States delivered a directive to the FDA to study institutional means for risk assessment (National Research Council, 1983). In response to this directive, and broadening the intent of the directive, the National Academy of Sciences, under contract to the FDA, developed *Risk Assessment in the Federal Government: Managing the Process*, commonly known as the Red Book (National Research Council, 1983). This has become the basis for our current concepts on risk assessment. In the Red Book, a paradigm for risk assessment was developed, consisting of four components: exposure assessment, hazard identification, dose–response assessment, and risk characterization. The Red Book also made some broad recommendations. The committee suggested that risk assessments should take full advantage of the scientific knowledge, in its entirety, available at the time of the assessment. They also recommended the creation of a mechanism that would ensure continuous review and modification of risk-assessment procedures as improvements in scientific understanding of the hazards occur. Finally, they recommended the standardization of analytic procedures among the Federal programs through uniform inference guidelines, as different agencies used widely differing procedures for risk assessment.

Partially in response to the recommendations for the development of uniform inference guidelines in the Red Book, the EPA published a series of assessment guidelines in 1986, including revisions to its interim cancer risk assessment guidelines, originally published in 1976. In its *Guidelines for Carcinogen Risk Assessment* (U.S. EPA, 1986), the EPA provided more specific details on the application of the weight-of-evidence cancer classification essentially adopted from the European International Agency for Research on Cancer (Albert, 1994; Sanner et al., 1996; Rhomberg, 1997). All four elements described in the Red Book, hazard identification, dose–response assessment, exposure assessment, and risk characterization, were included in the EPA's cancer guidelines (U.S. EPA, 1986; Albert, 1994). The EPA emphasized the incorporation of human data and provided two alternatives to low-dose extrapolation to replace the one-hit model used in the 1976 interim guidelines (U.S. EPA, 1976): linearized multistage or time-to-tumor models.

Although the EPA's *Health Assessment Document for Trichloroethylene* (1985) was published in 1985, the proposed Guidelines for Carcinogen Risk Assessment (accepted in 1986) were the basis for the assessment. Both qualitative and quantitative approaches to TCE cancer risk were attempted in the document. The qualitative weight-of-evidence approach adopted by the EPA resulted in a cancer classification for TCE of B2: probable human carcinogen based on sufficient animal data but insufficient or no human data.

Indeed, the EPA evaluated six epidemiologic studies for this assessment, none of which was considered adequate for a quantitative analysis. A quantitative risk assessment was completed, based on a rodent gavage bioassay in which an increased incidence in hepatocellular carcinomas was observed. Using the linearized multistage model, an upper-bound potency was determined to lie between 5.8×10^{-3} and 1.9×10^{-2} mg/kg/d, with a geometric mean of

1.1×10^{-2} mg/kg/d. These values were converted to a unit drinking water risk of 3.2×10^{-7} per μg/L. By this methodology, an adult weighing 70 kg, consuming 2 L of drinking water containing 3.1 μg TCE per liter each day, 350 days per year for 70 years, would have an associated excess cancer risk of one in one million. The upper-bound nature of this risk estimate suggests that the true risk is unlikely to exceed this value and actually may be lower (U.S. EPA, 1985).

What information did the EPA use to come to this conclusion? It was known that TCE was extensively metabolized in the body and that the major metabolites included chloral hydrate, trichloroethanol, trichloroethanol–glucuronide, and tricholoroacetic acid (TCA). Other metabolites found in the urine or exhaled breath were carbon monoxide, carbon dioxide, monochloro- and dichloroacetic acids, TCA–glucuronide, oxalic acid, N-(hydroxyacetyl) aminoethanol, and chloroform. Microsomal systems gave rise to TCE–epoxide, glyoxylic acid, and carbon monoxide. It was recognized at the time that chloroform may have been an artifact of the analytical methodology that would need verification (U.S. EPA, 1985).

Despite the presence of equivocal in vitro studies, the science at the time indicated that TCE in and of itself was not likely a direct-acting carcinogen. Therefore it was likely that a reactive intermediate was responsible for the TCE-induced cancers found in the rodent bioassays. With the presence of a double bond, it was hypothesized that TCE was oxidized to a reactive epoxide, which then could adduct to important macromolecules, including DNA and proteins.

The original *Health Assessment Document for Trichloroethylene* (U.S. EPA, 1985) considered primarily the oral route of exposure. By 1987, the EPA had sufficient information to publish a draft addendum to the *Health Assessment Document for Trichloroethylene: Updated Carcinogenicity Assessment for Trichloroethylene* (U.S. EPA, 1987) that dealt with the potential cancer risk of TCE inhalation exposures. In the 2 years that had passed since the publication of the original TCE health-assessment document, there had been some changes in the basic scientific understanding of the metabolism of TCE. The epoxide still was considered to be an important reactive intermediate. Two important metabolites of TCE, TCA and dichloroacetic acid (DCA), however, had been shown to be complete carcinogens. These chemicals also were shown to be peroxisome proliferators. The proposed mechanisms of action included effects of oxidative stress caused by unequal production of hydrogen peroxide–generating enzymes (20- to 30-fold increase) relative to hydrogen peroxide–degrading enzymes (two-fold increase) (Rao and Reddy, 1991). The renal metabolism of TCE and resulting effects were considered for the first time. In the section on oncodynamics, there was some discussion of the glutathione (GSH) conjugation pathway reported by Dekant et al. (1986). This was a novel and relatively minor pathway. The significance of this finding was the identification of a potential urinary metabolite that was both nephrotoxic and genotoxic. The existence of the GSH pathway did not enter into further characterization of risk for TCE (U.S. EPA, 1987).

Although this addendum included additional epidemiology studies, they all were considered inadequate to either demonstrate or refute the carcinogenic potential of TCE in humans. The draft addendum supported the original weight-of-evidence classification for TCE (B2). As in the 1985 document, an upper-bound risk level based on the linear multistage model was used to estimate cancer risk at low levels of exposure. The EPA established a cancer inhalation unit risk of 1.7×10^{-6} ($\mu g/m^3)^{-1}$ based on the incidence of mouse lung and liver tumors in inhalation bioassays. The upper-bound nature of this means that the true lifetime (70 years) carcinogenic risk from exposure to 1 $\mu g/m^3$ TCE, 24 hours per day, for an individual weighing 70 kg is unlikely to be greater than 1.7×10^{-6}, but it is very possibly less than 1.7×10^{-6} (U.S. EPA, 1987).

The EPA included the weight-of-evidence cancer classification and cancer slope potency factor for TCE in their Integrated Risk Information System in about 1987. Development of the reference concentration and dose for TCE was initiated but never completed. By 1989, the cancer slope potency factor was withdrawn, pending further review (U.S. EPA, 1999). The draft addendum to the 1985 health-assessment document was never published in a final form, presumably because of the controversy surrounding its classification. The B2 weight-of-evidence classification for TCE (probable human carcinogen) was sufficient for the EPA's Office of Drinking Water to require an automatic (unenforceable) maximum contaminant level (MCL) goal of 0 for TCE, and an enforceable MCL as close to the MCL goal as technologically and economically feasible. The MCL was set at 5 ppb. The MCL has been adopted by the regulators in the remediation community as their "applicable and relevant and appropriate requirements." Therefore this is the current clean-up value for groundwater at many state remediation sites and for most national Superfund sites.

From 1989 through 1995, the cancer classification for TCE was reexamined by a variety of agencies. The American Conference for Governmental Industrial Hygienists (ACGIH) published *Notice of Intended Change*: *Trichloroethylene* in 1992; it was adopted in 1993. The cancer classification was changed to A5: not suspected as a human carcinogen, because the substance has been demonstrated by well-controlled epidemiological studies not to be associated with any increased risk of cancer in exposed humans (ACGIH, 1992).

Trichloroethylene was revisited more recently by the International Agency for Research on Cancer (IARC), with a different result. Prior to the fall of 1995, TCE had been classified as a group 3 chemical: not classifiable as to carcinogenicity to humans. Review of data available to the IARC in Spring 1995 resulted in a reclassification of TCE as a 2A chemical: probably carcinogenic to humans: limited human evidence, sufficient evidence in experimental animals (IARC, 1995).

It is interesting to note that in this situation, the ACGIH and the IARC based their respective conclusions on a similar database. Unlike the ACGIH, the IARC performed an analysis of the aggregated results of the cohort studies at that time (Antilla et al., 1995; Axelson et al., 1994; Spirtas et al., 1991). The results of the IARC's analysis showed a statistically significant increase in liver and biliary-tract tumors and non-Hodgkin's lymphoma. None of the original authors concluded that exposure to TCE was associated with a significant increase in any cancer in his or her individual paper.

Finally, the National Toxicology Program (NTP) announced in the fall of 1997 its intent to include TCE in its *Report on Carcinogens* (9th edition) as a "reasonably anticipated human carcinogen" (NTP, 1997). As of August 1999, the 9th edition was in the final stages of review.

There are apparent differences in how the ACGIH, the NTP, and the IARC considered their decisions concerning TCE. The NTP and IARC are looking specifically at the hazard-identification component of the risk-assessment paradigm. There can be no question that TCE causes cancer in rodent bioassays. The question remains of what is the relevance of the rodent bioassays to humans. The ACGIH focused more on the human response at exposure levels likely to be associated with occupational exposures and incorporated this dose–response component of the risk-assessment paradigm into its decision-making process.

In the Spring of 1995, a meeting (referred to as the *Williamsburg meeting*) of many of the major players in TCE research was convened to discuss the current state of the science regarding TCE health-risk assessment. The group was provided with specific questions to address (Clewell and Andersen, 1995). Some of the questions considered included: What are the appropriate endpoints for a TCE cancer-risk assessment? Which data should be regarded as critical? What are the continuing uncertainties for the TCE cancer risk assessment? What approaches should be used for risk characterization? What are the ranges of opinion within the group? Are there immediate, short-term data gaps in which research would significantly improve confidence in the risk estimate?

There was general agreement that a new cancer-risk assessment for TCE should be conducted on a tissue-by-tissue basis, focusing on the target tissue correspondence between the animal bioassay and humans. The four tissues identified for evaluation were liver, kidney, lung, and the hematopoietic system, with the liver and kidney being most relevant to humans. The dilemma of how to evaluate the mouse lymphoma was raised. It was suggested that lymphomas should be identified in any future epidemiologic studies, and that an upper-bound estimate of potency for lymphoma be derived from epidemiologic studies.

There also was generalized agreement that sufficient physiologically based pharmacokinetic data existed to model the human liver cancers. Although it was not unanimous, many of the group thought that a nonlinear model or a benchmark-dose approach was appropriate to develop what was referred to as a *virtual threshold* for tumors and then apply appropriate safety factors for the liver as a target tissue.

Just as there was a general agreement on the specific approach to be taken with the liver, there was a general agreement that there were insufficient data available to make similar conclusions regarding either the kidney or the lung as a target tissue. Although the glutathione conjugation pathway was considered a low-production pathway, and therefore it may not be plausible that toxic products accumulate to sufficient levels to produce tumors, the need to more fully characterize the products of the cytochrome P450 and GSH-dependent pathway in the kidney was identified. In addition, it was concluded that the role of sulfoxidation had been insufficiently evaluated. A suggestion was made that an attempt to estimate the potency that the GSH pathway products, such as dichlorovinyl cysteine, would have to have to induce the observed tumor incidence should be made.

For the lung, the overall conclusion was that corresponding data between animal bioassays and humans were lacking, preventing an attempt at either a qualitative or a quantitative assessment.

The group as a whole felt that there were significant uncertainties in the TCE database. In the liver, three carcinogenic metabolites have been identified, one of which is also mutagenic. How does one apportion carcinogenic risk to each of the individual carcinogens? How does one quantitatively approach the mode of action possibly involving a potential for genotoxicity below the range of observable effects? How does one intersect one model for nonlinear mechanisms (cytotoxicity or mitogenicity) within the observable range with a linear model for genotoxicity below the level observation? Finally, the group was uncomfortable with the prospect that chloral, a genotoxic metabolite in both the lung and the liver, had not been sufficiently accounted for (Clewell and Andersen, 1995).

During the period from 1989 through 1995, the EPA remained quiet on the topic of TCE. If asked, the agency generally would respond that TCE was considered to be somewhere on a continuum between a B and C carcinogen (or somewhere between a possible carcinogen and probable human carcinogen). The fact that the EPA was quiet regarding TCE does not suggest that it was uninvolved. It was during this time that debate on the 1986 *Guidelines for Carcinogen Risk Assessment* was ongoing. When the EPA was ready to commit in 1996 to review all the recent research appropriate for a new health risk assessment for TCE, they agreed to do so in the spirit of the *Proposed Guidelines for Carcinogen Risk Assessment* (U.S. EPA, 1996). The proposed guidelines incorporated some of the comments from *Science and Judgment in Risk Assessment* by the NRC (1994) and recent innovations in the risk-assessment community in general.

Although the four basic aspects (hazard characterization, dose–response characterization, exposure characterization, and risk characterization) were to remain, hazard and dose characterization were expanded. Specifically, hazard characterization was altered to be more inclusive of all the available mechanistic data to evaluate the relevance of the animal cancer bioassay results to the human situation. Within the hazard characterization, more consideration would be given to both the route and the level of exposure in estimating the likelihood of a human hazard.

Dose–response characterization encompassed even greater changes. The new guidelines called for the utilization of all the available data to predict the likely shape of the dose–response curve. The dose–response characterization would be accomplished in two steps, starting with the development of a dose–

response curve in the observable range followed by extrapolation to a realistic potential human exposure range. Biologically based models were allowed, if available; otherwise a combination of curve fitting in the observable range with a benchmark-dose approach to develop an appropriate point of departure for extrapolating into the low-dose area would be taken. Without the availability of a biologically based model, alternative defaults to extrapolate to levels below the range of observation would incorporate information on the mode of action for the specific chemical. If the mode of action suggests that a chemical is genotoxic, a linear extrapolation from the appropriate point of departure through the origin would be appropriate. For those chemicals that can demonstrate a nongenotoxic mode of action, however, the EPA recommended adoption of the margin-of-exposure approach: The evaluation of the ratio between anticipated human exposures and exposures associated with tumors would be conducted and used for risk-management decisions.

Extrapolations into the area of low-dose exposures would be made from appropriate "points of departure." In the past, extrapolations to low doses relied on the linearized multistage model. As an alternative, the EPA would allow a benchmark-dose approach to cancer-risk assessment. In this approach, a dose–response curve would be developed only in the observable range of data and extrapolations made from a point of departure equivalent to 95% lower confidence level of an appropriate effective dose. Although what exactly is the appropriate effective dose on which to base this is a policy issue, it is likely that judgments on the severity of the effect will play a part in that decision. The appropriate point of departure will probably fall between the 1% and 10% effective dose.

Mode of action also will play a critical role in the evaluation of chemical carcinogenesis. The EPA is allowing for the possibility that not all chemical carcinogens act by interacting with DNA. If a chemical causes cancer by a nongenotoxic mode, then nonlinear modeling may be appropriate to predict effects from low-dose extrapolations, if sufficient data are available.

Finally, biologically based dose modeling is allowed in the proposed cancer guidelines, including physiologically based pharmacokinetic modeling. The advantages of such modeling include the ability to extrapolate not only from high dose to low dose but also from one route of exposure to another, and from one species to another. Physiologically based pharmacokinetic modeling may improve estimations of the effects in humans from rodent studies (U.S. EPA, 1996).

Representatives from the EPA's National Center for Environmental Assessment were in attendance at the 1995 Williamsburg meeting. Less that one year later (March 1996), the EPA announced its intent to revisit and possibly revise *Health Assessment Document for Trichloroethylene* (U.S. EPA, 1985, 1987). In responding to comments in *Science and Judgment in Risk Assessment* (NRC, 1994), the EPA declared a new process for the next risk assessment on TCE. As a part of this, the EPA indicated that the chemical-specific risk assessments would no longer be considered final documents, as an iterative approach would be applied in the future. Therefore, reevaluations of the risk assessments would occur as often as substantive information became available that would make a significant impact the outcome of the risk assessment.

The TCE health-risk assessment will be written to reflect the EPA's new cancer guidelines. The EPA has opened the process to give increased emphasis to external peer involvement and review. This document will be written in two sections. The first section will focus on state-of-the-science papers by experts from both inside and outside the EPA, many of whom are actively involve in TCE research. The goal of these papers will be a balanced and unbiased view representing plausible scientific interpretations of the results, along with consideration of the strengths and limitations of the scientific data.

The second section will be dedicated to a synthesis of the state-of-the-science papers into a risk characterization that will update the EPA's position on TCE, from both the qualitative and the quantitative points of view. In accordance with *Proposed Guidelines for Carcinogen Risk Assessment* (U.S. EPA, 1996), consideration will be given to mode of action and biologically based models. In addition, this risk assessment will include for the first time evaluations of noncancer endpoints (Maull et al., 1997).

Questions remain as to the relevance of the rodent bioassays to the induction of potential cancers in humans, especially in view of the lack of concordance of cancers in the different species. There is no single compelling mechanism that can be used reliably as the sole basis for estimating the dose–response relationship for human liver cancer. One key observation is the occurrence of liver cancer in mice and not rats, and the corresponding differences in the metabolism of TCE in these two species. Metabolism of TCE is saturated at lower concentrations in the rat relative to the mouse. The end result is circulating levels of TCA that are 5- to 10-fold higher in the mouse than the rat, given the same exposure level (oral dosing, 1000 mg/kg Prout et al., 1985; Larson and Bull, 1992). In addition, the mouse appears to be more sensitive to the effects of TCA, developing hepatic tumors at lower exposure levels (140 mg/kg/d, 82 weeks) than observed in the rat (378 mg/kg/d, 104 weeks, no liver tumor formation) (Pereira, 1996; DeAngelo and Daniel, 1992). Humans metabolize approximately 60 times less TCE on a body-weight basis than mice at similar exposure levels. In addition, TCA does not appear to induce peroxisomal proliferation in human hepatocytes (Geoptar et al., 1995).

The evidence surrounding kidney cancer, though limited, is reasonable on several levels. There are similarities between the sites and the histopathologic characteristics of the tumors observed in patients and rat bioassays (Vamvakas et al., 1993). The metabolites derived from the likely ultimate electrophilic intermediates of bioactivation of TCE are identical in humans and experimental animals (Birner et al., 1993). Based on levels of urinary metabolites of TCE, it appears that humans are more sensitive than rats to the development of the primary biochemical lesions leading to renal cancer (Birner et al., 1993). Finally, Dekant et al. (1986) have elucidated the molecular mechanisms of this type of nephrocarcinogenicity.

Although all this information supports the relevance of the rat kidney tumors to humans, there have been criticisms of these studies. One study

(Henschler et al., 1995) may have been initiated after the observation of a cancer cluster. Weiss (1996) was concerned about the possibility of increased disease surveillance because of a suspected cluster. In addition, potentially high levels of TCE exposure may have been encountered by workers without personal protection equipment (NTP, 1997).

The EPA has at its hands the tools for an improved health-risk assessment for TCE. Not only have the metabolic pathways for TCE been elucidated further, but the information has been integrated into physiologically based pharmacokinetic models to allow for both species and low dose extrapolation. The *Proposed Guidelines for Carcinogen Risk Assessment* (U.S. EPA, 1996) have built-in flexibilities that will allow the EPA to move away from the overly conservative approaches of the past, if they chose to do so. The journal *Environmental Health Perspectives* has agreed to publish the expert contributions in a special supplement this year. Finally, a qualitative and quantitative analysis of TCE, to include noncancer endpoints, is scheduled to be completed and included in the EPA's Integrated Risk Information System by the end of 1999.

REFERENCES

Albert, R. E. 1994. Carcinogen risk assessment in the U.S. Environmental Protection Agency. *Crit. Rev. Toxicol*, 24:75–85.

Agency for Toxic Substances and Disease Registy. 1997. *Toxicologic profile for trichloroethlyene (update)*. Atlanta: U.S. Department of Health and Human Services, Public Health Service.

American Conference of Governmental Industrial Hygienists. 1992. Notice of intended change: Trichloroethylene. *Appl. Occup. Environ. Hyg.* 7:786–791.

Anttila, A., Pukkala, E., Sallmen, M., Hernberg, S., and Hemminki, K. 1995. Cancer incidence among Finnish workers exposed to halogenated hydrocarbons. *J. Occup. Environ. Med.* 37:797–806.

Axelson, O., Selden, A., Andersson, K., and Hogstedt, C. 1994. Updated and expanded Swedish cohort study on Trichloroethylene and cancer risk. *J. Occup. Environ. Med.* 36:556–562.

Birner, G., Vamvakas, S., Dekant, W., and Henschler, D. 1993. Nephrotoxic and genotoxic N-acetyl. S-dichlorovinyl-L-cysteine is a urinary metabolite after occupational 1,1,2-trichloroethylene exposure in humans: Implications for the risk of trichloroethylene exposure. *Environ. Health Perspect.* 99:281–284.

Carson, R. 1994. *Silent Spring*. Houghton Mifflin.

Clewell, H. J., and Andersen, M. E. 1995. *Report on the Trichloroethylene Workshop, Williamsburg, Virginia, May 18–19, 1995*. Prepared for the U.S. Air Force, Armstrong Laboratory, Occupational and Environmental Health Directorate, Toxicology Division, Wright-Patterson AFB, OH.

DeAngelo, A. B., and Daniel, F. B. 1992. An evaluation of the carcinogenicity of the chloroacetic acids in the male F344 rat. *Toxicologist* 12:206.

Dekant, W., Metzler, M., and Henschler, D. 1986. Identification of S-1,2-dichlorovinyl-N-acetylcysteine as a urinary metabolite of trichloroethylene: A possible explanation for its nephrocarcinogenicity in male rats. *Biochem. Pharmacol.* 35:2455–2458.

Geoptar, A. R., Commandeur, J. N. M., van Ommen, B., van Bladeren, E. J., and Vermeulen, N. P. E. 1995. Metabolism and kinetics of trichloroethylene in relation to toxicity and carcinogenicity: Relevance of the mercapturic acid pathway. *Chem. Res. Toxicol.* 8:3–21.

Henschler, D., Vamvakos, S., Lammert, M., Dekant, W., Kraus, B., Thomas, B., and Ulm, K. 1995. Increased incidence of renal cell tumors in a cohort of cardboard workers exposed to trichloroethylene. *Arch. Toxicol.* 69:291–299.

Higginson, J. 1993. Environmental carcinogenesis. *Cancer* 72:971–977.
International Agency for Research on Cancer. 1979. *Monograph on the evaluation of the carcinogenic risk of chemicals to humans: Some halogenated hydrocarbons.* Lyon, France: World Health Organization.
International Agency for Research on Cancer. 1995. *Dry cleaning, some chlorinated solvents and other industrial chemicals*, volume 63, IARC Monographs on the Evaluation of Carcinogenic Risks to Humans. Lyon, France: World Health Organization.
Larson, J. L., and Bull, R. J. 1992. Species differences in the metabolism of trichloroethylene to the carcinogenic metabolites trichloroacetate and dichloroacetate. *Toxicol. Appl. Pharmacol.* 115:278–285.
Maull E. A., Cogliano, V. J., Scott, C. S., Barton, H. A., Fisher, J. W., Greenberg, M., Rhomberg, L., and Sorgen, S. P. 1997. Trichloroethylene health risk assessment: A new and improved process. *Drug Chem. Toxicol.* 20:427–442.
National Institute of Occupational Safety and Health. 1975. Current intelligence bulletin no. 2: Trichloroethlyene (TCE). In *NIOSH Current Intelligence Bulletin Reprints: Bulletins 1–18* (1975–1977). Website:http://www.cdc.gov/niosh/cibs2.html
National Research Council 1983. *Risk assessment in the Federal government: Managing the process*, Washington, DC: National Academy Press.
National Research Council. 1994. *Science and judgment in risk assessment.* Washington, DC: National Academy Press.
National Toxicology Program. 1997. Website: http://NTP:ntp-server.niehs.nih.gov/ NewHomeRoc/9thConsideration.html
Pereira, M. A. 1996. Carcinogenic activity of dichloroacetic acid and trichloroacetic acid in the liver of female B6C3F1 mice. *Fundam. Appl. Toxicol.* 31:192–199.
Prout, M. S., Provan, W. M., and Green, T. 1985. Species differences in response to trichloroethylene. *Toxicol. Appl. Pharmacol.* 79:389–400.
Rao, M. S., and Reddy, J. K. 1991. An overview of peroxisome proliferator-induced hepatocarcinogenesis. *Environ. Health Perspect.* 93:205–209.
Rhomberg, L. R. 1997. A survey of methods for chemical health risk assessment among federal regulatory agencies. *Hum. and Ecol. Risk Assess.* 3:1029–1196.
Sanner, T., Dybing, E., Kroese, D., Roelfzema, H., and Hardeng, S. 1996. Carcinogen classification systems: Similarities and differences. *Reg. Toxicol. Pharmacol.* 23:128–138.
Spirtas, R., Stewart, P., and Lee, S. 1991. Retrospective cohort mortality study of workers at an aircraft manufacturing facility: I. Epidemiological results. *Br. J. Indust. Med.* 48:515–530.
U.S. Environmental Protection Agency 1976. Interim procedures and guidelines for health risk and economic impact assessments of suspected carcinogens. *Fed. Regist.* 41:21402–21405.
U.S. Environmental Protection Agency 1985. *Health assessment document for trichloroethylene*, EPA/600/8-82/006F. Washington, DC: Author.
U.S. Environmental Protection Agency 1986. Guidelines for carcinogen risk assessment, *Fed. Reg.* 51:33992–34003.
U.S. Environmental Protection Agency 1987. *Addendum to the Health Assessment Document for Trichloroethylene: Updated carcinogenicity assessment for trichloroethylene* (review draft). EPA/600/8-82/006FA. Washington, DC: Author.
U.S. Environmental Protection Agency 1996. *Proposed guidelines for carcinogen risk assessment:Notice, Fed. Reg.* 61:17960–18011.
U.S. Environmental Protection Agency 1999. IRIS website: www.epa.gov/ngispgm3/iris/subst-fl.htm
Vamvakas, S., Dekant, W., and Henschler, D. 1993. Nephrocarcinogenicity of haloalkenes and alkynes. In *Renal disposition and nephrotoxicity of xenobiotics*, pp. 323–342. San Diego, CA: Academic Press.
Weiss, N. S. 1996. Cancer in relation to occupational exposure to trichloroethylene. *Occup. Environ. Med.* 53:1–5.

CHAPTER
EIGHTEEN

HISTORY OF METHYLENE CHLORIDE IN CONSUMER PRODUCTS: TRACING SCIENTIFIC KNOWLEDGE, REGULATIONS, AND PERCEPTIONS

Donna M. Riley and Paul S. Fischbeck

Department of Engineering and Public Policy and Department of Social and Decision Sciences, Carnegie Mellon University, Pittsburgh, Pennsylvania

Methylene chloride was first synthesized in the mid-1800s but was not produced on a large scale until the 1940s. One of its earliest uses was as a paint stripper, though it had applications ranging from refrigeration to anesthesia (Kirk-Othmer, 1949). Today it is commonly used in pharmaceutical processing, degreasing, decaffeinating coffee, and manufacturing photographic film and insecticides (Kirk-Othmer, 1993).

To provide an overview of the history of methylene chloride, Figure 18.1 shows how its production and sales rapidly grew from the 1940s through the 1960s, flattening out in the 1970s and early 1980s and then decreasing sharply after the mid-1980s when it became a suspect human carcinogen.

Somewhat correlated with the past 20 years of these production and sales trends are the workplace exposure standards. Figure 18.2 shows changes in these standards over this same time period. The American Conference of Govermental Industrial Hygienists (ACGIH) set an 8-hour time-weighted average standard of 500 ppm in 1946. This standard went unchanged until the mid-1970s, when the ACGIH lowered their standard to 100 ppm, though the Occupational Safety and Health Administration (OSHA) retained the 500-ppm standard. In the mid-1980s, the ACGIH lowered its standard from 100 ppm to 50 ppm, and OSHA began investigating the possibility of lowering its standard as well. After more than 10 years of debate over whether the standard should be 50 ppm or 25 ppm, OSHA finalized its rule in 1997, setting the new standard at 25 ppm (Federal Register, 1997).

Following behind these changes in the occupational exposure standards are the consumer literature and the information available to the public. Weekend home-repair enthusiasts are always looking for products that will make their

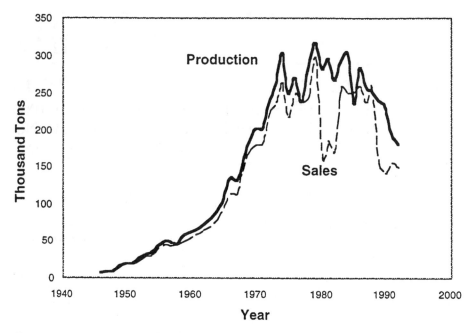

Figure 18.1 Methylene chloride production and sales data.

chores easy, effective, and affordable. How important is safety? How does the consumer literature take complex scientific findings and regulations and translate them into understandable, easy-to-read articles? What "facts" get stressed? How clear is the message? Is the information consistent? Is the advice well motivated? Can a reader understand why the risks are important and what can be done to reduce them?

Consumers make many decisions as to which products to buy and how to use them. Whether a particular risk-mitigation strategy is employed is directly tied to the consumer's appreciation of the risk and the effectiveness of the strategy. The brief and often tersely written warning label and instructions on the side of a can of paint stripper may not be the most salient sources of information for the public. Understanding the source of a consumer's knowledge is a critical step in designing better risk communications and warning labels and ultimately in reducing the risks that consumers face.

The remainder of this chapter is structured around four periods in the history of methylene chloride: The Early Years: 1944–1960, Better Things for Better Living: The 1960s, The Decline: 1970–1985, and The Cancer Era: 1985–Present. For each of these periods, the three themes of the chapter are traced: the progression of scientific knowledge about methylene chloride, the response from regulatory agencies, and the information presented in the

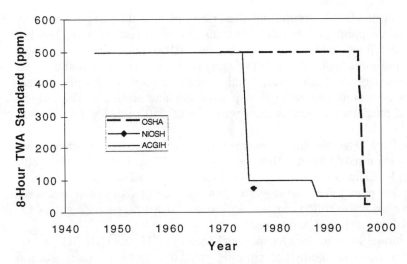

Figure 18.2 Methylene chloride standards. TWA, time-weighted average.

consumer literature. A conclusion section amplifies the importance of this type of research and points to follow-up work.

THE EARLY YEARS: 1944–1960

Though discovered decades earlier, it was during this time period that the many uses of methylene chloride were conceived, large-scale production began, and the first occupational exposure standards were established. Because of the popularity of the chemical in commercially available paint strippers, it is also during this period that the consumer literature begins to give advice as to how methylene chloride should be used. The known health concerns are explicitly delineated to the public in a straightforward though somewhat unmotivated manner.

Scientific Knowledge

The narcotic properties of methylene chloride have been known since the 1880s (NIOSH, 1976), and it was even marketed commercially in the 1920s and 1930s in Germany as the anesthetic Solästhin (Hirsch, 1927; Arrias, 1931; Domanig, 1930). Collier (1936) discussed injuries related to occupational exposure, documenting headaches, giddiness, irritability, rapid pulse, shortness of breath, poor coordination, and "stupidity" among workers. He cites the belief of the day that "with good ventilation its industrial use is practically harmless."

Heppel et al. (1944) reported on the effects of high daily exposures (5000 ppm and 10,000 ppm) on laboratory animals. No ill effects were observed at 5000 ppm for dogs, rabbits, or rats, but at 10,000 ppm, there were light anesthesia and some residual effects including pulmonary congestion and edema and fatty degeneration of the liver. Applications of methylene chloride directly to the ears of rabbits caused mild skin irritation and scaliness. The authors suggested a maximum allowable concentration of 500 ppm for 8-hour daily exposure.

Flinn (1946) suggested that humans should not be exposed to air in which the smell of chlorinated hydrocarbons is detectable; Heppel et al. (1944) cited a German study (Lehmann and Flury, 1938) in which methylene chloride could be detected at 310 ppm. Flinn also suggested that because of skin irritation and the potential for skin absorption, employees should "keep their hands out of the solvents." Gloves were not mentioned.

The National Institute for Occupational Safety and Health (NIOSH) in 1976 cited three reports of methylene chloride–related poisoning among workers from this era. First, Moskowitz and Shapiro (1952) reported four cases of acute exposure in a factory in which all four men became unconscious while working. One died and the other three suffered head injuries and irritation of the eyes, lungs, or respiratory tract. Hughes (1954) reported a case of pulmonary edema in addition to fatigue, sleepiness, lightheadedness, and nausea. Gerritsen and Buschmann (1960) reported a case of phosgene poisoning in a painter working in a room with a kerosene stove.

Regulatory Activity

There was relatively little regulatory activity on methylene chloride during this time period. In 1946 the ACGIH set an 8-hour daily workplace standard of 500 ppm for methylene chloride, based on the recommendation in Heppel et al. (1944; NIOSH, 1976).

Despite the lack of specific regulations pertaining to methylene chloride, during this period the groundwork was laid for future regulations with the passage of three important acts: the Food, Drug, and Cosmetic Act (FDCA) in 1938, the Federal Insecticide, Fungicide, and Rodenticide Act (FIFRA) in 1949, and the Federal Hazardous Substances Act (FHSA) in 1960. FIFRA (governing pesticides) and later FHSA (governing hazardous substances in general) included requirements for clear warnings on labels to protect public health, including information on how to prevent harm, and what to do in case of accidental exposure.

The FDCA included provisions for permitting and regulating the use of chemicals used in food processing. In 1959, methylene chloride was exempted from tolerances for fumigation of crops such as corn, rice, wheat, and barley under the FDCA (Federal Register, 1959). It was exempted because a petitioner argued that methylene chloride was not present at all in grains for human consumption and that the residues were not harmful to animals (or to humans who might eventually eat them).

Consumer Literature

In the 1940s and 1950s, the consumer literature warned consumers about risks from inhalation of methylene chloride. The risk warnings, dealing with the acute known physical effects of the chemical, were straightforward and demonstrated realism regarding safety concerns. The consumer literature from the 1940s and 1950s shows a surprisingly detailed consideration for safe-use practices for methylene chloride paint strippers. The chemical is seen as the safest alternative available, but articles caution about the importance of good ventilation, and one article went into such detail as to instruct its readers about how to ventilate properly (Haan, 1956):

> To avoid inhalation, a positive circulation of air is important. The current of air should flow away from the worker and out an open window or door. An exhaust fan of suitable size will assure enough ventilation.

Despite these instructions, the articles are not specific about the health effects resulting from overexposure to methylene chloride. The effects described are vague, such as "serious poisoning or collapse" (*Consumers' Research Bulletin*, 1946) or "their vapors may make you extremely ill" (Gladstone, 1951). The use of gloves and goggles is not mentioned at all in this time period, and workers are shown in photographs working without gloves. In one article, a worker is shown working indoors with apparently poor ventilation (Gladstone, 1951), as seen in Figure 18.3. This image contradicts warnings in the text of the article that stress the importance of good ventilation.

In the 1940s and 1950s, methylene chloride represented a real improvement in safety and performance among paint strippers. Table 18.1 shows the advantages and disadvantages of the available types of paint stripper as discussed in one article (*Consumers' Research Bulletin*, 1946). The article contained a careful and thorough evaluation of the advantages and disadvantages of alkaline, benzol, and methylene chloride paint strippers.

Lye (alkali) was considered the least safe paint stripper because of its caustic properties. It also was considered an inferior product because of its tendency to react with certain metals; its slowness; its tendencies to darken wood, raise the grain of wood, and dissolve furniture glue; and the necessity of an afterwash to neutralize the alkali. Benzol, the existing chemical alternative, worked faster than lye and did not stain wood or dissolve glue, but it still required an afterwash to remove the wax that was added to benzol to slow evaporation. The use of benzol raised the safety concerns of noxious fumes and flammability, though it was not caustic. Methylene chloride solved many problems associated with both lye and benzol. It did not react with metal, stain or bleach wood, or dissolve furniture glue; it required no afterwash; and it

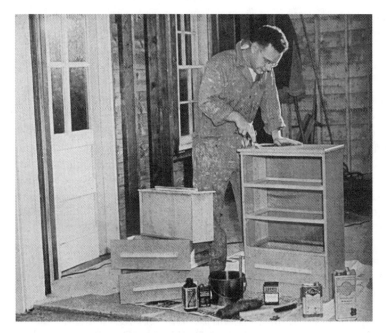

Figure 18.3 Working indoors without good ventilation or gloves. Note the open containers of paint stripper, the lack of gloves, and the closed windows and doors. Reprinted with permission from *Popular Science* magazine, copyright 1951, Times Mirror Magazines, Inc.

Table 18.1 1940s comparison of paint stripper types

	Alkali	Benzol	Methylene chloride
Performance	Reacts with non-ferrous metal	Nonreactive	Nonreactive
	Darkens, raises grain of wood, glue dissolves	Does not stain or bleach or dissolve glue	Does not stain or bleach or dissolve glue
	Slow	Faster	Fastest
	Afterwash needed to neutralize	Afterwash needed to remove wax	No afterwash needed
Safety	No noxious fumes	Noxious fumes	Noxious fumes, less toxic than benzol
	Eats through skin	—	—
	Nonflammable	Flammable	Nonflammable

Source: *Consumers' Research Bulletin*, 1946.

worked the fastest of all three types. It was not caustic; it came in nonflammable varieties; and, though it did release noxious fumes, they were considered less toxic than those of benzol.

The consumer literature in the 1940s and 1950s concluded based on these types of evaluations that methylene chloride was the preferred paint stripping alternative:

> Have you tried the new liquid paint removers that are nonflammable, have faster action and a deeper bite and do not require any "after wash" or neutralizing? If not, there's a distinct surprise in store for you! (Haan, 1956).

> [Solvent-based strippers] are easy to handle and they won't attack flesh and clothing like the corrosive, alkali types. (Gladstone, 1951).

> Modern removers based on methylene chloride are not nearly as toxic as benzol used in many older removers. (Haan, 1956).

In the 1940s and 1950s, with acute inhalation effects of primary concern in the consumer literature, risk communications found in popular magazines were relatively detailed, direct, and to the point. Methylene chloride was seen as safer than other types of paint removers, but the authors were practical about the risks that methylene chloride was believed to pose to consumers.

BETTER THINGS FOR BETTER LIVING: THE 1960s

The 1960s were the glory years for methylene chloride. Production and sales skyrocketed as few problems and many advantages for its use were found. The consumer literature amplified this optimism by extoling its virtues and minimizing its shortcomings.

Scientific Knowledge

Science in the 1960s seemed to uncover mostly good news about methylene chloride, especially relative to the other chlorinated hydrocarbons. It was found not to cause liver damage (Kutob and Plaa, 1962a; Kutob and Plaa, 1962b; Klaasen and Plaa, 1966) and to cause kidney damage only if doses reached lethal levels (Klaasen and Plaa, 1966; Plaa and Larson, 1965). Investigations into the metabolism of chlorinated hydrocarbons suggested explanations for why methylene chloride did not cause lipoperoxidation and necrosis of the liver, unlike carbon tetrachloride (Reynolds and Yee, 1967; Fowler, 1970, Garner and McLean, 1970). Dingell and Heimberg (1968) showed that though both methylene chloride and carbon tetrachloride combine with reduced cytochrome P450 causing a spectral shift, only carbon tetrachloride inhibited certain enzyme reactions.

One report of ill effects of methylene chloride came from Weiss (1967) who reported a case of toxic encephalosis (NIOSH, 1976).

Regulatory Activity

There was a significant amount of regulatory activity in the 1960s related to methylene chloride, but it mostly focused on establishing new uses for the chemical. In 1961, at the request of a spice company, a spice-extraction process involving methylene chloride and other chlorinated solvents was permitted under the FDCA. Concentrations of total chlorinated solvents were not to exceed 30 ppm (*Federal Register*, 1961). In 1962, methylene chloride was included in the labeling requirements for "economic poisons" under FIFRA (*Federal Register*, 1962). Certain phrases were required for labels containing methylene chloride including "harmful if swallowed," "avoid prolonged or repeated breathing of vapor," and "avoid prolonged or repeated contact with skin." These phrases reflect the primary negative health effects that had been reported by that time in the scientific literature.

In 1965 methylene chloride was approved for use as a solvent of hops for beer production in response to a petition filed by the Hops Extract Corporation of America (*Federal Register*, 1965). The hops extract was required to not exceed 2.2% residual methylene chloride, and the extract was required to be added to the beer before or during the cooking process. In 1969 a new process was approved for "modified hop extract," with a new standard of 5 ppm residual methylene chloride allowed in the extract (*Federal Register*, 1969). In 1967 methylene chloride was approved for use in the decaffeination of coffee, limiting the allowable methylene chloride residue to 10 ppm in roasted coffee or instant coffee (*Federal Register*, 1967).

Consumer Literature

In the 1960s, risk communication was not a focus of articles, and safety advice was shortened to simple general statements such as "ventilate well," though no specifics were identified as to how a consumer should ventilate well, or how much ventilation was considered sufficient. *Consumer Reports* (1961) advised, "Use adequate ventilation and don't take chances with fire. Avoid inhaling the fumes."

The safety concerns mentioned in the consumer literature in the 1960s focused primarily on flammability of paint strippers. *Consumer Reports* (1961) called attention to inconsistencies in the Federal regulatory definition for "flammable." *Consumer Reports* argued for stricter definitions for labeling purposes, and flammability tests were conducted by brand to identify which would burn the easiest.

Gloves appeared for the first time in text and photos, as the 1961 *Consumer Reports* piece contained a warning about skin irritation and featured a photo of a man using gloves as he worked (Fig. 18.4). However, *Consumer Reports* was ahead of its time, as other articles in the 1960s did not discuss these concerns and actually advised consumers to touch the sludge to see if it were ready to be scraped (Hand, 1966), as in Figure 18.5.

Alkali strippers were not considered a viable alternative for paint stripping in the 1960s consumer literature and were mentioned only in passing as an inferior type of stripper. "Its only advantage is economy in large quantities... It is extremely caustic and is considered dangerous to use" (Hand, 1966). Table 18.2 shows the three stripper types considered in a 1966 *Popular Science* article. Benzol and two types of methylene chloride strippers are considered in depth,

METHYLENE CHLORIDE 243

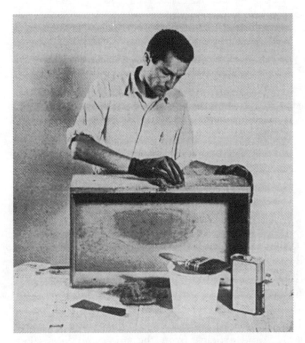

Figure 18.4 Gloves are shown being used for the first time. Copyright 1961 by Consumers Union of the U.S., Inc., Yonkers, NY. Reprinted by permission from *Consumer Reports*, 1961.

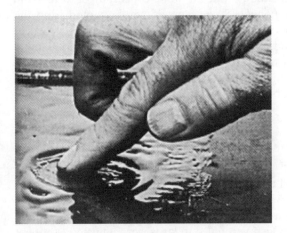

Figure 18.5 Ready for scraping? Note that a gloveless finger is used to test the paint stripper to see if the paint is ready for scraping. Reprinted with permission from *Popular Science* magazine, copyright 1966, Times Mirror Magazines, Inc.

Table 18.2 1960s comparison of paint stripper types

	Benzol/acetone mix	Methylene chloride/ acetone mix	Methylene chloride
Performance	Cheapest	More expensive	Most expensive
	Slow	Faster	Fastest
	Afterwash needed to remove wax	No additional solvents	Water wash, no scraping
Safety	—	Harmful vapors	—
	—	Cannot be swallowed	Cannot be swallowed
	Extremely flammable	Flammable	Nonflammable

Source: Hand, 1966.

but alkalis are not discussed as an alternative. In this piece, there is less information about the safety concerns than in the 1946 article. Speed, price, and convenience are the main criteria for consideration, with flammability being the only safety concern that receives much attention.

Popular Science concluded that methylene chloride without acetone was the safest and most effective product. "The key ingredient in the better removers is methylene chloride. It is the best, fastest-working of the solvents. Moreover, it is a fire retardant" (Hand, 1966). Some articles from the mid- and late 1960s glossed over the hazards associated with methylene chloride paint strippers that previous articles had focused on. They offered little or no instruction to consumers who would actually use the product at home concerning how to avoid or reduce their risks. The 1966 *Popular Science* piece merely quoted from the labels of cans as an indication of hazards. A 1967 *Popular Mechanics* article (Howard, 1967), though it showed users with gloves, only discussed flammability as a risk in the text. A table that rated strippers had "low toxicity" as a criterion for comparison, but there was no explanation of what was meant by the term. Both methylene chloride strippers and a "paste" stripper were listed as having "low toxicity."

THE DECLINE: 1970–1985

The optimism of the 1960s faded during the next decade, as research uncovered cardiovascular risks associated with methylene chloride use. Health concerns that had been raised previously were now explained with direct evidence and a well-understood biologic model. Occupational standards were adjusted to reflect this new understanding, and the consumer literature became more critical of methylene chloride use.

Scientific Knowledge

A major change in scientific knowledge occurred in 1972 when an article published in the journal *Science* (Stewart et al., 1972a,b) found that methylene chloride was linked to elevated levels of carboxyhemoglobin (COHb); in fact, the then-current standard of 500 ppm would produce COHb loadings in the body that exceeded the standard for carbon monoxide. Stewart et al. (1972b) also found evidence of central nervous system depression at 1000 ppm, a level allowed in industry for shorter time periods. Stewart et al. called attention to the special concerns of the elderly and people with cardiovascular disease, because elevated COHb levels were known to stress the cardiovascular system. Moreover, methylene chloride was found to be stored in the body and metabolized later, maintaining COHb loadings for more than twice as long as was observed with carbon monoxide inhalation.

A series of articles investigated the effect of methylene chloride on the heart. Clark and Tinston (1973) examined cardiac sensitization to adrenaline; Reinhardt et al. (1973) found no cardiac arrhythmias in dogs because the dose that they were given produces anesthesia first; Aviado and Belej (1974) reported that methylene chloride both produces cardiac arrhythmias and sensitizes the heart to epinephrine; and Belej et al. (1974) suggested that the hazard of methylene chloride use is, therefore, increased in people with heart disease.

Then, in 1974, Ratney et al. proposed a lower threshold limit value standard for methylene chloride, so that COHb loading after methylene chloride exposure would not exceed those observed at maximum allowable CO concentrations. Because the standard for carbon monoxide also was being lowered at the time from 50 ppm to 35 ppm, it was suggested the target for methylene chloride should be 75 to 100 ppm, set to keep the COHb load below 5% after 8 hours in nonsmokers. Ratney et al. also pointed out that smokers start out with a load of 4.5%, and therefore this standard would not protect them.

By 1976 there was proof of the methylene chloride link to heart attacks in the case of an elderly man who had suffered three consecutive heart attacks while working with paint stripper (Stewart and Hake, 1976). Stewart and Hake took the Consumer Product Safety Commission, the Environmental Protection Agency, and paint-stripper manufacturers to task for not having corrected this problem since 1972 when the first discovery was made. Similar sentiments were expressed by Langehennig et al. (1976), who noted that apparently COHb loadings caused by methylene chloride caused the same anoxic symptoms but did not cause the same CO poisoning symptoms because CO from methylene chloride was not entering blood plasma.

The carboxyhemoglobin issue continued to dominate the medical literature on methylene chloride through the late 1970s with Benzon et al. (1978) and Fagin et al. (1980) reporting cases of occupational exposure related to high COHb loads, and Barrowcliff and Knell (1979) discussing the possible long-term effects of elevated COHb levels if alveolar exchange also is impaired, including brain damage, dementia, memory loss, difficulty speaking, and loss of coordination.

Other articles in the 1970s dealing with other aspects of methylene chloride toxicity include those by Weinstein et al. (1972), who revisited the issue of liver damage in mice with more powerful microscopy and found some liver damage, as well as mice developing tolerances for the chemical; Loyke (1973), who found that methylene chloride reduces high blood pressure in rats; and Ballantyne et al. (1976), who found corneal swelling, intraocular tension, and conjunctivitis as a result of splash contamination of the eyes.

In the late 1970s, studies began to show evidence of mutagenicity and cell transformation (Simmon et al., 1977; Price et al., 1978; Nestmann et al., 1981), and the National Toxicology Program (NTP) initiated a study to determine the carcinogenicity of methylene chloride (Nestmann et al., 1981).

Long-term occupational studies reported no health problems from long-term industrial exposure (Friedlander et al., 1978; Cherry et al., 1981). Wells and Waldron (1984) reported a case of severe skin burns from exposure to methylene chloride in an open vat.

Regulatory Activity

According to OSHA (*Federal Register*, 1997), the ACGIH responded in 1975 to the findings in the literature from 1972 through 1974 by lowering its recommended workplace standard to 100 ppm for the 8-hour time-weighted average. Otson et al. (1981), however, report that in 1979 the ACGIH adopted an 8-hour standard of 200 ppm with a notice of an intended change to 100 ppm. NIOSH (1976) concurred with this lowering and set its recommended standard at 75 ppm in 1976. These values reflect those recommended by Ratney et al. (1974) to keep the carboxyhemoglobin levels below what was then considered safe for direct exposure to carbon monoxide. OSHA did not change its standard at this time, leaving the 8-hour time weighted average at 500 ppm.

In 1978, in response to suggestions in the literature that methylene chloride might be carcinogenic, testing was recommended to determine several unknown possible effects of the chemical, including carcinogenicity, mutagenicity, teratogenicity, and other chronic effects (*Federal Register*, 1978). In 1981 a proposed test rule reiterated the need for these studies and laid out a plan for which agencies would perform the necessary tests (*Federal Register*, 1981).

Consumer Literature

In the 1970s, the consumer literature began to view methylene chloride more critically, and the general philosophy was articulated that "a chemical mixture potent enough to remove paint can also harm you" (*Consumer Reports*, 1972). A 1972 *Consumer Reports* article said,

> Paint removers are among the most dangerous products used in the home.... If indeed, there were a good, safe alternative to chemical paint removers, we wouldn't test such a dangerous product [methylene chloride].... Alas, there isn't an alternative that [Consumer's Union] believes people would readily turn to. (p. 147)

It is interesting to note the philosophy that Consumer's Union would not even test a product that it considered to be "dangerous" as long as alternatives were available. This approach seems to stay with *Consumer Reports* through the 1990s.

The 1972 article offers a comprehensive list of hazards from paint stripper from skin contact, eye contact, ingestion, and inhalation and recommends ventilation, gloves, goggles, and total coverage with clothing. Descriptions of health effects are vague in some places ("They can sicken with their noxious fumes") but direct in others ("If accidentally ingested, they can blind or kill"). The article still did not give as detailed a description about how to achieve good ventilation as in the 1950s, but it did recommend the use of a fan, and it was thorough in naming the broad range of potential health effects and general precautionary measures. *Consumer Reports* again offers much more detail than other publications of the time.

The popular press had differing reactions to the news about methylene chloride's link with heart attacks. *Science Digest* (1976) advised consumers to use paint strippers without methylene chloride, which it said were "hard to find." *Consumer Reports* (1976), on the other hand, gave explicit safety instructions advising good ventilation, including the use of a fan. It emphasized the risk to retired hobbyists, who were at greater risk for heart attacks. These articles focused directly on this one health effect of using methylene chloride but did not describe other effects.

In the mid-1970s, alternatives to chemical stripping were emerging with heat-based and mechanical tools to strip paint. The heat gun originally was considered quite dangerous because it used an open flame; the improved flameless heat gun, however, received rave reviews. "I'd have to rate it as one of the best paint removers I've ever used. The safety this tool gives, coupled with the fact that the substrate isn't scorched when the paint is burned off, has earned [it] a permanent niche in my toolbox" (Wicks, 1975).

Another invention was the rotary stripper, which was not accepted in the consumer literature as an effective tool because of the damage it caused to wood. "It is [our] opinion that a tool of this kind should never be used for cleaning the surfaces of fine furniture or veneer woods" (*Consumers' Research*, 1978).

These mechanical alternatives now were compared with chemical strippers in the consumer literature, placing them in the spotlight. In the 1960s, they had received only brief mention as an inferior method. In contrast, *Sunset* (1978) now offered a thorough discussion of different types of chemical strippers and reviewed two kinds of mechanical strippers as well (see Table 18.3). Users of methylene chloride were advised to ventilate, protect their skin with gloves specified by material type (i.e., neoprene), and be careful of flammability in some brands. Again these comparisons were not as thorough as the one from the 1940s, though several different options were covered in the article. The discussion of health effects in the article was spotty; for example, risks of lead dust were mentioned for rotary-stripper use but not for heat-gun use. Skin burns and toxic fumes were mentioned for the strippers containing only methylene chloride, but not for the acetone-mixture or water-rinse types.

Table 18.3 1970s comparison of paint stripper types

	Methylene chloride	Methylene chloride, water rinse	Methylene chloride, acetone	Heat gun	Rotary stripper
Performance	—	Dissolves glue	Less effective	Slower, but removes more layers	Gouges wood
	—	Raises wood grain	—	Must use Methylene chloride for last layer	Only works on flat or convex surfaces
Safety	Toxic fumes	—	—	—	—
	Skin burns	—	—	—	Lead dust
	Nonflammable	Flammable	Extremely flammable	—	—

Source: *Sunset*, 1978.

In the late 1970s and early 1980s a difference of views emerged over which chemical was safer for stripping paint, with a surprising return to lye as an option. Once viewed as the least safe alternative, lye was touted in a 1979 *Popular Mechanics* article as the home-grown solution to expensive chemical strippers. The article misrepresented safety concerns in its claims about alkali paint strippers, saying, "It's the same lye grandma used to make soap" (implying that if it was safe enough for grandma, then it is safe enough for the reader). It warned about the hazards of methylene chloride—"Most strippers contain methylene chloride and other solvents that force the manufacturer to put them in containers aglow with warning notices"—but made no mention of the warning labels on lye containers. "Lye has no toxic fumes. It's nonflammable, so it won't explode in your face if you get near a flame." Though this is true, it wrongly implies that methylene chloride would explode in your face if you get near a flame. As an afterthought, the author warns, "Do be careful not to splash it [lye] on your skin, though." Despite this warning, the article contains a photo (Fig. 18.6) with gloveless hands stirring lye over a hot stove, with a caption that reads, "Stir as you add lye; then get it piping hot."

Subsequently the article did mention lye's performance disadvantages such as killing grass, dissolving furniture glue, darkening wood, and raising the grain of the wood, but these did not weigh heavily in the product considerations.

A more balanced article from *Consumer Reports* (1982) described the safety concerns with paint strippers based on lye as follows: "They can burn eyes and skin irreparably, and they are harmful or lethal if swallowed. Using the products calls for goggles, gloves, and a dust mask to keep the powder out of your nose and throat." Though *Consumer Reports* carefully called for these protective measures, a *Popular Science* article (Scott, 1982) on lye advised only gloves.

Some articles of the time seemed to view lye strippers as safer than methylene chloride. It is important to note that this was before any studies

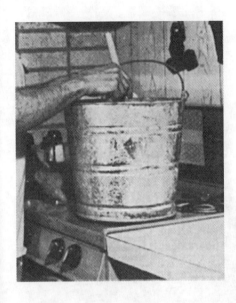

Figure 18.6 "Stir as you add lye. Then get it piping hot." Reprinted from *Popular Mechanics* (November, 1979). Copyright the Hearst Corporation. All rights reserved.

speculated about the cancer risk of methylene chloride. Somehow the perception of effectiveness also changed between the 1940s and 1950s and the 1980s. Though negative performance characteristics were described (bleaching wood, raising the grain of wood), they were not considered as problematic (relative to the safety benefits) as in the 1950s. *Consumer Reports* (1982) declared that the hazards of lye "are somewhat easier to deal with than those associated with solvent paint removers" and "because these alkalis don't create the noxious fumes that are typical of organic solvents, they would be better to use indoors."

Other articles in the late 1970s and early 1980s, however, continued to advocate the use of methylene chloride. A 1979 article in *Family Handyman* called methylene chloride the "key to safety" because of its fire-retardant properties. The article also contained warnings about heart attacks and stressed the importance of ventilation. Though the article advised users to wear gloves, the photos did not match the advice, as gloveless hands were shown painting, scraping, and hosing.

A 1983 article in *Popular Mechanics* offered perhaps the best-ever risk communication on methylene chloride in the consumer literature, providing a careful discussion of the potential health effects of methylene chloride and detailed safety instructions including the use of a fan and an air-supplied respirator. Consider Figure 18.7, which features a man donning goggles, gloves, a long-sleeved shirt, and an air-supplied respirator to strip paint. In fact, the article's title ("Paint Strippers: Beware the Hidden Hazard") demonstrates how safety has become a main focus. This article specifies the protective equipment one needs and not only advises the use of a fan but also explains in significant detail what kind of ventilation is required, including suggested air changes per hour and the minimum air delivery rating for an adequate exhaust fan. It

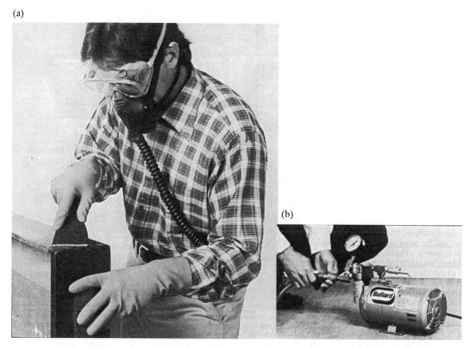

Figure 18.7 Outfitted for paint stripping: goggles and gloves (*A*) and respirator (*B*). Reprinted from *Popular Mechanics* (October, 1983). Copyright the Hearst Corporation. All rights reserved.

includes a thorough description of the health effects of methylene chloride (including "light-headedness, nausea, mental confusion and irritation of the eyes and respiratory tract. Methylene chloride also has been known to contribute to heart attacks."). This is the first time such a thorough discussion appeared in the consumer literature.

Few articles in the early 1980s focused on more than one way to strip paint, however. Whether they reviewed lye or methylene chloride, articles tended to consider only one product or one method for stripping paint and mention others only in passing as negative comparisons. This is quite different from articles in the 1940s and 1950s that thoroughly compared at least three different types of paint strippers across different performance and safety characteristics. Up to this point, cancer concerns associated with methylene chloride had not yet emerged and risk communication focused only on acute effects.

THE CANCER ERA: 1985–PRESENT

The concerns about methylene chloride greatly increased with research that showed a link to cancer.

Scientific Knowledge

The NTP study of methylene chloride initiated in the early 1980s was completed and reported in 1986, finding evidence of animal carcinogenicity and labeling methylene chloride a probable human carcinogen. Specifically, inhalation exposure increased prevalence of both malignant and benign tumors in mice and benign tumors in rats. The International Agency for Research on Cancer (1986) monographs reported, based on a review of the existing literature, that there was sufficient evidence for methylene chloride's carcinogenicity in animals and "inadequate evidence for carcinogenicity in humans." This evidence was based largely on the NTP report, because other studies cited by the agency involving drinking-water exposure (Serota et al., 1986a,b) and intraperitoneal injection (Theiss et al., 1977) were negative.

Data on occupational exposure in humans continued to be gathered; Hearne et al. (1987) reported no increased risk for ischemic heart disease, liver cancer, or lung cancer in workers exposed to methylene chloride and followed for as long as 30 years. Data did show increased incidence of pancreatic cancer among these workers (Mirer et al., 1988), but further reports with additional data (Hearne et al., 1990) made these observances not statistically significant. It is noted (International Programme on Chemical Safety, 1996) that these workers were all not permitted to smoke at work, which may have lowered the incidence rates compared with the general population, particularly for lung cancer and heart disease.

A 1983 study by Ott et al. evaluated long-term health effects in workers at a fiber production plant. Though there was no increase in mortality rate in the study, the authors did find a significant increase in the risk of ischemic heart disease among white men. Ott's study was not designed to evaluate cancer mortality, but a follow-up study (Lanes et al., 1990) reported a significant increase in biliary and liver cancer. A more recent follow-up (Lanes et al., 1993) reported no additional cancer deaths, but the increase was still significant with the new data. Gibbs (1992) reported on workers (who were not allowed to smoke at work) in a different fiber plant, finding increased rates of prostate cancer especially among men with high methylene chloride exposure (> 350 ppm), and increased rates of cervical cancer among women with low exposure to the chemical (50–100 ppm) (no dose–response relationship was found). Mortality rates from lung, biliary, liver, and pancreatic cancer were not found to be significant.

The proposed change in OSHA's 8-hour workplace standard from 500 ppm to 25 ppm raised some controversy in the scientific community. Some scientists argued that the new standard should be 50 ppm and that 25 ppm was unnecessarily low. Soden et al. (1996), for example, argued on the basis of elevated carboxyhemoglobin levels that 50 ppm was sufficient to prevent adverse effects in humans.

Regulatory Activity

In 1985 the release of the study by the NTP (1986) raised the question of methylene chloride's carcinogenicity and sparked several policy evaluations in government agencies. The CPSC reviewed methylene chloride's presence in paint strippers, spray paints, and adhesive removers. The Food and Drug Administration reviewed methylene chloride's presence in cosmetic aerosol products and decaffeinated coffee. OSHA began a review of its 40-year-old workplace standards.

In 1988 the ACGIH officially lowered its recommended 8-hour workplace standard to 50 ppm. At that time, OSHA considered adopting this standard; however, in the final rule (*Federal Register*, 1997), OSHA explains that it did not adopt this standard because "OSHA standards must eliminate significant risks to the extent feasible, whereas the ACGIH sets limits under which it is believed that nearly all workers may be repeatedly exposed day after day without adverse health effects." OSHA further points out that it is required to perform quantitative risk assessments and the ACGIH is not.

Food and Drug Administration. The Food and Drug Administration (FDA) risk assessment resulted in the removal of methylene chloride from aerosol cosmetics. This decision was strongly motivated by the predicted occupational exposure to beauty-industry workers; the estimated cancer risk was between 1 excess case in 1000 and 1 excess case in 100 as reported in Lecos (1986). The products were voluntarily removed from the market when the FDA proposed a ban of methylene chloride in hair spray in 1987, and the ban was made official in 1989 (*Federal Register*, 1989).

An article in *FDA Consumer* from 1986 (Lecos, 1986) that covers the FDA's activity on methylene chloride perpetuates misconceptions about how a consumer can protect him- or herself from the chemical. Figure 18.8 shows a hair stylist using hair spray and wearing a dust mask, as though the dust mask would protect him from the chemical.

The FDA also considered the risk to consumers of decaffeinated coffee, because methylene chloride is used in the decaffeination process and leaves a residue. By 1986, consumers were reported to be spending 30% to 40% more on water-decaffeinated coffee to avoid methylene chloride (Reed, 1986). But in 1986, the FDA allowed methylene chloride to stay in coffee after judging the worst case risk to be one cancer death in one million for a lifetime decaffeinated coffee drinker. This was the first application of the de minimis legal principle to the 1958 Delaney Clause of the Food Additives Amendment to the FDCA. The Delaney Clause stated that any food product shown to cause cancer in animals or humans would be considered unsafe, but the de minimis principle states that the law does not concern itself with trivial matters, so that if the cancer risk is "regarded as remote," a product may be considered safe (Lecos, 1986). Even *Consumer Reports* (1987) supported the FDA's decision not to ban, calling the controversy "much ado about nothing." Despite this, the fear of methylene

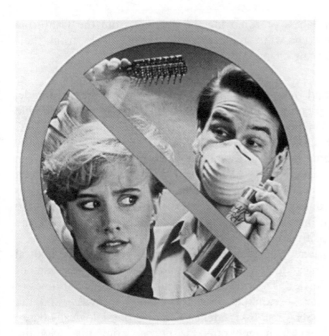

Figure 18.8 Protection from methylene chloride? Reprinted with permission from *FDA Consumer* magazine, copyright 1986.

chloride is still being used to sell water-decaffeinated coffee in 1997, with Starbucks offering both kinds of coffee and informational literature about the risks of methylene chloride.

CPSC. The CPSC's risk assessment for paint stripper in 1985 found three excess cancer cases per 1000 people using a worst-case assumption of people using paint stripper once a year from age 25 through 70 years (a 3-hour job in a closed work room). The consumer literature reported that this was the highest cancer risk the CPSC had ever calculated. A 1985 article from *Consumer Reports* showed that concern about methylene chloride had increased: "Several solvents used in consumer products are known or suspected carcinogens. One of the worst, and most commonly used, is methylene chloride."

The CPSC ruled methylene chloride a toxin to be regulated under the FHSA in 1987 and required labeling of all products with greater than 1% methylene chloride content (*Federal Register*, 1990).

There was a great deal of legislative and legal activity around methylene chloride in consumer products in the late 1980s and early 1990s. California passed Proposition 65, which listed a set of state-identified carcinogens that required labeling identifying them as such. In 1990 the Environmental Defense Fund and the Sierra Club sued several paint-stripper formulators under this law, calling their products "cancer in a can." Companies were given the choice of adding warnings to their labels or removing the product from the California market. Some companies chose to remove methylene chloride from their products altogether, and many changed their labels.

OSHA. OSHA's review and rule-making process spanned more than a decade, as initial studies led to a proposed rule in 1991 that sparked considerable controversy and a long comment period before the final rule in January 1997 (*Federal Register*, 1997). The rule proposed in 1991 (*Federal Register*, 1991) included a suggested 8-hour workplace standard of 25 ppm. The change from 500 ppm was long overdue, as groups like NIOSH and the ACGIH had been recommending figures in the 75 to 100 ppm range as early as the mid-1970s because of COHb-related risks. It is unclear why OSHA did not lower the standard in the 1970s, but once the possibility of carcinogenicity was raised, the debate and pressure intensified.

Discussions of methylene chloride's carcinogenicity, appropriate medical models, the economic impact of new standards, and OSHA's risk-assessment techniques became more heated. The rule making was reopened several times to allow for commentary from researchers, industry, small businesses, and the public. This was the first OSHA risk assessment to employ physiologically based pharmacokinetic modeling, which generated response from the scientific community. The haggling that ensued for the next 6 years was over whether the standard should be OSHA's suggested 25 ppm, or 50 ppm as recommended by many researchers and industry groups. Fifty parts per million is reportedly low enough to avoid adverse effects from COHb (Soden et al., 1996); this debate was focused on working through the possible cancer risks and associated uncertainties. OSHA submitted its final rule in 1997, setting the new 8-hour workplace standard at 25 ppm.

Consumer Literature

Despite all this activity in government agencies, consumer magazines continued to cover methylene chloride paint strippers and their alternatives.

In 1986 the last popular magazine article that we could find with detailed instructions for safe use of methylene chloride paint strippers was published (Williams, 1986). It reviewed the research on the carcinogenicity of methylene chloride and also discussed a case of an acute exposure in which a professional painter, using only air conditioning for ventilation, experienced numbness around her face and mouth and suffered persistent memory problems and permanent damage to her nervous system. The article warned people about the importance of ventilation, including the use and placement of a fan, advised frequent breaks, and warned against using dust masks as a means to reduce exposure.

In 1989 alternative chemical formulations began to appear on the market and in the consumer literature. Safest Stripper, by 3M, dominated the consumer literature in 1989, garnering rave reviews:

Look Ma, no gloves! Here's a revolutionary new paint stripper that's gentle to your hands, has almost no smell, and can't catch on fire. And yes, it really strips paint. (Collier, 1989)

It pours out looking like white frosting and emits no odors or fumes. Because it is nonflammable and contains no methylene chloride, you can use it indoors and you don't even have to wear gloves. (Lees, 1989)

[It's] nonflammable, it won't burn or irritate your skin and it emits no harmful fumes. It's so mild, you don't even need to wear gloves and it cleans up with water. (Capotosto, 1989)

Safety and performance were weighed against each other, viewed as competing qualities in the consumer literature that compared methylene chloride with alternative chemical strippers. In the 1940s and 1950s, methylene chloride seemed to outdo the other stripper alternatives in both safety and performance; it was not necessary to sacrifice one for the other. In 1991, however, a *Consumer Reports* article discussed safety and performance as trade-offs and landed squarely on the side of safety first. The article stated on the one hand that methylene chloride was versatile, able to dissolve a variety of tough finishes, and was not flammable, and that the new products were both "slow" and "expensive" by comparison. But these differences were considered small when "the safety factor [is] paramount." They recommended alternative strippers for all projects to be undertaken indoors and recommended professionals handle any projects that could be moved outdoors: "If you can carry the item to be stripped outdoors, you should keep going—all the way to a professional paint remover, who's likely to do a better job" (*Consumer Reports*, 1991). The same article article offered a thorough comparison of paint removers, including methylene chloride, safer formulations, and heat guns (see Table 18.4).

Table 18.4 1990s Comparison of paint stripper types

	Methylene chloride	"Kinder chemicals"	Heat gun
Performance	Less expensive	More expensive	Cheap after initial expense
	Fast	Slow, dries out	Fastest
	Wide range of finishes	—	Does not work on single layer, varnish, or metal
	Multiple applications	Multiple applications	Only go over an area once
Safety	Harmful vapors causes cancer, kidney disease, heart attack	No odor	Lead dust hazard
	Skin, eye damage	Less likely to irritate skin	Skin burns
	Nonflammable	Flammable	Fire hazard

Source: Consumer Reports, 1991.

Reviews of paint-stripping products focused on safer strippers in the 1990s. A 1992 *Consumer Reports* article did a comparative test of alkali strippers versus the new chemical formulations, and methylene chloride was not even discussed. Alkali strippers outperformed the alternative chemical formulations in this test. The alkali stripper was "fastest, easiest to use, and most effective," but it darkened the wood.

CONCLUSIONS

Tracing the historical path of preferences reflected in the consumer literature, a complete cycle of recommendations can be seen: Most recently, in the 1990s, alkalis have come out on top as the improved product over "safer strippers," which in the late 1980s were the improved product over methylene chloride, which in the 1950s was the improved product over benzol, which in the 1940s was the improved product over... alkalis. This confusion is further exacerbated by the fact that the tests presented in the consumer literature comparing the various alternatives have not always been comprehensive, with only a few types of paint stripper being examined. This means that product recommendations often have been made without full information about the complete set of alternatives. As we have demonstrated, much of the consumer literature would now be classified as incomplete based on the more recent scientific and medical findings. It should be noted, however, that the even the "best" information on the carcinogenicity of methylene chloride is controversial (Kaiser, 1996).

What is interesting is that despite methylene chloride's disappearance from the consumer literature, increased regulation, and negative exposure in the press, it is still very popular among consumers. The majority of strippers available on the shelf in a typical home improvement center contain methylene chloride. This is not to say that there have not been improvements in the competing products as well: consider the shift from the open flame to flameless heat gun, or the emergence of Peel Away, a lye-based paint remover that comes spread on strips of paper, reducing the risk of skin burns and eye splash injuries among users. To put the strength of consumers' preference for methylene chloride into perspective, in a 1995 article in *Chemical and Engineering News*, a marketing executive from Monsanto, makers of an alternative formulation of stripper, credits the regulation of methylene chloride for the success (albeit limited) of his products: "The government is my best salesman." This executive believes that without regulation, his products would not sell, because their performance is inferior. "Nothing is better than methylene chloride to strip paint."

The bottom line is that consumers still are buying methylene chloride products, despite its recent lack of recommendations (or even exposure) in the consumer literature. This leads to several questions: If consumers buy methylene chloride paint strippers, do they understand the associated risks and pathways of exposure? If they are aware of the risks, how great is their concern? What are the sources of their risk information? Do they take the necessary precautions to reduce their exposure? What actual exposure levels do consumers face when they strip paint? Are they at risk? Are there ways that risk communications can be targeted to better inform consumer decisions about paint stripper? If they are choosing methylene chloride over safer formulations, are they doing this with knowledge of the risks? Why is the recent consumer literature silent about methylene chloride paint strippers? Is this "silent approach" effective in reducing exposure levels? Future research needs to investigate the consumer's perspective of this problem. Only by answering these questions can effective regulations and risk-communication protocols be developed.

REFERENCES

Arrias, E. 1931. Narcosis "a la reine" with Solästhin. *Nederland. Tijdschr. Geneeskunde.* 75:3130–3132.
Aviado, D. M., and Belej, M. A. 1974. Toxicity of aerosol propellants on the respiratory and circulatory systems: I. Cardiac arrhythmia in the mouse. *Toxicology* 2:31–42.
Ballantyne, B., Gazzard, M. F., and Swanston, D. W. 1976. The ophthalmic toxicology of dichloromethane. *Toxicology* 6:173–187.
Barrowcliff, D. F., and Knell, A. J. 1979. Cerebral damage due to endogenous chronic carbon monoxide poisoning caused by exposure to methylene chloride. *J. Soc. Occup. Med.* 29:12–14.
Belej, M. A., Smith, D. G., and Aviado, D. M. 1974. Toxicity of aerosol propellants on the respiratory and circulatory systems: IV. Carditoxicity in the monkey. *Toxicology* 2:381–395.
Benzon, H. T., Claybon, L., and Brunner, E. A. 1978. Elevated carbon monoxide levels from exposure to methylene chloride. *JAMA* 239:2341.
Capotosto, R. 1989. Super safe paint stripper. *Popular Mechanics*, May:146.
Chemical and Engineering News. 1995. Methylene chloride hard to beat. Sept. 25:45.
Cherry, N., Venables, H., Waldron, H. A., and Wells, G. G. 1981. Some observations on workers exposed to methylene chloride. *Br. J. Indust. Med.* 38:351–355.
Clark, D. G., and Tinston, D. J. 1973. Correlation of the cardiac sensitizing potential of halogenated hydrocarbons with their physiochemical properties. *Br. J. Pharmacol.* 49:55–357.
Collier, H. 1936. Methylene dichloride intoxication in industry. *Lancet* i:594–595.
Collier, K. 1989. Safe stripper and more. *Family Handyman*, February:16.
Consumer Reports. 1961. Paint, varnish, and lacquer removers. 26:558–562.
Consumer Reports. 1972. Paint removers. 37:144–147.
Consumer Reports. 1976. Paint removers: The danger of heart attack. 41:434.
Consumer Reports. 1982. Powdered paint removers: An alternative to solvents. 47:333–334.
Consumer Reports. 1985. Indoor Air Pollution. 50:600–603.
Consumer Reports. 1987. Ground coffee. 52:527–533.
Consumer Reports. 1991. Paint removers: New products eliminate old hazards. 56:340–343.
Consumer Reports. 1992. Slow but safer chemicals to strip paint. 57:353.
Consumers' Research Bulletin. 1946. Paint, varnish, and shellac removers. 17:12–14.
Consumers' Research Magazine. 1978. Rotary paint strippers. 61:35.
Dingell, J. V., and Heimberg, M. 1968. The effects of aliphatic halogenated hydrocarbons on hepatic drug metabolism. *Biochem. Pharmacol.* 17:1269–1278.
Domanig, E. 1930. Modern methods of narcosis. *Wiener Klin. Wochschr.* 43:1026–1031.
Fagin, J., Bradley, J., and Williams, D. 1980. Carbon monoxide poisoning secondary to inhaling methylene chloride. *Br. Med. J.* 281:1461.
Federal Register. 1959. Exemption from requirement of tolerance for residues of methylene chloride. 24:5242.
Federal Register. 1961. Food additives. 26:2403–2404.

Federal Register. 1962. Interpretation with respect to warning, caution and antidote statement required to appear on labels of economic poisons. 27:2267–2277.
Federal Register. 1965. Food additives. 30:6.
Federal Register. 1967. Food additives. 32:12605.
Federal Register. 1969. Food additives. 34:13414.
Federal Register. 1978. Toxic substances control: Second report of the Interagency Testing Committee. 43:16684–16688.
Federal Register. 1989. Methylene chloride in consumer products. 55:32282.
Federal Register. 1991. Occupational exposure to methylene chloride: Proposed rule. 56:57036.
Federal Register. 1997. Occupational exposure to methylene chloride: Final rule. 62:1494.
Flinn, F. 1946. Industrial exposures to chlorinated hydrocarbons. *Am. J. Med.* 1:388–394.
Fowler, J. S. L. 1970. Chlorinated hydrocarbon toxicity in the fowl and duck. *J. Comp. Pathol.* 80:465–471.
Friedlander, B. R., Hearne, T., and Hall, S. 1978. Epidemiologic investigation of employees chronically exposed to methylene chloride. *J. Occup. Med.* 20:657–666.
Garner, R. C., and McLean, A. E. M. 1969. Increased susceptibility to carbon tetrachloride poisoning in the rat after pretreatment with oral phenobarbitone. *Biochem. Pharmacol.* 18:645–650.
Gerritsen, W. B., and Buschmann, C. H. 1960. Phosgene poisoning caused by the use of chemical paint removers containing methylene chloride in ill-ventilated rooms heated by kerosene stoves. *Br. J. Indust. Med.* 17:187–189.
Gibbs, G. W. 1992. The mortality of workers employed at a cellulose acetate and triacetate fibers plant in Cumberland, MD: A 1970 cohort followed, final report to Hoechst Celanese Corporation. Alberta: Hoechst Celanese.
Gladstone, B. 1951. What you should know about paint removers. *Popular Science*. 158:186–188.
Haan, E. R. 1956. Easier and safer paint removal. *Popular Mechanics*. 105:205–207.
Hahner, J. 1979. Paint removers: How to choose and use them. *Family Handyman*. 29:38–40.
Hand, A. J. 1966. Paint removal: How to do it right. *Popular Science*. 188:150–155.
Hearne, F. T., Grose, F, Pifer, J. W., Friedlander, B. R., and Raleigh, R. L. 1987. Methylene chloride mortality study: Dose-response characterization and animal model comparison. *J. Occup. Med.* 29:217–228.
Hearne, F. T., Pifer, J. W., and Grose, F. 1990. Absence of adverse mortality effects in workers exposed to methylene chloride: An update. *J. Occup. Med.* 32:234–240.
Heppel, L. A., Neal, P. A., Perrin, T. L., Orr, M. L., and Porterfield, V. T. 1944. Toxicology of dichloromethane (methylene chloride). *J. Indust. Hyg. Toxicol.* 26:8–16.
Hirsch, C. 1927. Solästhin narcosis in ear, nose, and throat surgery. *Deutsche Med. Wochschr.* 53:409–410.
Howard, S. J. 1967. Picking the right paint remover. *Popular Mechanics*. 128:164–166.
Hughes, J. P. 1954. Hazardous exposure to some so-called safe solvents. *JAMA* 156:234–237.
International Agency for Research on Cancer. 1986. *IARC monographs on the evaluation of the carcinogenic risk of chemicals to humans: Some halogenated hydrocarbons and pesticide exposures*, pp. 43–75. Lyon, France: Author.
International Programme on Chemical Safety. 1996. *Methylene chloride*. Geneva: World Health Organization.
Kaiser, J. 1996. New data help toxicologists home in on assessing risks. *Science* 272(5259):200.
Kirk-Othmer Encyclopedia of Chemical Technology. 1949. 1st ed., vol. 3, pp. 749–750.
Kirk-Othmer Encyclopedia of Chemical Technology. 1993. 4th ed., vol. 5, pp. 1041–1050.
Klaasen, C. D., and Plaa, G. L. 1966. Relative effects of various chlorinated hydrocarbons on liver and kidney function in mice. *Toxicol. Appl. Pharmacol.* 9:139–151.
Kutob, S. D., and Plaa, G. L. 1962b. A procedure for estimating the hepatotoxic potential of certain industrial solvents. *Toxicol. Appl. Pharmacol.* 4:354–361.
Kutob, S. D., and Plaa, G. L. 1962a. Assessment of liver function in mice with bromsulphalein. *J. Appl. Physiol.* 17:123–125.

Lanes, S. F., Cohen, A., Rothman, K. J., Dreyer, N. A., and Soden, K. J. 1990. Mortality of cellulose fiber production workers. *Scand. J. Work Environ. Health* 16:247–251.
Lanes, S. F., Rothman, K. J., Dreyer, N. A., and Soden, K. J. 1993. Mortality update of cellulose fiber production workers. *Scand. J. Work Environ. Health* 19:426–428.
Langehennig, P. L., Seeler, R. A., and Berman, E. 1976. Paint removers and carboxyhemoglobin. *N. Engl. J. Med.* 295:1137.
Lecos, C. 1986. Cancer, the law, and methylene chloride. *FDA Consumer* 20:15–17.
Lees, A. 1989. Super stripper. *Popular Science*. April:152.
Lehmann, K. B., and Fury, F. 1938. *Toxikologie und Hygiene der technischan Losungsmittel*. Berlin: Julius Springer Publishers.
Loyke, H. F. 1973. Methylene chloride and chronic renal hypertension. *Arch. Pathol.* 95:130–131.
Mirer, F. E., Silverstein, M., and Park, R. 1987. Metylene chloride and cancer of the pancreas. *J. Occup. Med.* 30:475–476.
Moskowitz, S., and Shapiro, H. 1952. Fatal exposure to methylene chloride vapor. *Arch. Indust. Hyg. Occup. Med.* 6:116–123.
National Institute for Occupational Safety and Health. 1976. *Criteria for a recommended standard: Occupational exposure to methylene chloride*, pp. 76–138. Washington, DC: U.S. Department of Health, Education, and Welfare.
National Toxicology Program. 1986. *Toxicology and carcinogenesis studies of dichloromethane (methylene chloride) in F344/N rats and B6C3F1 mice (inhalation studies)*. Technical report no. 306. Research Triangle Park, NC: U.S. Department of Health and Human Services.
Nestmann, E. R., Otson, R., Williams, D. T., and Kowbel, D. J. 1981. Mutagenicity of paint removers containing dichloromethane. *Cancer Lett.* 11:295–302.
Otson, R., Williams, D. T., and Bothwell, P. D. 1981. Dichloromethane levels in air after application of paint removers. *Am. Indust. Hyg. Assoc. J.* 42:56–60.
Ott, M. G., Skory, L. K., Holder, B. B., Bronson, J. M., and Williams, P. R., 1983. Health evaluation of employees occupationally exposed to methylene chloride. *Scand. J. Work Environ. Health* 9(suppl. 1):1–16.
Plaa, G. L., and Larson, R. E. 1965. Relative nephrotoxic properties of chlorinated methane, ethane, and ethylene derivatives in mice. *Toxicol. Appl. Pharmacol.* 7:37–44.
Price, P. J., Hassett, C. M., and Mansfield, J. I. 1978. Transforming activities of trichloroethylene and proposed industrial alternatives. *In Vitro* 14:290–293.
Ratney, R. S., Wegman, D. H., and Elkins, H. B. 1974. In vivo conversion of methylene chloride to carbon monoxide. *Arch. Environ. Health.* 28:223–226.
Reed, J. D. 1986. Coffees you can sleep on. *Money*. August:93–97.
Reinhardt, C. F., Mullin, L. S., and Maxfield, M. E. 1973. Epinephrine-induced cardiac arrhythmia potential of some common industrial solvents. *J. Occup. Med.* 15:953–955.
Reynolds, E. S., and Yee, A. G. 1967. Liver parenchymal cell injury: V. *Lab. Invest.* 16:591–603.
Rhine, C. 1979. How to make your own paint remover. *Popular Mechanics* 152:187–188.
Science Digest. 1976. Paint remover cardiacs. 79:22.
Scott, D. 1982. Peel-off paint stripper. *Popular Science* 220:114.
Serota, D. G., Thakur, A. K., Ulland, B. M., Kirschman, J. C., Brown, N. M., Coots, R. G., and Morgareidge, K. 1986a. A two-year drinking water study of dichloromethane on rodents: I. Rats. *Food Chem. Toxicol.* 24:951–958.
Serota, D. G., Thakur, A. K., Ulland, B. M., Kirschman, J. C., Brown, N. M., Coots, R. G., and Morgareidge, K. 1986b. A two-year drinking water study of dichloromethane on rodents: II. Mice. *Food Chem. Toxicol.* 24:959–963.
Simmon, V. F., Kauhanen, K, and Tardiff, R. G. 1977. Mutagenic activity of chemicals identified in drinking water. In *Progress in genetic toxicology*, eds. D. Scott, B. A. Bridges, and F. H. Sobels, pp. 249–258. Amsterdam: Elsevier/North-Holland Biomedical Press.
Soden, K. J., Marras, G., and Amsel, J. 1996. Carboxyhemoglobin levels in methylene chloride-exposed employees. *J. Occup. Environ. Med.* 38:367–371.
Stewart, R. D., and Hake, C.L. 1976. Paint-remover hazard. *JAMA* 235:398–401.

Stewart, R. D., Fischer, T. N., Hosko, M. J., Peterson, J. E., Baretta, E. D., and Dodd, H. C. 1972. Carboxyhemoglobin elevation after exposure to dichloromethane. *Science* 176:295–296.

Stewart, R. D., Fischer, T. N., Hosko, M. J., Peterson, J. E., Baretta, E. D., and Dodd, H. C. 1972. Experimental human exposure to methylene chloride. *Arch. Environ. Health* 25:342–348.

Sunset. 1978. When paint needs stripping: Chemicals or tools? 960:158–159.

Theiss, J. C., Stoner, G. D., Shimkin, M. B., and Weisburger, E. K. 1977. Test for carcinogenicity of organic contaminants of United Sates drinking waters by pulmonary tumor response in strain A mice. *Cancer Res.* 37:2717–2720.

Triuni, J. 1983. Paint strippers: Beware the hidden hazard. *Popular Mechanics* 160:65.

Weinstein, R. S., Boyd, D. D., and Back, K. C. 1972. Effects of continuous inhalation of dichloromethane in the mouse: Morphologic and functional observations. *Toxicol. Appl. Pharmacol.* 23:660–679.

Weiss, G. 1967. Toxic encephalosis as an occupational hazard with methylene chloride. *Zentralbl. Arbeitsmed.* 17:282–285.

Wells, G. G., and Waldron, H. A. 1984. Methylene chloride burns. *Br. J. Indust. Med.* 41:420.

Wicks, H., 1975. Flameless paint peeler. *Popular Mechanics.* 143:138.

Williams, G. III. 1986. Methylene chloride: Controversy cloaks a powerful stripper. *Home Mechanics.* Oct:85.

CHAPTER
NINETEEN

RISK ASSESSMENT AND RISK MANAGEMENT IN REGULATORY DECISION MAKING: RECOMMENDATIONS OF THE COMMISSION ON RISK ASSESSMENT AND RISK MANAGEMENT

Gail Charnley and the Members of the Commission on Risk Assessment and Risk Management

HealthRisk Strategies, Washington, DC

The Commission on Risk Assessment and Risk Management was mandated by Congress in the 1990 amendments to the Clean Air Act. The commission was asked to address risks that are regulated under the many laws aimed at protecting the environment and the health and safety of the American people from potentially dangerous exposures to chemicals and other hazardous substances in air, water, food, the workplace, and consumer products. Of the 10 members of the risk commission, six were appointed by the majority and minority leaders of the House and Senate, three by the president, and one by the president of the National Academy of Sciences.

The commission's mandate is summarized in the following phrases:

- Assess uses and limitations of risk assessment
- Evaluate exposure scenarios used to characterize current or potential risks
- Determine how to describe and explain uncertainties
- Enhance strategies for risk-based management decisions
- Review desirability of consistency across Federal programs

Gail Charnley was formerly Executive Director, Commission on Risk Assessment and Risk Management.

Members of the Commission on Risk Assessment and Risk Management were Gilbert S. Omenn (chair), University of Michigan; Alan C. Kessler (vice-chair), Buchanan Ingersoll; Norman T. Anderson, American Lung Association; Peter Y. Chiu, Kaiser Permanente and Stanford University Medical School; John Doull, University of Kansas Medical Center; Bernard D. Goldstein, Environmental and Occupational Health Sciences Institute; Joshua Lederberg, Rockefeller University; Sheila M. McGuire, Iowa Health Research Institute; David Rall, formerly of the National Institute of Environmental Health Sciences; and Virginia V. Weldon, Monsanto Company.

In addition to its legislative mandate, the commission was asked by both Congress and the Administration to evaluate the appropriate roles of peer review, economic analysis, and judicial review in risk-management decision making.

The commission's two-volume final report was released in early 1997. Volume 1 focuses exclusively on the characteristics and implementation of the commission's framework for environmental health risk management, launching a major new era in environmental and health protection. We are hopeful that this framework will achieve common usage, becoming for risk management what the National Academy of Sciences' "Red Book" framework was for risk assessment more than a decade ago. Our framework puts particular risks in public health and ecologic context, involves stakeholders from the earliest stages, and moves beyond the one-chemical, one-risk, medium-by-medium approach of most current regulation. Volume 2 addresses ways to improve risk communication and risk management, provides guidance on how to approach risk assessment, provides complementary guidance for analysis of the options and costs of potential risk reduction actions, makes recommendations about the roles of peer review and of judicial review in risk assessment and risk management, and provides recommendations for specific federal regulatory agencies and programs. The report's executive summary is provided here. The final report can be obtained from the commission's home page on the Internet at http://www.riskworld.com or ordered from the Government Printing Office by calling (202) 512-1800 and asking for document #055-000-00567-2 (Volume 1, $6.00) or #055-000-00568-1 (Volume 2, $ 19.00).

RISK COMMISSION REPORT EXECUTIVE SUMMARY

Public opinion polls have consistently shown strong support throughout the United States for effective environmental stewardship and for identifying and addressing risks to the environment, public health, and worker health. At the same time, many citizens and local officials are demanding greater attention to priorities and costs. There is an emerging national vision of sustainable development for our environment, our economy, and our society, which this commission shares. Regulatory agencies, businesses, environmental and public health advocates, and communities deserve credit for well-documented gains in air quality, water quality, habitat protection, worker health and safety, product safety, waste disposal, recycling, and pollution prevention achieved over the past 25 years. The commission values and seeks to sustain such gains. Our findings and recommendations reflect an increasing need to recognize and capitalize on lessons learned and our intent to stimulate even more effective, more efficient, risk-based means of protecting public health and the environment.

The Commission on Risk Assessment and Risk Management was mandated by Congress in the Clean Air Act Amendments of 1990 "to make a full investigation of the policy implications and appropriate uses of risk assessment and risk management in regulatory programs under various Federal laws to prevent cancer and other chronic human health effects which may result from exposure to hazardous substances." The Commission began meeting in May 1994 and held hearings across the country, obtaining information and insights that made important contributions to our deliberations and to our findings and recommendations. We issued a draft report for public review and comment in June 1996 and introduced a framework for making risk-management decisions. Based on the 130 formal comments that we received, on comments made at public meetings and scientific meetings, and on numerous informal discussions with stakeholders, we refined our recommendations to produce this final report to Congress and the President of the United States. Volume 1 of our two-volume final report focuses solely on our risk-management framework and its implementation. It is a reader-friendly document explaining the framework, the process of putting problems in public health context, and the strategies that can be used to stimulate effective stakeholder involvement. It has many real-world examples.

In volume 2 we have revised the entire draft report to update our findings. We make recommendations about the uses and limitations of risk assessment, economic analysis, risk management, and regulatory decision making, and we address selected activities of specific regulatory agencies and programs.

A New Risk-management Framework

The Commission has adopted a unique risk-management perspective to guide investments of precious public-sector and private-sector resources in risk-related research, risk assessment, risk characterization, and risk reduction. We recognize that it is time to modify the traditional approaches to assessing and reducing risks that have relied on a chemical-by-chemical, medium-by-medium, risk-by-risk strategy. Although risk assessment has been growing more complex and sophisticated, the output of risk assessment for the regulatory process often seems too focused on refining assumption-laden mathematic estimates of small risks associated with exposure to individual chemicals rather than on the overall goal: risk reduction and improved health status. Scientists, federal agencies, the National Academy of Sciences and National Research Council, and many other organizations have issued many reports with recommendations for improving health-risk assessment. Despite many years of managing risks, however, there have been few systematic attempts to examine the role of risk assessment itself in risk management and health and environmental protection. No generally accepted framework or principles for making risk-management decisions has emerged.

We propose a systematic, comprehensive framework that can address various contaminants, media, and sources of exposure, as well as public values, perceptions, and ethics, and that keeps the focus on the risk management goal. The new risk-management framework comprises six stages (see Fig. 19.1):

- Formulate the problem in broad context
- Analyze the risks
- Define the options

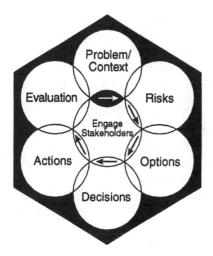

Figure 19.1 The commission's risk-management framework.

- Make sound decisions
- Take actions to implement the decisions
- Perform an evaluation of the effectiveness of the actions taken

The framework explicitly embraces collaborative and early involvement of stakeholders; the process can be refined and its conclusions can be changed as important new information is acquired. The framework requires that a potential or current problem be put into a broader context of public health or environmental health and that the interdependence of related multimedia problems be identified. The framework focuses on cumulative risks to human and environmental health and on addressing the benefits, costs, and social, cultural, ethical, political, and legal dimensions of risk reduction options. Our framework is described in great detail in volume 1.

The commission's framework can help to improve the cumbersome, fragmented risk-management approach often used by the Federal regulatory agencies—an approach that resulted from the patchwork of Congressional statutes that have been enacted over the past 25 years to address individual risks. Coordination within and among agencies and among Congressional committees and subcommittees can advance the more comprehensive proposed framework without a new, overarching environmental statute. When individual environmental statutes are reauthorized, they can be modified to reflect the comprehensive nature of the framework. The framework is also applicable to risk-management activities carried out by public and private entities at the state, regional, and local levels and through Federal/state performance partnerships. Despite potential obstacles, we believe that implementation of this framework will enable the country to manage risks more effectively and more efficiently and to make progress toward the goal of sustainable development.

Risk Management and Regulatory Decision Making

Risk managers use information from risk assessment and economic analysis, together with information about public values and statutory requirements, to make decisions about the need for and methods of risk reduction. The wide array of statutes and their implementing regulations have resulted in different definitions of negligible and unacceptable risk.

Improvement of Risk Communication. In communicating with various audiences about risks, risk assessors and risk managers must seek a two-way interaction, learning about patterns of exposure, gaining an understanding of the different perceptions people have of what is a negligible risk and what is an unacceptable risk, and describing risks and uncertainties openly and understandably. Relying on overly precise single estimates of risk is unjustified.

We support the use of comparisons of specific risks related to a proposed action. Such comparisons are most understandable and helpful if they involve chemically related agents, different sources of exposure to the same agents, different agents to which humans might be exposed in similar ways, and different agents that produce similar effects. Such context can help all stakeholders, including risk assessors, to understand the potential benefit of reducing exposures to an agent. We recommend that such risks be expressed in terms of potential adverse effects per year in a given community or exposed population, as well as per hypothetical lifetime.

We also recommend the identification and evaluation of a common metric to assist comparative risk assessment and risk communication related to both carcinogens and noncarcinogens. We have moved this recommendation from the toxicity-assessment section to the risk-communications section of the final report.

Bright Lines. *Bright lines* are specific exposure concentrations that are meant to provide a clear distinction between what is considered safe and what is not. Bright lines can be useful as guideposts or goals for decision making but should not be applied inflexibly, because of uncertainty about risks and variation in susceptibility. We support the use of sets of bright lines to protect both the general population and specific populations potentially at higher risk, such as children and pregnant women. We recommend that Congress not legislate particular bright lines. In response to comments, we have clarified the differences between bright lines for measurable emissions, exposures, and contaminant concentrations and attempts to use bright lines for estimated low levels of probabilistic risks, which cannot be measured.

Standards for Judicial Review. We recommend that judicial review be limited, as now, to final agency action, and that the existing arbitrary-and-capricious standard be retained.

Uses and Limitations of Risk Assessment

The commission considers risk assessment a useful analytic process that provides valuable contributions to risk management, public health, and environmental policy decisions. Risk assessment was developed because Congress, regulators, and the public require scientists to go beyond scientific observations of the relationships between exposures to chemicals and pollutants and their effects on people, the environment, or test systems, and to rely on many scientific inferences and assumptions to answer social questions about what is unsafe. Sophisticated and complex risk assessments, however, cannot substitute for basic knowledge about the chemical's toxicity to humans. We recommend that the performance of risk assessments be guided by an understanding of the issues that are important to manager's decisions and to the public's understanding of what is needed to protect public health and the environment.

Use of Scientific Advances in Toxicity Assessments. The commission recognizes that important advances are being made in the scientific basis for risk assessment. Further developments will improve the recognition and estimation of risks to humans associated with chemical and other exposures in the environment and provide biologic markers for measuring exposure, early effects, and variation in susceptibility. We recommend the use of all relevant peer-reviewed information about a chemical's mode of action in evaluating the weight of the scientific evidence supporting its toxicity in humans. We support current agency efforts to distinguish more clearly between experimental findings in rodent or other bioassays that are predictive for humans and findings that are not. We recognize that risks for microbial and radiation exposures, not just chemical exposures, need to be addressed.

Use of Realistic Scenarios in Exposure Assessments. The commission supports basing risk-management decisions on exposure assessments derived from realistic scenarios. Agencies should continue to move away from using the hypothetical "maximally exposed individual" to evaluate whether a risk exists, toward more realistic assumptions based on available scientific data, as they have done in recent analyses. We recommend use of analytic methods that, if data permit, combine the many characteristics of probable exposure into an assessment of the overall population's exposures. If possible, exposure assessments should include information about specific groups, such as infants, children, pregnant women, low-income groups, and minority-group communities with exposures influenced by particular cultural or social practices. Stakeholders can provide information about patterns and sources of exposure that otherwise might be neglected.

Recognition of Risk Associated with Chemical Mixtures. We agree with testimony that we need data and risk estimates about chemical mixtures and combined chemical–microbe–radiation exposures, because people are exposed to multiple hazards. We recommend direct toxicity assays of environmental mixtures.

Uses and Limitations of Economic Analysis

The commission supports the use of economic analysis as a consideration, but not as the overriding determinant of risk-management decisions. Both human health and ecologic benefits should be accounted for when the consequences of actions to reduce emissions, exposures, and risks are being evaluated. We call for explicit descriptions of the assumptions, data sources, sources of uncertainty, and distributions of benefits and costs across society associated with economic analyses, in parallel with the descriptions associated with risk assessments.

The Role of Peer Review

We support efficient use of peer review, with care to exclude financial conflicts, for both risk assessment and economic analysis. Overall quality and effectiveness of peer-review practices should be evaluated periodically by the agencies. We urge Congress to match resources to its demands on agencies for research, risk assessment, and economic analysis and to allow the agencies considerable discretion in allocating resources for peer review.

Recommendations for Agencies

The commission developed findings and recommendations about several Federal agencies and programs in order to illustrate our general recommendations, address inconsistencies, and assist Congress and the agencies on particular matters. As agencies begin to comply with the Government Performance and Results Act of 1993, these recommendations may be helpful in identifying performance indicators.

Environmental Protection Agency. In the 1990 amendments to the Clean Air Act, Congress mandated that this commission review and make recommendations on the analysis and management of residual risk associated with section 112 hazardous air pollutants after the completion of the current technology-based risk-reduction program. We present a tiered approach to set priorities for this huge effort and emphasize the critical need for more and better emissions and exposure data before meaningful analyses are possible. We recommend that residual risks associated with hazardous air pollutants be considered in the context of risks associated with the same pollutants from other sources, in the context of other air pollutants, and in the context of other risks to health. We have clarified the tiered scheme presented in the draft report.

We recommend more frequent determinations of future land use at the start of Superfund site risk assessments, and we endorse a comprehensive watershed management approach to managing risks under the Clean Water Act.

We are pleased that our recommendations were accommodated in the 1996 Safe Drinking Water Act.

Occupational Safety and Health Administration. We recommend establishing guidelines for agency risk assessments and a streamlined process for developing permissible exposure limits for air contaminants in the workplace. We also endorse greater cooperation between the Occupational Safety and Health Administration and the National Institute for Occupational Safety and Health.

Food and Drug Administration. We recommend a substantial modification of the "Delaney Clause" to a standard of reasonable certainty of no harm of all population groups, as was enacted in the Food Quality Protection Act of 1996. We endorse international harmonization of risk assessment and clinical trial protocols for pharmaceuticals, and restoration of the Food and Drug Administration's authority to require scientific evidence supporting health claims for dietary supplements.

Department of Agriculture. We recommend that risk assessment and benefit–cost analysis be performed early in the rule-making process instead of at the decision stage for both microbial and chemical hazards.

Department of Energy and Department of Defense. We support further development and evaluation of risk-based approaches to priority setting and budget making for cleanup of contaminated sites at Federal facilities.

Conclusion

After the final report was released, the commission remained active until September 1997 to assist the Congress, the Administration, and various other interested parties in considering these recommendations and finding common ground with relevant proposals from others. The commission believes that our risk-management framework will prove to be far more useful and effective than traditional regulatory approaches to solving common multimedia risk problems and, along with the other recommendations in our final report, will help improve risk-management decision making as we tackle the problems of the 21st century.

CHAPTER
TWENTY

RISK ASSESSMENT AND RISK MANAGEMENT: PATHWAYS TOWARD PROCESS ENHANCEMENT

Eugene J. Olajos and Harry Salem

U.S. Army Edgewood Chemical and Biological Center, Aberdeen Proving Ground, Maryland

The theme of this chapter is that synergy between the scientific and regulatory communities, the integration of pacing and cutting-edge technologies, and clearly articulated regulatory goals can greatly enhance risk-assessment and risk-management processes. Traditionally, health-risk assessment was based on experimental data, a system of safety factors, probabilistic evaluation, and judgmental evaluation. This process evolved as a more quantitative process exploiting mathematic models for extrapolation, mechanistic studies, refinement in analytic methodology (e.g., dose–response and dosimetry models), and weight-of-evidence criteria. Currently, the trend is toward a multisource, multimedia, multichemical, and multirisk context—as recently advocated by the Presidential/Congressional Commission on Risk Assessment and Risk Management (1997). As stated in that report, the risk paradigm must go "beyond the narrow context that considers just one chemical, one environmental medium, one risk at a time." Health-risk assessment is but one area of risk assessment, which predicts the likelihood of unwanted effects. It is a multifaceted process comprising the input of scientific, social, political, and economic issues that forms the basis of informed regulatory decisions and risk management. The ultimate goal is to make realistically achievable a comprehensive risk assessment (of single or aggregate risks). Despite inroads in viewing the risk-assessment process as integrative and multidisciplinary, with perspectives from both the scientific and nonscientific communities, the prevailing view in health-risk assessment is that scientific issues often play a predominant role. Consequently, this places the challenge on the scientific community to continually improve the risk-assessment paradigm through innovative concepts and the utilization of

---

The views of the authors do not purport to reflect the position of the Department of Defense. The use of trade names does not constitute an official endorsement or approval of the use of such commercial hardware or software.

emerging or pacing technologies. The challenge is also on the regulatory communities in their role in the facilitation and acceptance of new scientific methods, which assures continuity in the process from conceptualization to acceptance and continued progress in risk assessment. Relatively recently, regulatory decisions were complicated in part by the necessity of predicting future technologic progress. This could continue to be a burden in future regulatory decision making and risk assessments, unless there is incorporation of validated cutting-edge and pacing technologies in a more timely manner. There is no question that the inclusion of cutting-edge technologies is one of several ways in which a more transparently derived regulatory decision can be attained.

Among the various scientific disciplines involved in health-risk assessment, toxicology has an integral role. The toxicology community and allied health sciences, through basic and applied research, develop data on chemical agents that the regulatory community must assess in terms of potential adverse (unwanted) health effects to the human population or subpopulations. The assessment of toxicological data, as a basis for predicting health risks from chemical exposures, is not of recent origin (Weil, 1972) and closely parallels the U.S. Environmental Protection Agency (EPA), Occupational Safety and Health Administration, and Food and Drug Administration developments in risk assessment. This is not altogether surprising, because major impetus for conducting risk assessments originates from Federal legislation. Over the years, the assessments have improved because of the incorporation and use of new techniques in assessment. Examples include low-dose extrapolation models coupled with advances in scientific methodologies (i.e., biomarkers of sufficient sensitivity and specificity to assess subtle toxicant-induced effects), modeling techniques (e.g., physiologically based pharmacokinetic modeling, uptake models of absorption), improved dosimetry (e.g., macromolecular adducts, dosimetry modeling), mechanistic approaches, improved analytic measures of exposure, and improved exposure-assessment techniques (i.e., biomarker technology). The use of improved exposure assessments and low-dose extrapolation models in itself has greatly impacted the risk-assessment process—thus, since the 1980s occupational health standards and environmental regulations have been based on the results of low-dose extrapolation models and exposure assessments (Munro and Krewski, 1981; Rodricks et al., 1987). Risk-assessment methods have been used to set standards for environmental pollutants, workplace exposures, pharmaceuticals, food additives, pesticide residues, contaminants in consumer products, drinking-water standards, and ambient air standards. As a final introductory note, one cannot help but notice that a number of initiatives and drivers from within and outside the scientific and regulatory communities has led to novel approaches as well as enhancements and improvements in the risk-assessment process. Many of these are listed here:

1. Need to reduce the uncertainty in risk assessment
2. Need for greater degree of quantification
3. Need to focus away from single issues
4. Need for greater emphasis on noncancer endpoints

5. Need to develop databases on environmentally relevant exposures
6. Need to develop databases on multiple pathways/multiple exposures/ chemical mixtures
7. Need to focus on long-term low-level exposure
8. Need for harmonization and linkage
9. Socioeconomic and political demands
10. Need to increase public trust and confidence in risk assessment and risk prediction

RISK MANAGEMENT

Risk management is one of two distinct elements in the regulatory process, the other being risk assessment (National Academy of Sciences, 1983). Risk management is not a scientific process per se; however, in practice there is a considerable gray area between the processes of risk assessment and risk management. It is that part of the regulatory process that invokes the evaluation of a wide range of factors (risk-assessment outcome, extrascientific factors, socioeconomic issues, and political aspects) to ultimately protect human health and assure environmental quality. Hallenbeck (1986) defined risk management in the following terms: "Risk management refers to the selection and implementation of the most appropriate regulatory action based upon the results of risk assessment, available control technology, costs, benefit analysis, acceptable risk, acceptable number of cases, policy analysis, and social and political factors." This description is relevant and applicable today because it draws attention to the complexity, breath, and scope of the process. A contemporary definition of risk management by the Presidential/Congressional Commission on Risk Assessment and Risk Management (1997) is as follows: "Risk management is the process of identifying, evaluating, selecting, and implementing actions to reduce risk to human health and ecosystems." The conceptual steps in hazard management as described by Lave nearly 20 years ago (Lave, 1982) are essentially still valid today. The focus was on hazard identification and risk assessment, and contemporary concerns still gravitate to these two processes. With regard to regulatory decision making, Lave identified four steps toward improving the regulatory decision: (1) clarification of an agency's goals, (2) improving scientific information, (3) structuring the decision process such that the data are correctly interpreted, and (4) exploring and pursuing alternatives. Again, these are as relevant today as they were nearly two decades ago. The components of risk management and its relationship to risk assessment have been described (National Academy of Sciences, 1994).

RISK ASSESSMENT

Risk assessment is a scientific process that characterizes risk and assesses the likelihood of its occurrence. In his overview on the practice of health risk assessment, Paustenbach (1995) stressed the criticality of quantitative risk assessment and the ongoing need for improvements in the risk-assessment process, with outcomes that address public concerns regarding adverse and unwanted health effects. Physiologically based pharmacokinetics, low-dose extrapolation modeling, and the weight-of-evidence approach are illustrative of high-profile advances that represented important refinements in the risk-assessment process and are now mainstream processes in risk assessment. In addition to the previously mentioned developments, ongoing efforts focus on the development and application of emerging concepts and new or refined techniques related to biomarker methodologies, statistical modeling, mixtures assessment, and hormesis as tools in improving the risk-assessment paradigm. These are discussed in greater detail elsewhere in this book and in this chapter. Risk assessment (for some synonymous with quantitative risk assessment) is the characterization of potential deleterious health effects of human exposure to chemical, biologic, and physical stressors. It has been practiced in the United States and other industrialized nations for nearly 20 years and is the framework for most environmental and many occupational health regulations in the United States and abroad. Contemporary health risk assessment processes have their origins most notably within the Food and Drug Administration and the EPA and are integral parts of Federal and state regulatory activities and legislation. Approaches to risk assessment have varied and are best described in wording by the National Academy of Sciences (NAS) (1983) as follows: "The different structures, procedures, and histories of the agencies responsible for regulating toxic substances have produced diversity in their approaches to risk assessment but common patterns can be discerned." There has been a considerable degree of intra- and interagency activity directed at establishing guidelines for risk assessment. The EPA and European Economic Community have published risk-assessment guidelines for cancer and noncancer endpoints (U.S. EPA, 1984, 1986a,b, 1988a,b, 1994a,b, 1996; EEC, 1994).

Conceptually, health-risk assessment is a process wherein toxicologic information compiled from human and animal studies as well as epidemiologic findings are integrated with exposure data to quantitatively predict the likelihood that an adverse effect (response) will be noted in some human subpopulation (NAS, 1994). The presidential commission defined risk assessment as "an organized process used to describe and estimate the likelihood of adverse health outcomes from environmental exposure to chemicals" (Presidential Commission, 1997). To more fully understand the approaches and techniques involved in enhancing the risk-assessment process, one needs to outline the steps in the risk assessment process, initially described by the NAS (1983). The risk-assessment paradigm consists of hazard identification, dose–response assessment, exposure assessment, and risk characterization. One needs to define these various steps. The following definitions are those that appeared in a 1993 Center for Risk Analysis publication entitled *Risk Assessment in the Federal Government: Questions and Answers*:

Hazard identification is the qualitative process of determining whether an agent might pose a threat to human health.

Exposure assessment is the process of determining the magnitude and duration of human exposures to the agent in a defined population.

Dose–reponse evaluation is the process of using the existing toxicity information from human or animal studies to identify risks at various dose levels.

Risk characterization is the process of combining information about hazard, exposure, and dose–response in a way that effectively communicates the nature and the magnitude of the risk.

HAZARD IDENTIFICATION

Hazard identification involves an evaluation of available data to determine whether or not there is a causal relationship between exposure to compound and certain adverse (unwanted) health effects. In dealing with noncancer endpoints, an important aspect of hazard identification is the characterization of the spectrum of treatment-related effects (primary and secondary effects).

EXPOSURE ASSESSMENT

Exposure assessment is an integral part of the risk-assessment process that links chemical exposure to toxicologic manifestation or disease outcome. It is a process that addresses the probability of uptake from the environment by any combination of oral, inhalation, and dermal routes of exposure, and EPA guidelines for estimating exposures have been developed (U.S. EPA, 1986c, 1992). Exposure assessment, as defined by Fowle (1989), is "the process of measuring or estimating the magnitude, frequency, duration, and route of contact with a chemical or physical agent in the environment." There are many factors (e.g., route, duration of exposure, intermittent versus continuous exposure, target populations, sensitive subpopulations) to be considered. The complexities increase if one goes beyond the context of a one environmental medium–one chemical–one exposure route to a multichemical–multipathway context (see Preuss and Ehrlich, 1987). Fowle (1989) categorized exposure-assessment methodologies into three categories: direct (actual measurement of xenobiotics), predictive (measures of ambient exposure and mathematic modeling), and reconstructive (body burden of xenobiotic and biomarkers). More recently, Simonsen et al. (1996) have highlighted the multiplicity of approaches utilized in estimating the exposure or the actual dose acquired. Estimates can be obtained directly by biologic monitoring or indirectly by use of models for source release, for exposure, and for uptake (physiologically based toxicokinetic models for toxic effects are promising tools in this context [Anderson, 1989; Conolly, 1990]). Exposure assessment is a two-fold process consisting of exposure-estimate development and characterization of the "interface" of that estimate with human populations to attain an appropriate perspective concerning the significance of potential exposures (Cote et al., 1994). An exposure assessment relies on a combination of monitoring data on the target pollutant (in one or more environmental media) and on environmental fate data or assumptions. The exposure estimate is linked to available epidemiologic data and extrapolations from animal data to characterize the risk or hazard (risk characterization) to obtain a meaningful perspective regarding the significance of an exposure. Characterization of the interface with human populations, the second step in the process, provides an estimation of the extent of human exposure. There are uncertainties in the exposure-assessment process —the lack of human exposure data is the most notable reason for the uncertainty in exposure assessment. Of the various approaches to improving the science and utility of exposure assessment, the approaches considered the most promising are highlighted: advances in exposure marker methodologies (biomarkers) and advances in uptake models and dosimetry.

DOSE–RESPONSE EVALUATION

The dose–response assessment component of the risk-assessment process involves the quantitative relationship between exposure and the occurrence of health effects. It requires an extrapolation from high-dose animal exposures to exposures expected from human contact with a chemical in an occupational or environmental setting. The principal approaches in dose–response assessment include the safety (uncertainty-factor) approach and the mathematic modeling approach. Improvements in both of these areas of risk assessment have provided a more scientific basis for the risk-assessment process, with outcomes producing a risk assessment with greater predictability and less uncertainty. Salient advances in the dose–response evaluation component of risk assessment are highlighted.

RISK CHARACTERIZATION

Risk characterization is the summary and interpretation of the information collected. It identifies limitations in databases and data sets and uncertainties. It is the final step in the risk-assessment process. Results of the dose–response assessment are combined with the result of the exposure assessment to obtain a quantitative estimate of risk, which compares the estimated level of risk with the acceptable level.

BIOMARKERS AND HEALTH-RISK ASSESSMENT
Biomarkers: General Overview

One area that has generated immense interest and research activity in the toxicology and risk-assessment communities is that of biomarkers. This heightened activity is based on a multiplicity of factors: (1) the fact that current environmental protection strategies are all too often inadequate, (2) the need for detecting early adverse effects of toxicants or pollutants, (3) the need to relate biomarker response to a particular degree of altered physiology, (4) the need to address insidious long-term pollutant effects, (5) the notion that biomarkers can provide an integrated view of health status, and (6) the utility of biomarkers as predictors of higher-level effects. Numerous biomarkers have been developed and utilized successfully to quantify toxicant-induced changes in biochemical processes and pathways, physiologic functions, and structure or morphology in the laboratory (Fig. 20.1). Biomarkers augment current strategies (e.g., conventional toxicity tests, structure–activity relationships approach). Furthermore, biomarkers are powerful tools for detecting and documenting exposure to and effects of chemical exposure in the occupational or environmental settings. The applications of biomarkers in the various components of risk assessment have included hazard identification, exposure assessment/biomonitoring, dose–reponse assessment, high- to low-dose extrapolation, animal to human extrapolation, and biologic variability in response. There is no question that contemporary biomarker approaches have the potential to greatly enhance the health-risk assessment of chemical, biologic, and physical stressors. Paramount among the challenges facing the scientific and regulatory communities is their integration into the current test paradigms and their practical application to the risk-assessment process. Additional concerns associated with the research and application of biomarkers are (1) the establishment of biochemical and physiologic "norms"; (2) defining biomarker variability; and (3) careful evaluation, validation, and proper use. Contemporary biomarker approaches represent the scientific community's endeavor to utilize "tiered" biomarker assays, to establish linkage between various biomarkers, to improve the sensitivity and specificity of the measures, and to recognize their emerging importance in regulatory decision and policy making. An indicator of the latter is the incorporation of the biomarker concept into regulatory guidelines (i.e., the EPA [1996] guideline on carcinogen risk assessment). The greatest future utility of biomarkers may be in quantification of effects and the fact that biomarkers provide an integrated view of health status.

The notion of measuring a biologic parameter as an indicator of the physiologic state, health status, or well-being of an organism is well established. Biomarkers are used extensively in medicine, in the evaluation of occupational health risks, and as previously indicated as a tool for environmental protection. Biomarker approaches potentially are applicable over a broad range of species —more importantly over the entire range of biologic organization from molecular to community levels (see Fig. 20.2). Broadly defined, biomarkers are indicators signaling events in biologic systems. The definition used by the NAS (1989) is as follows: "A biomarker is a xenobiotically-induced variation in cellular or biochemical components or processes, structures, or functions that is measurable in a biological system or sample." One definition that we feel is highly relevant to contemporary theory and practice of risk assessment is that of

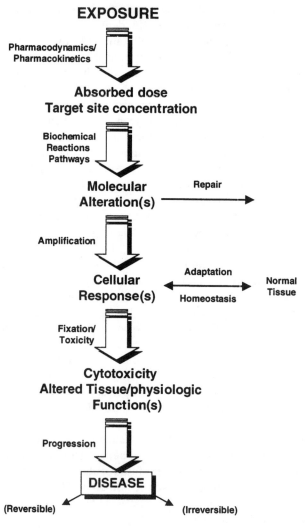

Figure 20.1 Diversity and level of biologic processes involved in the expression of chemically induced health effects. Adapted from Anderson, 1995.

Mayer et al. (1992), which defines biomarkers as "quantifiable biochemical, physiological, or histological measures that relate in a dose- or time-dependent manner the degree of dysfunction that the contaminant has produced." Depledge (1994) has broadened the definition of biomarkers to account for the increasing concern for the total environment: "An ecotoxicological biomarker is a biochemical, cellular, physiological, or behavioral variation that can be measured in tissue or body fluid samples or at the level of the whole organism (either individual or populations) that provides evidence of exposure to and/or effects

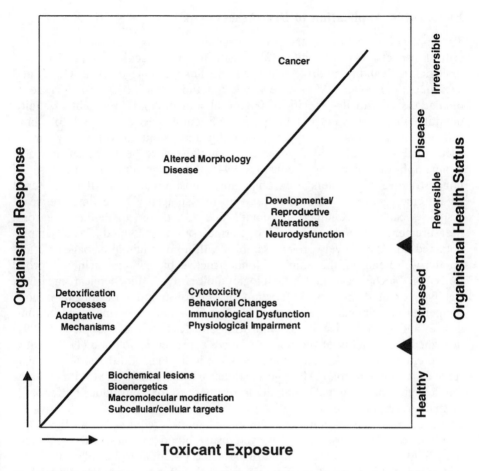

Figure 20.2 Conceptual representation of biologic responses to toxicant exposure and linkage to health status. Adapted from McCarthy et al., 1989.

of one or more chemical pollutants (and/or radiations)." Biomarkers may be categorized as nonspecific or specific; specific indicators may be classified further as organ- or toxicant-specific. The NAS (1987) classification scheme has served well both conceptually and in practice; it classifies biomarkers as markers of exposure, markers of effect, or markers of susceptibility. Consistent with the NAS definitions, a biomarker of exposure can be a foreign substance or its metabolite or the product of an interaction between a xenobiotic and a target molecule. Biomarkers of effect are measurable biochemical, physiologic, or histologic alterations that signal cellular, tissue, or organ dysfunction, health impairment, or disease. A biomarker of susceptibility is an indicator of decreased ability (inherent or acquired) to respond to the challenge of a chemical, biologic, or physical stressor.

Biomarkers: Application to Risk Assessment

The application of biomarkers to risk assessment has its basis on the following critical aspects: (1) reliability, (2) sensitivity and specificity (chemical and biologic), (3) validity, and (4) relevance and linkage. Hugget et al. (1992) and subsequently Peakall (1994) have advocated the following criteria for use of biomarkers: sensitivity, specificity (chemical and biologic), reliability, validity, quantifiability, and interpretability. Peakall emphasized the need for more validated biomarkers, and in terms of utility the extent to which they can be used nondestructively. Nondestructive biomarkers have been the subject of a monograph by Fossi and Leonzio (1994). The arguments for the use of nondestructive biomarkers are compelling—most notable are that (1) serial measurements can be made on the same test subject, (2) the time course of response can be examined in detail, and (3) there are ethical reasons. Measurements in body fluids (blood, urine, saliva, etc.) and tissue samples obtained nondestructively provide samples with no or minimal damage or effect on the well-being of the animal. Nondestructive biomarkers include a broad range of biochemical and physiologic indices (e.g., biochemical measures signifying organ damage or dysfunction, oxygen consumption or utilization, body temperature, pulmonary parameters, cardiac function, endocrine perturbations, growth and reproductive status, and urine and feces output). Depledge (1994) described the benefits of the nondestructive approach as follows: (1) Repeated measurements can be conducted on the same individual, and the individual may serve as its own control; (2) long-term studies may be conducted; (3) it facilitates the detection of individual variability in response to toxicant-induced effects; (4) biomarker responses can be assessed more accurately in relation to toxicant challenge; and (5) it minimizes the number of animals required for a study. Most nondestructive biomarkers are assayed using blood samples, although other body fluids and tissues are utilized or have the potential to be relevant source material for bioassays. Considerable research efforts are being devoted to improve bioassay methodologies in blood and other tissues. A synopsis of commonly used biomarkers and their assay potential in blood and other tissues is presented in Table 20.1.

Biochemical Markers

Toxicants manifest their effects at different levels of biological organization; perturbations at the biochemical/molecular level are sensitive indices of effect and exposure and in many instances usually the most immediate (first detectable) quantifiable response to toxicant exposure. Changes in biochemical systems and pathways underlie effects at higher levels of biologic organization. Current efforts at the forefront of biochemical biomarker research include (1) enhancing the practical value by developing biomarker responses that are detectable in advance of deleterious and unwanted responses, (2) efforts related to establishing linkage between a biochemical change and subsequent biologic effects, (3)

Table 20.1 Common biomarkers: Assay utility in blood and other tissues

Biomarker/category[a]	Tissue of choice	Assayable potential in blood	Comment
Biomarkers of exposure			
δ-Aminolevulinic acid dehydratose	Blood	+	Tissue of choice
Adduct formation	Wide range	+	Hemoglobin is good surrogate for DNA
Acetylcholinesterase inhibition	Neural	+/?	Effects in blood transient, red blood cells can be used
Porphyrins	Liver	+/?	Advances enabling use in plasma
Stress proteins	Wide range	?	Some database using erythrocytes
Metallothioneins	Liver, kidney	−	Associated with storage in organs
Biomarkers of effect			
Sister chromatid exchange	Wide range	+	Blood lymphocytes suitable for assay
DNA strand breakage	Wide range	?	Potential using blood lymphocytes
Neurotoxic esterase	Neural	+/?	May be assayed in blood
Immunotoxicity	Bone marrow, lymphatics	−	Limited assays available for blood
Biomarkers of susceptibility			
Cytochrome P450 and isozymes	Liver	+/?	Genetic polymorphism basis for use as susceptibility marker, immunoassays routine
Glutathione-S-transferase and ioszymes	Liver	−	Tissue of choice

Source: Modified from Peakall, 1994.
[a] Some biomarkers may be considered in more than one category; however, prevailing viewpoint regarding categorization is used for classification.

efforts toward adaptation from laboratory to field (biomonitoring potential), and (4) development of biomarker technologies that have practical application to risk assessment. Biochemical markers may be nonspecific, as in the case of stress proteins or specific (organ-specific, e.g., p-aminohippurate clearance by the kidney; or toxicant-specific, e.g., cytochrome P450 induction, UDP-glucuronosyl transferase induction, metallothionein synthesis, perturbations involving heme/porphyrin pathway). Biochemical changes are extremely diverse and range from measures of enzyme activity (acetylcholinesterase [AChE]) to indicators of reactant moieties with macromolecules (DNA and hemoglobin adducts). Of the many advances in biomarker technology and approaches (cytochrome P450 induction, stress proteins, oxidant-mediated responses, heme and porphyrins), P450 induction and stress protein response are highlighted as

Table 20.2 Characteristics and utility of various biochemical indices

	Exposure biomarker	Effects biomarker	Integration/ linkage	Sensitivity	Specificity Chemical	Biologic	Reliability
Cytochrome P450	+	+	+	High	Polycyclic/halogenated hydrocarbons	Vertebrates	High
Conjugating (postoxidation) enzymes	+	?	+	Low	Polycyclic/halogenated hydrocarbons	Vertebrates	High
Heme and porphyrins	+	?	+	Moderate	Metals	Eukaryotes, prokaryotes	High
Metallothioneins	+	?	+	High	Metals	Eukaryotes	High
Stress proteins	+	?	+	High	Metals, inorganics, organics	Eukaryotes, prokaryotes	Not validated
Oxidative damage	+	+	+	High	Oxidants	Broad	High

Adapted from: Stegeman et al., 1992.

illustrative of technical refinements and advances that have enhanced or improved the risk-assessment process. The reader is referred to an authoritative review on biochemical components as indices of chemical exposure and effect by Stegeman et al. (1992). The characteristics and utility of various biomarkers are summarized in Table 20.2.

Cytochrome P450 Monoxygenases

Mixed function oxidases are coupled electron transport systems comprising a cytochrome and a flavoprotein that is involved in the bioconversion of xenobiotic chemicals. Most research has focused on the cytochrome component, implicated as a terminal oxidase in the metabolism of drugs and xenobiotics and inducible by various chemicals. Cytochrome P450 monoxygenases exist in multiple forms —neither precisely "3-MC-type" or "PB-type"—with differing but overlapping specificities and inducibilities (Nebert, 1979; Lu and West, 1980). Cytochrome P450 and P450 isozymes have considerable potential for detecting exposure and early effects through P450 and P450 isozyme induction. Cytochrome P450 induction or modulation is involved in oxidative and conjugation metabolism and may be directly involved in toxicant-induced injury. Altered oxidative and conjugation metabolism are clear consequences of P450 induction; however, other consequences of P450 induction are of more recent revelation (i.e., altered steroid metabolism). Cytochrome P450 enzymes are involved in the bioconversion of organic chemicals rendering in some cases nontoxic moieties ("detoxification") and in others transformation leading to enhanced toxicity ("toxification") (Armstrong, 1987; Buhler and Williams, 1988). The P450 family of enzymes is inducible by various hydrocarbons (e.g., organochlorines, polyaromatic hydrocarbons). Induction of P450 enzymes is well documented and linked to chemical inducers in the environment—for reviews see Ortiz de Montellano (1986), Payne et al. (1987), and Parke (1990). Cytochrome P450 induction has been utilized as a biomarker of exposure and in biomonitoring applications. Methods for determining P450 induction have evolved from utilization of measures of enzyme activity (AHH) to utilization of DNA probes (i.e., c-DNA). Noncatalytic assay procedures were prompted by findings that analysis of P450 activity alone might not indicate the occurrence of induction, whereas immunochemical-based assays provided evidence for P450 induction (Gooch et al., 1989). In fact, Foster et al. (1986), in a study on the distribution/localization of P450 in tissues, advocated the utility of immunochemical techniques in ascertaining P450 induction in tissues not readily measurable by other techniques. Cytochrome P450 induction now can be reliably detected and measured by use of a set of specific probes; assay methods for cytochrome P450 induction are highlighted in Table 20.3.

Stress Proteins and Metallothioneins

The stress-protein response, initially referred to as *heat-shock response*, is widely exhibited in the animal kingdom (Lindquist, 1986). It can be viewed as a

Table 20.3 Assay methods for cytochrome P450 induction

	Measurement	Probes	References
Catalytic			
Ethoxyresorufin-O-deethylase	Enzyme activity	Benzo[a]pyrene	Nebert and Gelboin (1968), Schenkman et al. (1977), Guengerich (1982)
Aryl hydrocarbon hydroxylase		Ethoxyresorufin	Burke and Mayer (1974), Klotz et al (1984)
Immunochemical			
Western blot immunoassay	Protein levels	Moncolonal/polyclonal antibodies	Forster et al. (1986), Anderson et al. (1987), Forkert et al. (1988, 1989), Gooch et al. (1989), Smolowitz et al. (1991) Baron et al. (1981), Moody et al. (1983), Ratanasavanh et al. (1986).
Northern blot immunoassay	mRNA levels	DNA probe (i.e., cDNA)	Haasch et al. (1989), Kloepper-Sams and Stegeman (1989)

manifestation of altered gene expression ("environmental response machinery") to chemical and physical stressors (Schlesinger et al., 1982; Moromoto et al., 1990). It is characterized by the induction of stressor-specific proteins, with concomitant reduction in synthesis of the proteins transcribed prior to toxicant challenge (Welch et al., 1989). The stress proteins are divided into two groups, namely heat-shock protein—discovered on exposure to elevated temperatures— and glucose-regulated proteins. The induction of glucose-regulated proteins is thought to be a consequence of a glucose- or oxygen-deprived milieu or conditions of disrupted calcium homeostasis. There are many similarities between these families of stress proteins (Welch et al., 1989; Welch, 1990). The stress-protein response is a useful, sensitive biomarker, because it reflects the cellular physiologic state and may reflect the lowest level of adverse effect. The stress-protein response, as in the case of P450 induction, signals that exposure has taken place and is an excellent biomarker of exposure. It also may be valid as a biomarker of susceptibility; however, the utility of the stress-protein response as a biomarker of effect is difficult to evaluate presently because the molecular biology of the stress response and its relationship to higher levels of organization requires further exploration. The stress-protein response is elicited by a variety of chemical and physical agents including hormetic agents such as heavy metals and antibiotics. Chemical and physical inducers include heavy metals (Hammond et al., 1982; Caltabiano et al., 1986), xenobiotics (Sanders, 1990); teratogens (Bournias-Vardiabasis et al., 1983; Bournias-Vardiabasis and Buzin, 1986); liver carcinogens (Carr et al., 1986); anoxia (Spector et al., 1986); and oxidative perturbations (Kapour and Lewis, 1987).

Alterations in metallothioneins and heme oxygenase may be regarded as indicative of stress-protein responses (Kagi and Nordberg, 1978; Keyse and Tyrrell, 1989). The role of metallothioneins as biomarkers and their application are addressed only briefly—see reviews of metallothionein chemistry, biochemistry, and function (Garvey, 1984; Hamer, 1986; Kagi and Kojima, 1987; Engel and Brouwer, 1989). Metallothioneins are low molecular weight proteins involved in sequestration and metabolism of heavy metals. Extensive knowledge and available highly sensitive methods for measuring metallothionein induction provide evidence of induction at environmental levels of pollutants. Despite incompleteness in our understanding of the physiologic function of metallothioneins, their induction is a credible biomarker of exposure, confirmation of exposure, and indication of metal stress. A wide variety of agents can induce metallothonein synthesis, most notably heavy metals (Bracken and Klaassen, 1987). Endogenous biochemical components also have been demonstrated to induce metallothionein synthesis, including glucocorticoids, progesterone, catecholamines, interleukin 1, and interferon (Karin, 1985; Bremner et al., 1981; Brady and Helvig, 1984; Cousins and Leinart, 1988; Friedman and Stark, 1985). As with any biochemical biomarker, one may ask the following questions: (1) What is the relevance of the measure to health and disease? (2) Can a linkage be established between the response and physiological or functional change at higher levels of biologic organization? (3) To what extent can the biomarker be utilized in the risk-assessment paradigm? Using stress-protein response as a case example, we address these questions.

The current view is that stress proteins serve a protective function, and, within limits, the cellular physiology and function are preserved. The protective function of stress proteins is of great interest, in terms of not only the mechanistic perspective but its relationship to the hormetic response. The hormetic response, an increasingly important yet controversial aspect of evaluating toxicant-induced effects at low-level exposures, and its integration into the risk-assessment process are discussed in a subsequent section of this chapter and elsewhere. If exposures result in this protective function being overwhelmed, subsequent biologic events occur, leading to more serious biologic dysfunction, which may be reversible or irreversible in nature. The underlying biochemical events (mechanisms or pathways) involved are as yet poorly understood; however, ongoing and future research at the molecular and mechanistic level should clarify the relationship between these events and initiation of dysfunction or disease. Subjeck and Shyy (1986) have advanced the notion that heat-shock and glucose-regulated proteins may be involved in the protection, enhancement of longevity, and restoration of normal cellular functions in cells responding to environmental variables. In addressing the second question, linkage (mechanistic pathways, alterations in the organism's biochemical and physiologic processes, physiologic or functional change at higher levels of biologic organization) can be established for the stress-protein phenomenon. An interesting postulate pertaining to stress proteins and linkage to the hormetic response was proposed by Smith-Sonneborn (1992). Essentially, it was postulated that the hormetic response may operate through the stress-protein response. According to Smith-Sonneborn, this hypothesis is supported by the following findings: (1) Agents identified as hormetic also induce the stress response; (2) hormetic agents having molecular interactions/responses common to heat shock response can induce thermotolerance; (3) the stress response includes preferential synthesis of moieties (products) that repair both protein and DNA, resulting in outcomes enhancing longevity; and (4) alterations in chromatic structure could facilitate depression of growth-promoting products or provide pathways to DNA repair.

Finally, some discussion is needed pertaining to whether an outcome is considered an indicator or biomarker of stress or a biomarker of adaptation. DePledge (1994) discusses issues concerned with this question: When is a biochemical or physiologic response to xenobiotic exposure considered an indicator of stress or a manifestation of an adaptation response? This has considerable implication as to the hormetic-response concept, and hormetic-response data sets are utilized in the risk-assessment and management paradigms.

Organ- and Toxicant-specific Biomarkers

As previously stated, biomarkers are utilized to document exposure and effects and are classified into broad categories of nonspecific and specific biomarkers.

Specific indicators are further categorized as either organ-specific or toxicant-specific. Organ-specific biomarkers for the detection—and in many cases for the evaluation—of toxicant-induced dysfunction or injury exist for all of the organ systems. The array of useful biomarkers, sensitivity, diagnostic effectiveness, utility across species, and predictive value varies considerably. Thus, among organ systems useful and reliable indicators of hepatic dysfunction or injury outnumber those identifiable as useful and reliable indicators of endocrine dysfunction. In general, organ-function tests, organ-specific enzymes or biochemical constituents, and histopathologic alterations represent the various approaches and techniques that relate to organ-specific biomarkers. Organ- and toxicant-specific biomarkers have been intensively researched, the subject of numerous workshops and symposia, and extensively dealt with in the toxicology and health risk assessment literature. In this much-condensed overview, however, we focus on biomarkers indicative of hepatic and renal dysfunction or injury by highlighting developments illustrative of approaches and techniques that have enhanced the detection or evaluation of organic-specific damage or dysfunction and thus improved the risk-assessment process.

As an organ system, the liver demonstrates marked vulnerability to chemically induced dysfunction or damage. Detection and evaluation of liver dysfunction or injury has been approached from an integrative perspective as including biochemical, physiologic, and morphologic components, concomitant with the recognition of the need for linkage to other biologic events and higher-order processes. This paradigm also has served as a model for other organ systems. Mechanistic approaches have contributed significantly to understanding the processes involved in toxicant-induced dysfunction or injury and in the development of reliable indicators of exposure or effect. Of parallel importance is the recognition that the development of biomarker technology and its application to the detection and assessment of liver dysfunction or injury has directed attention to the difficulties encountered in the development and selection of appropriate indicators of toxicant-induced dysfunction or injury. This is particularly evident if one considers organ systems that are characterized by considerable diversity in functional activity and multiplicity of response to chemical or physical stressors and prone to changes in the homeostasis or functional integrity of another organ system. Although it is difficult to select appropriate tests and assays to ascertain functional and morphologic changes involving the hepatic system, various tests have been developed that are highly useful in the detection and evaluation of liver dysfunction/injury in both mammalian and nonmammalian systems (Galen, 1975; Kachmar and Moss, 1976; Gingerich and Weber, 1979; Plaa and Charbonneau, 1994; Stonard and Evans, 1994). Assays utilized in the detection/evaluation of hepatic dysfunction/injury include the following: (1) serum enzyme assays, (2) hepatic clearance/excretion assays, (3) assessment of changes in endogenous constituents, and (4) histologic assessment of liver injury. The determination of hepatic enzyme activity in plasma, made possible by the release of tissue enzyme into the blood by the damaged liver, is a very useful tool in the detection and assessment of hepatotoxicity. Considerable emphasis is placed on the use of plasma enzymes as indicators of organ damage, and a number of enzyme-based assays are available to assess liver dysfunction or injury. These assays may be grouped as follows: (1) enzyme assays that are somewhat nonspecific because these activities are also found in extrahepatic tissues (e.g. lactate dehydrogenases, transaminases); (2) assays based on enzymes localized mainly in the liver (i.e., alanine aminotransferase); and (3) assays based on enzymes exclusively associated with the liver (e.g., sorbitol dehydrogenase). Alanine aminotransferase commonly is used as a sensitive indicator of hepatotoxicity, although it does lack some specificity. Sorbitol dehydrogenase, a liver-specific enzyme found in the cytoplasm, has been demonstrated to be a very reliable indicator of hepatic injury (Asada and Galambos, 1963). Isoenzyme patterns also have been utilized as a basis for the detection of tissue/organ damage (Wilkinson, 1970). For example, serum isoenzyme patterns of lactate dehydrogenase activity have been used successfully as an indicator of hepatic and nonhepatic tissue damage in animals and humans (Cornish et al., 1970). Other enzyme assays, for example alkaline phosphatase and in particular leucine aminopeptidase (LAP), have been developed specifically to detect impaired biliary excretion or obstructive liver injury (Plaa and Charbonneau, 1994). Several dye-clearance assays have been used as indicators of hepatic dysfunction. Bromosulfothalein and indocyanine green, commonly used cholephilic dyes, have been utilized to detect and assess hepatic function (Kachmar and Moss, 1976; Stonard and Evans, 1994). A synopsis of organ-specific and toxicant-specific biomarkers related to hepatic dysfunction/injury is given in Table 20.4.

The renal system is multifunctional (e.g. regulation of extracellular fluid volume, electrolyte composition, hormonal functions) and is critical in the control and regulation of homeostasis. As is the liver, the kidney is vulnerable to chemically induced dysfunction or damage. Evaluation of the effects of an exogenous substance on the renal system can be achieved using in vivo or in vitro methodologies (Foulkes, 1993; Davis and Berndt, 1994; Tarloff and Goldstein, 1994). Assessment of nephrotoxicity can be accomplished via serum chemistry, urinalysis, clearance procedures, and histopathologic analysis. A number of biochemical measures have been utilized as indicators of chemically induced renal dysfunction or injury. Enzyme activities in blood or urine indicative of kidney dysfunction or disease include lactate dehydrogenase, N-acetyl-β-glucosaminidase (NAG), alkaline phosphatase, and maltase. The assessment of maltase activity has been demonstrated as a reliable index of kidney dysfunction (Stroo and Hook, 1977). Urinary excretion of proteins also is a reliable indicator of renal dysfunction or damage: Excretion of high molecular weight proteins (e.g., albumin) is suggestive of glomerular damage and excretion of low molecular weight proteins (i.e., β_2-microglobulin) is indicative of tubular injury (Christensen and Nielsen, 1991). Clearance procedures to evaluate glomerular filtration rate are conducted via monitoring the renal handling of inulin, creatinine, or p-aminohippurate. Glomerular function also may be assessed by monitoring blood urea nitrogen levels. A summary of organ-specific and toxicant-specific biomarkers related to kidney dysfunction or injury is presented in Table 20.4.

Table 20.4 Organ- and toxicant-specific biomarkers

Organ and function	References	Enzyme	References	Toxicant-specific	References
p-Aminohippurate, clearance by kidney	Kachmar and Moss 1976; Miller, 1981; Foulkes, 1993; Davis and Berndt, 1994	Alkaline phosphatase	Kachmar and Moss, 1976; Plaa and Charbonneau, 1994	Acetylcholinesterase	Weiss, 1965; Holland et al., 1967; Voss and Sachsse, 1970; Grue et al., 1983; St Omer and Rottinghaus, 1992
Sulfobromophthalein indocyamine green, clearance by liver	Kachmar and Moss 1976; Patton, 1978; Gingerich and Webber, 1979; Plaa and Charbonneau, 1994	Creatinine phosphokinase	Mayer et al., 1992		
		Lactate dehydratase	Cornish et al., 1970; Kachmar and Moss, 1976; Plaa and Charbonneau, 1994	δ-Aminolevulinic acid dehydratase	Hodson et al., 1977; Scheuhammer, 1987
		Lysosomal enzymes	Saundermann and Horak, 1981; Nogawa et al., 1986	Cytochrome P450	Lu and West 1986; Payne et al., 1987; Parke, 1990; Stegeman et al., 1992
		Maltase[a]	Davis and Berndt, 1994	Glucose-6-phosphatase	Recknagel and Glende, 1973
		Sorbitol dehydrogenase[b]	Asada and Galambos, 1963	Metallothioneins	Garvey, 1984; Hamer, 1986; Engel and Bremner, 1989
		Transaminases	Wroblewski and La Due, 1956; Kachmar and Moss, 1976; Gingerich, 1982		

[a] Enzyme specific for kidney.
[b] Enzyme specific for liver.

Histopathologic alterations also have been used as biomarkers of chemically induced organ toxicity. Histopathologic biomarkers (e.g., organelle changes, accumulation of cytoplasmic inclusions, lipid accumulation [vacuole formation], changes in cell and nuclear volume, glycogen depletion, cellular swelling; refer to Trump et al., 1980; Hinton et al., 1992) are higher-level responses that reflect prior biochemical and physiologic alterations. Generally, concerns pertaining to morphologic indicators of toxicity are directed at the subjective nature of morphologic assessments and distinguishing toxicant-induced alterations from those caused by natural toxins, infectious disease, or normal physiologic variation. The subjective nature of morphologic assessments has contributed to the difficulty in correlating and linking morphologic alterations with other more quantitative endpoints. Considerable progress has been made, however, as a result of (1) more quantitative assessment of organ lesions, (2) improved techniques to detect "early" pathologic lesions, (3) generation and acquisition of more quantitative morphologic data by utilization of computer software, (4) utilization of in vitro systems, and (5) improved cytotoxicity bioassays.

ENHANCING THE EXPOSURE-ASSESSMENT PROCESS

The use of biomarkers as a means to enhance the quantitative character of the exposure-assessment component of risk assessment originated over a decade ago through the innovative efforts of Osterman-Golkar and Ehrenberg and colleagues (Osterman-Golkar et al., 1976; Ehrenberg et al., 1983). The EPA has come forth with a decision model for development of exposure biomarkers (U.S. EPA, 1989). To better and more fully understand current and future trends in the development and application of exposure biomarkers, one needs to examine both the issues and challenges confronting exposure biomarker research. There are two underlying issues that impact heavily on exposure biomarker research development and application: (1) The biologic event/biomarker must be evident prior to manifestation of an adverse (unwanted) effect; (2) the biomarker should provide a means to quantitate the extent of exposure and perhaps exposure duration. With regard to challenges confronting biomarkers of exposure, the following points of discussion are offered. One challenge to future biomarker research is the need to distinguish between biomarkers of exposure and those of effect. This challenge favors a construct that requires a rigid distinction between biomarkers of effect and of exposure, which may be difficult to attain as measures of biologic events and responses become increasing sensitive. Moreover, the distinction between exposure and effect markers is not absolute. Alternatively, the challenge is one of attaining better quantification and linkage. Stevens et al. (1991) have stated, "The ultimate aim of biomarker research is to develop markers, which can be quantitatively related to both exposure and effect." Advances in biomarker (biomonitor, molecular epidemiology) technology, the integration of biomarker data into pharmacokinetic and pharmacodynamic models, the utilization of exposure biomarkers as dosimeters, and dosimetry modeling represent the more promising developments that can be applied towards improving the science and utility of exposure assessment. Biomarkers of exposure include a wide array of indices and measures that can be catalogued generally as follows: (1) presence or level of exogenous substance or metabolite in body fluids, tissues, excreta, and so forth; (2) interactive products (adducts) between toxicant and endogenous components (e.g., DNA, proteins); and (3) events or processes in the biologic system related to toxicant exposure (e.g., enzmye inhibition, enzyme induction, altered isozyme patterns, elevated serum enzymes, hormone perturbations, reproductive alterations, heightened immune system response). Recently, biomarkers have been advanced to improve estimates of internal dose thereby, providing a means towards improving exposure and dose–response assessment. Stevens et al. (1991), in developing a decision model for exposure markers, have defined certain characteristics of exposure markers as a requisite for utility as dosimeters: They must (1) demonstrate a linear relationship to exposure over a wide range of doses, (2) possess a high specificity for chemicals of interest, and (3) exhibit a well-established relationship between biomarker response and an adverse health effect. Also, dosimetry modeling has been advocated as a means to significantly improve the exposure and dose–response components of the risk-assessment process. Indeed, dosimetry modeling has led to a reshaping and rethinking of our approaches to dose–response assessment (Jarabek, 1995).

Exogenous Materials or Their Metabolites as Exposure Biomarkers

The measurement of foreign substances and their metabolites and degradation products has been used successfully in exposure assessment and for routine biomonitoring, particularly for organophosphate and carbamate insecticides. Exposure to xenobiotic chemicals that are not or poorly metabolizable (persistent) such as polychlorinated biphenyls are assayed by direct measurement of the intact xenobiotic. Exposure to xenobiotics that undergo metabolic conversion (e.g., organophosphates [Eto, 1974]; carbamates [Fukuto, 1972]; aromatic amines [Thorgeirsson et al., 1983]; and polynuclear aromatic hydrocarbons [Thakker et al., 1985]), however, can be assessed only via measurement of metabolites or degradation products. Thus, depending on the foreign substance, the metabolic conversion may generate readily analyzable moieties and therefore can be used as biomarker of exposure of the parent compound. Metabolic products of a xenobiotic may be analyzed in a number of body fluids or tissues because they may accumulate in these various compartments; however, in most cases the urine is the preferred sample source for analysis of metabolites. Additionally, because highly reactive metabolites may interact with cellular macromolecules, measurement of these complexes (adducts) are also indicative of exposure. It is reasonable to view the measurement of macromolecular reaction products as a progression in the measurement of metabolites—a highly useful tool in the quantitative exposure assessment of mutagenic and carcinogenic chemicals (discussed further in a subsequent section). To have utility as an exposure biomarker, the relationship between a metabolite and the parent compound must be known and the analysis procedures must be of sufficient sensitivity and specificity. The aforementioned criteria are adequate if one desires only to ascertain that exposure has taken place; however, in developing a quantitative estimate of exposure a further requirement, namely, characterization of the kinetics of elimination and excretion, must be met.

The measurement of metabolic products derived from organophosphate and carbamate bioconversion processes serves to illustrate how the evolution and application of a novel approach can result in the enhancement of exposure assessment and biomonitoring. The metabolic conversion of organophosphates and carbamates has been researched extensively in mammalian systems and to a lesser degree in nonmammalian systems. Pesticides belonging to these two classes are metabolized readily, and the products of bioconversion are excreted readily in the urine (Fukuto, 1972; Eto, 1974). The relationship between exposure levels of organophosphates and carbamates and urinary metabolite excretion has been studied in both experimental animals and humans (Comer et al., 1975; Bradway et al., 1977; Franklin et al., 1981, 1986). Additional research has indicated that urinary metabolites—particulary those derived from organophosphates—can be detected in the absence of altered cholinesterase activity or overt clinical manifestations of toxicity (Shafik and Bradway, 1976; Franklin et al., 1981; Kraus et al., 1981). This exemplifies success in attaining a critical objective in exposure biomarker development, namely, a measure that is evident prior to manifestation of adverse effects. The use of urinary metabolites of organophosphates (likewise carbamates) as indicators of exposure has been advocated strongly (Shafik and Bradway, 1976; Moseman and Oswald, 1980; Shafik, 1980; Duncan and Griffith, 1985; Coye et al., 1986; Franklin et al., 1986; Lavy and Mattice, 1986; Vasilic et al., 1987). In fact, the concept of biologic monitoring of pesticides was expanded to include measurement of urinary metabolites (World Health Organization, 1982). The World Health Organization protocol served as a model for the development of exposure monitoring of pesticides by the U.S. EPA (1987) and by the U.S. National Agricultural Chemicals Association (Honeycutt, 1986; Mull and McCarthy, 1986). Although sensitive and specific analytical procedures have been developed for measuring metabolites of organophosphates and carbamates, emerging technologies (e.g., immunochemical assays, particularly monoclonal antibody technology) for metabolite identification and quantitation have been and continue to be developed for pesticide metabolite and residue detection (Hammock and Mumma, 1980; Hammock et al., 1987; Mumma and Brady, 1987; and Vanderlaan et al., 1988). The immunochemical assays ultimately may provide a highly reliable methodology that is rapid, can be automated, and adapted for field use. Generally, at least for organophosphates, the measurement and monitoring of urinary metabolites has been transitioned from cutting edge and pacing technologies to routine procedures providing quantitative estimates of exposure.

Macromolecular Adducts as Exposure Biomarkers

Macromolecular adducts have emerged as highly useful biomarkers of exposure for a variety of reactive xenobiotics and have great potential as molecular dosimeters. Research on adduct formation dates back to the 1970s: The formation of polycyclic aromatic hydrocarbons and DNA adducts has been reported in many systems (Philip and Sims, 1979). The development and of macromolecular adduct methodology application to risk assessment have been discussed in great detail elsewhere (Farmer and Bailey, 1989; Skipper and Tannenbaum, 1990; Chang et al., 1994; DeCaprio, 1997) and need not be elaborated here. The conception and application of macromolecular adducts as potential dosimeters are relatively recent; however, this is gaining greater acceptance as a useful tool in developing more accurate and quantitative exposure assessment and is a subject discussed in greater detail by Stevens et al. (1991) and DeCaprio (1997). A brief synopsis pertaining to macromolecular adducts in risk assessment is presented.

Macromolecular adducts, the products of the interaction between reactive xenobiotics or their metabolites and DNA, RNA, or proteins, are useful indicators of exposure and utility as molecular dosimeters. The covalent bonding of electrophilic intermediates to DNA, RNA, or proteins is considered to be the "biochemical lesion" underlying such processes as cellular necrosis, mutagenicity, and carcinogenicity. Miller and Miller (1981, 1985) have viewed the covalent bonding to DNA by electrophilic moieties as the "critical event" in the process of chemical carcinogenesis. The utilization of DNA adducts in exposure and dose–response assessment has flourished mainly because of the requirement for more quantitative assessments and because assays for levels of cancer-causing agents in body fluids or tissues have not always provided an accurate estimate of the "biologically effective dose." The biologically effective dose (defined as "the amount of activated agent that has reacted with critical cellular targets" [Perera, 1987]) is a critical concept in the development of more quantitative risk assessments.

Biochemical interactions of reactive metabolic intermediates are not limited to genetic material and also include bonding with proteins resulting in the formation of protein adducts. Protein adducts (protein alkylation) have been advocated as exposure biomarkers for chemical carcinogens (Calleman et al., 1978). Theoretically, any protein could be used for monitoring protein adducts; however, hemoglobin is favored as a target protein for the following reasons: (1) good correlation between protein binding and DNA binding (Pereira et al., 1981, Ehrernberg et al., 1983; Murthy et al., 1984); (2) long lifetime, (3) stability of hemoglobin adducts throughout the life span of hemoglobin (Segerback et al., 1978; Tannebaum et al., 1983), (4) good accessibility, and (5) abundance. Thus hemoglobin adducts have demonstrated their utility not only as readily accessible surrogates for DNA adducts but as highly useful markers of exposure for both acute and repeated-dose scenarios (Pereira and Chang, 1981).

In conclusion, it can be said that although a vast amount of research has been dedicated to macromolecular adduct technology, there are continuing needs to develop this technology for more categories of chemicals, to validate emerging macromolecular adduct techniques, to research the biologic significance of DNA and protein adduct levels, and to consider the role and impact of background exposures.

Enzyme Systems as Exposure Biomarkers

The use of enzymes as exposure biomarkers is well established and supported by extensive databases. Research in this arena continues to progress, particularly as related to comparable biochemical markers in feral and nonmammalian systems. The aim of this is to develop a better risk assessment through the utilization of sound comparative databases comprising experimental animal, human, and nonmammalian data. Xenobiotic interactions and outcomes with enzyme systems can be characterized as follows: (1) direct enzyme inhibition, (2) enzyme induction, (3) elevated serum enzyme levels, and (4) altered enzyme activity caused by changes in metabolic fluxes or pathways. The assessment of enzyme activity has been demonstrated as a useful indicator of pollutant exposure, particularly if the interaction is toxicant-specific (e.g., organophosphate or carbamate inhibition of acetylcholinesterase/cholinesterase activities [St. Omer and Rottinghaus, 1992], lead inhibition of δ-aminolevulinic acid dehydratase [Hodson et al., 1977; Hammond and Belile, 1980]). Enzyme induction (i.e., P450 monooxygenases) by environmental pollutants is representative of well-established biomarkers of exposure (Kleinow et al., 1987; Payne et al., 1987; Stegeman et al., 1992). Measurement and monitoring of serum enzyme activities have emerged as highly useful indicators of chemical exposure and are outgrowths of accomplishments made in the biomedical era relevant to monitoring serum enzyme levels as indicators of tissue or organ damage or dysfunction. Chemical or physical stressors and disease states can lead to the release of cellular enzymes into the vascular system. Serum enzyme activities or profiles have been used extensively as simple yet accurate measures of damage and dysfunction at the cellular, tissue, and organ levels (e.g., prostate [acid phosphatase], heart and liver [transaminases], and kidney [lysosomal enzymes]). Furthermore, in many cases the relationship between serum enzyme levels and organism-level effects is well documented. The usefulness of serum enzymes as biomarkers of exposure has been amply demonstrated, and the trend toward utilization of a suite of serum enzymes can only improve exposure characterization. Serum transaminase activity, for example, has been used extensively as a biomarker of organ dysfunction in mammalian toxicity studies (Galen, 1975) and also has been researched using feral and nonmammalian species to improve the overall environmental risk assessment process. Serum transaminase activity, particularly aspartate aminotransferase, a cytosolic and mitochondrial enzyme found in various tissues, and alanine aminotransferase, a cytosolic enzyme normally associated with hepatic tissue, have been used effectively as biomarkers of chemical exposure and effects. Measurement of serum lysosomal enzymes, particularly N-acetyl-β-D-glucosaminidase (NAG), is potentially a very useful biomarker of exposure, especially if one considers their critical role in metabolic and pathologic processes. Elevated NAG levels or altered NAG isozyme patterns have been linked to a number of human diseases including cadmium-induced nephrotoxicity (Tucker et al., 1980; Ackerman et al., 1981; Nogawa et al., 1986).

Physiological Indices (Endocrine and Immunologic) as Exposure Biomarkers

Measures of endocrine perturbations may serve as indicators of exposure to chemical stressors. Measures of circulating levels of plasma hormones may be used to assess the impact of pollutants on metabolism, growth, and reproductive function. The following hormones have potential application as exposure biomarkers: corticosteroids, reproductive steroids, growth hormone, and thyroid hormones.

The immune system is highly sensitive to disruptions in physiologic homeostasis and is a target of toxic substances (Asher, 1978; Sharma, 1981; Sharma and Tomar, 1992; Bick, 1982). A wide variety of chemicals, including metals, carbamates, organophosphates, polynuclear aromatic hydrocarbons, and organochlorines, alters immune function (Vos, 1977; Dean et al., 1985, Rodgers et al., 1992; Thomas and House, 1995). Xenobiotics either directly or indirectly effect the immune system. Direct effects result from interactions with molecular, humoral, and cellular components of the immune system. Indirect effects are the result of the influence of other organ systems whose physiologic function or homeostasis also may have been altered by the toxicant—in particular the neuroendocrine system. Chemically induced alteration of immune function also may be viewed in terms of nonspecific versus specific immunity. Xenobiotics can modify nonspecific immunity (e.g., inflammation and phagocytosis) and specific immunity (e.g., cell-mediated immunity [CMI] and humoral-mediated immunity [HMI]). Generally, it can be said that impaired host defense most typifies the nonimmunologist's view of toxicant-induced damage to the immune system. Not as readily recognized is that a xenobiotic can elicit an inappropriate response or intensify a normal immune response to a level at which certain immune functions are characteristically pathologic and not protective (Vos, 1977; Luster et al., 1987; Weeks et al., 1992).

Despite our lack of fully understanding the complexities of such an elaborate physiologic system and the realization that relationships with adverse effects are not straightforward, biomarker methodologies have been developed to assess xenobiotic-induced perturbations of the immune system. Assays have been developed to assess immune function (e.g., antibody production, formation of antibody-producing cells, rosette formation, tests for inflammatory and allergic mediators, mucosal tissue infiltration by immune cells, assays for macrophage function [i.e., Ia expression]). Because of the complexity of the immune system and the fact that a single aspect or integrated aspects of the immune system might be under examination, a tiered system of testing immune-system responses or effects has been implemented (Vos, 1980; Luster et al., 1988; CDC/ATSDR, 1990). A number of methodologies appear promising as exposure or effect biomarkers, and Weeks et al. (1992) and Vogt (1991) have reviewed and discussed the application and utility of immunologic biomarkers as tools in enhancing health-risk assessment.

DOSE–RESPONSE EVALUATION: ENHANCING THE PROCESS

Historically, the uncertainty-factor method was utilized for both carcinogenic and noncarcinogenic compounds, but it is now used exclusively in the risk assessment of noncancer causing agents. Mathematic modeling techniques, generally used for assessing carcinogenic risks, is being increasingly utilized in the risk assessment of non-cancer causing agents. The safety or uncertainty factor approach is based on the "safe" dose concept. The safety- or uncertainty-factor method has been extensively reviewed (Munro and Krewski, 1981; Krewski et al., 1984; Dews, 1986; Lu, 1988; Kimmel, 1990; Shoaf, 1991; Dourson et al., 1996). Depending on the regulatory agency, various descriptors have been used to denote the "safe" dose (e.g., acceptable daily intake [ADI], reference dose [RfD], reference concentration, tolerable concentration, minimal risk level). The ADI, first introduced by Lehman and Fitzhugh (1954), remains a frequently used approach in dose–response assessment. The concept of ADI—its inception, development, and application in risk assessment—has been thoroughly reviewed (Lu, 1988; Lu and Sielken, 1991; Truhaut, 1991). The RfD approach, predominantly used by the EPA, is highlighted to illustrate advances in this arena and its impact in health risk assessment.

The RfD approach, an adaptation of the ADI approach, is the EPA's principal technique for assessing health risks from noncancer effects; for a detailed review refer to Barnes and Dourson (1988). The RfD is a dose operationally derived from the no-observed-adverse-effect level (NOAEL) by the application of uncertainty factors and in some instances a modifying factor. The RfD serves as a reference point in establishing the probability or as some prefer the likelihood of adverse effects to humans. A number of uncertainty factors are applied in the derivation of the RfD, which include adequacy of data base, animal-to-human extrapolation, subchronic-to-chronic, LOAEL-to-NOAEL, and sensitive subpopulations. The RfD is determined as

$$RfD = NOAEL/(UF \times MF)$$

where UF is the uncertainty factor and MF is the modifying factor. The technical sophistication underpinning uncertainty factors in noncancer risk assessment has progressed considerably beyond the use of the conventional default value of 10. Jarabek (1994) presents examples in which scientific development and research has resulted in a reduction in the use of default factors. There is a greater utilization of science-based (data-derived) uncertainty factors as opposed to the use of default values of 10-fold. For detailed discussions on the scientific underpinnings of uncertainty factors, the reader is referred to the literature (Dourson et al., 1992; HERA, 1995; TERA, 1996; Dourson et al., 1996). The trend is to incorporate more scientific data into the dose–response assessment (e.g., mechanisms/modes of action, toxicokinetics/toxicodynamics, interspecies and intraspecies sensitivity). The most significant benefit that results from the use of databased uncertainty factors—instead of the 10-fold default value—is a risk assessment characterized by a higher degree of confidence.

Despite research advances in the development of scientifically based uncertainty factors, there are limitations to the approach deriving the RfD from the NOAEL. Concerns related to the current RfD approach stem from the assumption that there is a threshold for critical effect and furthermore also may depend on the choice of a critical effect (i.e., adverse, unwanted). The limitation of the current RfD paradigm is that it focuses only on the NOAEL and essentially disregards the shape of the dose–response curve, other data, data variability, and homeostatic or compensatory mechanisms. The risk associated with doses at or above the NOAEL is not made explicit. Consequently, a number of alternate approaches—most notably the use of the benchmark dose (BD) as an alternative to the NOAEL in the derivation of an RfD. This paradigm was proposed initially by Crump (1984) and has been advocated as a basis for deriving the RfD for developmental toxicity (Kimmel and Gaylor, 1988; Gaylor, 1989). Its role in quantitative risk assessment has been reviewed and discussed (Kimmel, 1990). Recently, its use and application in risk assessment has been revisited (Barnes et al., 1995). The BD generally is defined as the lower confidence limit on a dose corresponding to an increase in the incidence of an effect at a particular level (Kimmel and Gaylor, 1988) or, stated another way, the lower confidence limit of the effective dose that causes an α-percent increase in risk. Uncertainty factors then may be applied to the BD to derive the RfD. Utilization of the BD as a starting point in the derivation of an RfD has distinct advantages: The BD approach utilizes data from the entire dose–response curve, it takes data variability into account, and it permits the estimation of risk at given exposure levels. The proposed use of a BD may represent a simple yet significant improvement in the dose–response assessment process. An extension of this is the confidence-profile method (CPM) of Jarabek and Hasselblad (1991) as an improvement on the RfD approach. The CPM expands the BD concept and considers total distribution, whereas the BD is associated with a particular confidence level. The CPM is discussed further under dose–response modeling.

Mathematic Dose–Response Modeling

Dose–response modeling is a mathematic description of the relationship between biologic effects and exposure to toxicant. Ideally, by utilizing appropriate mathematic modeling one can arrive at a precise and reproducible prediction of risk. The choice of model depends on the intent of the risk assessment. Thus, for example, an empirical curve-fitting model is used if the risk at a dose level within the experimental range is desired or a mechanistic model is used in predicting risk at low levels below the range of data points. Commonly employed mathematic models can interpolate data with reasonable exactness; however, they only can extrapolate to a limited degree outside the experimental data with an acceptable level of uncertainty. There is significant divergence in the estimates derived from various models if extrapolating from substantially outside the experimental data. Furthermore, there is a lack of consensus in the selection of low-dose extrapolation models. Therein lies the challenge, because the assessment of more environmental risks requires low-dose extrapolation to assess the risks from low-level exposures that are characteristic of environmental and occupational settings.

A number of approaches, suitable for mathematical dose–response modeling, have been developed to deal with the low-dose extrapolation problem: (1) the "maximum likelihood" approach, (2) the "control tolerance" approach, (3) the "z-zone" approach, and (4) the "metaanalysis" approach. The maximum likelihood approach is a commonly employed statistical procedure used in the benchmark approach as well as to describe cancer dose–response relationships. It is considered to be an improvement on the technique of using the NOAEL or LOAEL for derivation of the RfD. The control-tolerance approach, proposed by Gaylor and Slikker (1990, 1992), is a method that compares the variability in data sets between control and measured effect to estimate risk. The principal advantage of this approach is that control variability is clearly characterized. This approach is useful in instances in which the background incidence represents a major factor in the risk assessment. The z-zone approach, developed by Dews (1980), is based on the distribution of point estimates from various independently determined dose–effect functions to estimate the probability of an effect. The advantage of the z-zone approach is its applicability to most types of effects including quantal dose–response data. The metaanalysis approach (Hedges and Olkin, 1985; Chalmers, 1991) is based on the utilization of a variety of statistical techniques to analyses of data derived from separate studies. This approach is an attempt to estimate outcomes via the utilization of information from multiple studies because of data limitations of each individual study. The CPM and "categoric regression analysis" are representative of the metaanalysis approach and are the focus of recent research within the EPA on improving noncancer risk-assessment methodology.

The CPM has been developed to reduce the uncertainty and enhance the quantitative character of the dose–response evaluation component of risk assessment. It provides for the combining of databases from multiple sources and the incorporation of subjective judgment and expert views concerning critical parameters. It allows the utilization of both Bayesian and non-Bayesian statistical approaches. The key advantage of the CPM is the utilization of the entire distribution of likely values for a particular parameter. Jarabek and Hasselblad (1991, 1992) have applied the CPM to improve upon the RfD/reference concentration approach.

Categoric regression analysis has been developed by the EPA and continues to be refined. This approach offers considerable advantages in addressing non-cancer related health effects and has been reviewed in detail (Hertzberg and Miller, 1985; Hertzberg, 1989; Guth et al., 1991). Greatly oversimplified, this approach involves the assignment of noncancer health effects into various severity categories (e.g., NOAEL, adverse-effect level, lethality). A regression model then is used to quantify the relationship between severity and the time–concentration dimension. The analysis is conducted on the entire data set or may be differentiated into specific endpoints. The output of the analysis is expressed as the likelihood that a given severity category will be exceeded by a particular time–concentration combination. There are multiple advantages of the categoric regression analysis approach: (1) It permits the incorporation of quantal and quantitative data sets; (2) it permits the simultaneous analysis of many studies; (3) it can serve as an alternate to formal multivariate analysis; (4) it provides a concentration–time profile for any desired probability level, which is particularly useful in short-term exposure assessment; and (5) it provides for a reduction in interspecies uncertainty if human data are available.

Risk Assessment of Chemical Mixtures

Rarely is human exposure to xenobiotics limited to a single chemical, yet the vast bulk (about 95%) of toxicologic databases has been derived from single-chemical studies (Yang, 1994). Recently, public and regulatory concerns over multiple chemical exposures have escalated and have dictated the need for integrative approaches in the assessment of the toxicity of chemical mixtures. The paramount issue concerning health effects of chemical exposure is exposure to chemical mixtures and the resulting health consequences. Characterizing the toxicity of chemical mixtures and the development of realistic risk assessments are expanding functions of both the scientific and regulatory communities, as evidenced by the numerous publications in the field (Calabrese, 1991; Mauderly, 1993; Mumtaz et al., 1993, 1994; Feron et al., 1995; Fay and Feron, 1996; El-Masri et al., 1997; Cassee et al., 1998). It is understandable that the Presidential/Congressional Commission on Risk Assessment and Risk Management (1997) considered the risk assessment of mixtures to be a matter of considerable concern and importance.

Historically, toxicity evaluation of chemical mixtures has focused on mixtures containing relatively few components or on specific interaction studies. Overall, exposure and toxicity data for most chemical mixtures are fragmentary, and conventional toxicity-testing approaches are inadequate in addressing chemical-mixture issues. The EPA (1986d, 1990) over the years has recognized the importance, the complexities, and the technical difficulties associated with the toxicologic evaluation of chemical mixtures and has developed guidelines for the risk assessment of mixtures. The National Research Council of the NAS also has addressed the issues, concerns, and approaches related to the toxicity assessment of chemical mixtures (NAS, 1988). Considerable strides have been made in chemical-mixture toxicity evaluation and assessment. A number of studies has been conducted to evaluate the toxicity of combinations of chemicals of up to nine components (Jonker et al., 1990, 1993; Groten et al., 1994).

Toxicity studies on mixtures of groundwater contaminants also have been conducted (NTP, 1993). Whole-mixture toxicity testing of highly complex mixtures, containing hundreds of chemicals (e.g., diesel exhaust and other emissions), also has been performed. However, the general consensus within the scientific and regulatory communities is that systematic in vivo toxicity testing of chemical mixtures is impractical and unattainable because of the large number of combinations involved, ethical issues, and economic and resource considerations. In light of this, toxicity evaluation and risk assessment of chemical mixtures present formidable challenges to the scientific and regulatory communities. Two challenges of comparable significance are the development of databases derived from sources other than in vivo testing, and the utilization of integrative approaches (e.g., physiologically based pharmacokinetic modeling, and statistical/mathematic methodologies such as response surface methodology, median effect principle, and mechanistic-based studies). The utilization and integration of these approaches towards a better toxicologic characterization and a more predictive, realistic risk assessment have been discussed in several highly informative papers (El-Masri et al., 1997; Cassee et al., 1998).

Hormesis and Risk Assessment

The tenets that the dose makes the poison and that greater toxicities are manifested with increasing doses of chemical and physical agents provide the framework for assessing the hazard potential of chemicals. With the exception of carcinogens and certain immunotoxicants, it is generally recognized that there is a threshold dose below which toxic manifestations do not appear. Alternatively conceptualized, a given chemical is not interactive in a biologically meaningful way below the toxic threshold. The notion that a chemical or physical stressor is "inactive" below the toxic threshold, however, may not be an accurate description of the events occurring in the bioorganizational hierarchy from cells to the whole animal at "subtoxic" exposure levels. The hormesis concept may be understood best, both in terms of theory and relevance, if viewed as a composite of two phenomena, namely, the low-dose stimulatory effect and the adaptive response. Some authors have elected to place emphasis on one or the other of these two in describing the horemeis response. Low-dose stimulatory effect is the basis of the Arndt-Schulz law, which states that poisons are stimulatory at low doses. Nearly a century later, Stebbing (1982) defined hormesis in this context: "Hormesis is the stimulatory effects caused by low levels of toxic agents." There are many examples of hormetic and stimulatory effects on biologic processes following low-dose radiation or chemical exposure (Fritz-Niggli, 1995; Stebbing, 1985; Calabrese et al., 1987; Furst, 1987; Bailer and Oris, 1998).

The notion that hormesis is an adaptative response or mechanism originated from observations on the biologic effects of exposure to low-level radiation or to chemical agents. Representative topics of the many publications on inducible hormetic mechanisms include the following: low-level radiation (Sagen, 1989), free radical–generating systems (Utley and Mehendale, 1989, 1990a,b), and herbicide-induced stimulatory effects (Ries, 1976). Thus, the hormesis concept (the "two-stage" concept of toxicity) as currently viewed states that numerous chemical and physical stressors have the potential to initiate varying biologic events, including stimulatory action, at doses below the toxicity threshold. Hormesis is relevant to and has many implications for risk-assessment and risk-management processes and regulatory decision making. This is addresssed only briefly in this chapter, because it is covered in much greater detail in Chapter 10.

There is rigorous debate within the scientific and regulatory communities as to the validity and application of the hormesis concept. The implications for risk assessment as well as scientific issues must be addressed before hormesis can be integrated into risk-based regulations. Several of the more profound implications of hormesis involve the risk-assessment/risk-management paradigm (Paperiello, 1998; Sielken and Stevenson, 1998), derivation of RfDs (Calabrese and Baldwin, 1998), the development of regulatory limits (Foran, 1998), and risk perception and communication (Renn, 1998). The potential impacts of hormesis on risk assessment and suggested changes to the risk assessment process were discussed at length by Sielken and Stevenson. Some of the various ways in which hormesis could impact risk assessment are (1) a paradigm shift to facilitate the identification of the hormetic component of the dose–response relationship, (2) the inclusion of data sets indicative of salutary effects in low-dose risk characterization, and (3) a fuller characterization of the distribution of actual doses on exposure not limited to just upper bounds. Despite evidence for the hormetic response and the profound implications for risk assessment, the hormesis concept is as yet not "mainstream" in risk-assessment and regulatory processes. Regulatory agencies view the hormesis phenomenon as unproved or deem it irrelevant in regulatory decision making. This perspective stems from a number of factors: (1) The hormetic response may be not easily quantifiable and in some instances nondemonstrable; (2) beneficial effects such as hormesis have not been the focus of regulatory activities; and (3) regulatory interpretation of the mandates has seen them as the protection of the human population or the environment from health risks and not an endorsement of positive health effects; (4) hormetic-effects data sets have not been integrated into the risk-assessment paradigm, and their value is still under debate; and (5) there has been a contrast between public perception of risk and scientific rationale. Thus, the challenge is not simply addressing the scientific issues surrounding the hormesis phenomena but viewing the hormesis concept seriously to improve risk assessment and health-risk prediction in humans.

REFERENCES

Ackerman, W. G., Pott, G. Voss, B., Muller, K. M., and Gulach, U. 1981. Serum concentration of procollagen III peptide in comparison with the serum activity of N-acetyl-glucosaminidase for diagnosis of the activity of liver fibrosis in patients with chronic active liver disease. *Clin. Chim. Acta*. 112:365–369.

Anderson, L. M., Ward, J. M., Park, S. S., Jones, A. B., Junker, J. L., Gelboin, H. V., and Rice, J. M. 1987. Immuno-histochemical determination of inducibility phenotype with a monoclonal antibody to a methylcholanthrene-inducible isozyme of cytochrome P-450. *Cancer Res.* 47:6079–6085.

Anderson, M. E. 1989. Physiological modeling of tissue dosimetry. *CITT Activities* 9:2–8.

Anderson, M. E. 1995. What do we mean by ... dose? *Inhalation Toxicol.* 7:909–915.

Asada, M., and Galambos, R. J. 1963. Sorbitol dehydrogenase and hepatocellular injury: An experimental and clinical study. *Gastroenterology* 44:578–587.

Armstrong, R. N. 1987. Enzyme-catalyzed detoxication reactions: Mechanisms and stereochemistry. *CRC Crit. Rev. Biochem.* 22:39–888.

Asher, I. M. 1978. Inadvertent modification of the immune response: The effects of foods, drugs, and environmental contaminants. In *Proceedings of the 4th FDA Science Symposium, U.S. Naval Academy, Aug 28–30*. Washington, DC: FDA.

Bailer, A. J., and Oris, J. T. 1998. Incorporating hormesis in routine testing of hazards. *Belle Newsletter* 6(3):2.

Barnes, D. G., Daston, G. P., Evans, J. S., Jarabek, A. M., Kavlock, R. J., Kimmel, C. A., Park, C., and Spitzer, H. L. 1995. Benchmark dose workshop: Criteria for use of a benchmark dose to estimate a reference dose. *Regul. Toxicol. Pharmacol.* 21:296–306.

Barnes, D. G. and Dourson, M. 1988. Reference dose (RfD): Description and uses in health risk assessments. *Reg. Toxicol. Pharmacol.* 8:471–486.

Baron, J., Redick, J. A., and Guengerich, F. P. 1981. An immunohistochemical study on the localizations and distributions of phenobarbital- and 3-methylcholanthrene-inducible cytochromes P-450 within the livers of untreated rats. *J. Biol. Chem.* 256:5931–5937.

Bick, P. H. 1982. Immune system as a target organ for toxicity. *Environ. Health Perspect.* 42:2–7.

Bournias-Vardiabasis, N., and Buzin, C. H. 1986. Developmental effects of chemicals and the heat shock response in drosophila cells. *Teratogen. Carcinogen. Mutagen.* 6:523–536.

Bournias-Vardiabasis, N., Teplitz, R. L., Chernoff, G. F., and Seecof, R. L. 1983. Detection of teratogens in the drosophila embryonic cell culture test: assay of 100 chemicals. *Teratology* 28:100–122.

Bracken, W. M. and Klaassen, C. D. 1987. Induction of metallothionein in rat primary hepatocyte culture: Evidence for direct and indirect induction. *Toxicol. J. Environ. Health.* 22:163–174.

Bradway, D. E., Shafik, T. M., and Lores, E. M. 1977. Comparison of cholinesterase activity, residue levels, and urinary metabolite excretion of rats exposed to organophosphate pesticides. *J. Agric. Food. Chem.* 25:1353–1358.

Brady, F. O. and Helvig, B. S. 1984. Effect of epinephrine and norepinephrine on zinc thionein levels and induction in rat liver. *Am. J. Physiol.* 247:E 318–322.

Bremner, I., Williams, R. B., and Young, B. W. 1981. Effects of age, sex, and zinc status on the accumulation of (copper-zinc) metallothionein in rat kidneys. *J. Inorg. Biochem.* 14:135–146.

Buhler, D. R., and Williams, D. E. 1988. The role of biotransformation in the toxicity of chemicals. *Aquat. Toxicol.* 11:19–28.

Burke, M. D., and Mayer, R. T. 1974. Ethoxyresorufin: direct fluorometric assay of a microsomal O-dealkylation which is preferentially inducible by 3-methylcholanthrene. *Drug Metab. Dispos.* 2:583–588.

Calabrese, E. J. 1991. *Multiple Chemical Interactions*, Chelsea, MI: Lewis Publishers.

Calabrese, E. J., and Baldwin, L. A. 1998. Hormesis as a defalult parameter in RfD derivation. *Belle Newsletter* 7 (1):13–17.

Calabrese, E. J., McCarthy, M., and Kenyan, E. 1987. The occurrence of chemically-induced hormesis. *Health. Physics* 52:531–542.

Calleman, C. J., Ehrenberg, L., Jansson, B., Osterman-Golkar, S., Segerback, D., Svensson, K., and Wachtmeister, C.A. 1978. Monitoring and risk assessment by means of alkyl groups in hemoglobin in persons occupationally exposed to ethylene oxide. *J. Environ. Pathol. Toxicol.* 2:427–442.

Caltabiano, M. M., Koestler, T. P., Poste, G., and Greig, R. G. 1986. Induction of 32 and 34 –kDA stress proteins by sodium arsenite, heavy metals, and thiol-reactive agents. *J. Biol. Chem.* 261:13381–13386.

Carr, B. I., Huang, T. H., Buzin, C. H., and Itakura, K. 1986. Induction of heat shock gene expression without heat shock by hepatocarcinogens and during hepatic regeneration in rat liver. *Cancer Res.* 46:5106–5111.
Cassee, F. R., Groten, J. P., van Bladeren, P. J., and Feron, V. J. 1998. Toxicological evaluation and risk assessment of chemical mixtures. *Crit. Rev. Toxicol.* 28(1):73–101.
Centers for Disease Control (CDC)/ Agency for Toxic Substances and Disease Registry (ATSDR). 1990. *Internal report on biomarkers of organ damage and dysfunction for the renal, hepatobiliary, and immune systems*. Atlanta, GA: Subcommittee on Biomarkers of Organ Damage and Dysfunction of CDC/ATSDR, Centers for Disease Control.
Center for Risk Analysis. 1993. *Risk assessment in the Federal government: Questions and answers (Oct 1993)*. Cambridge, MA: Center for Risk Analysis, Harvard School of Public Health, Harvard University.
Chalmers, T. C. 1991. Problems induced by meta-analysis. *Stat. Methods* 10:971–980.
Chang, L. W., Hsia, S. M., Chan, P., and Hsieh, L. L. 1994. Macromolecular adducts: Biomarkers for toxicity and carcinogenesis. *Annu. Rev. Pharmacol. Toxicol.* 34:41–67.
Christensen, E. I., and Nielsen, S. 1991. Structural and functional features of protein handling in the kidney proximal tubule. *Semin. Nephrol.* 11:414–439.
Comer, S. W., Staiff, D., and Armstrong, J. 1975. Exposure of workers to nnnnnnnn. *Bull. Environ. Contam. Toxicol.* 13:385–391.
Conolly, R. B. 1990. Biologically-based models for toxic effects: Tools for hypothesis testing and improving health risk assessments. *CIIT Activities*. 10:1–8.
Cornish, H. H., Barth, M. L., and Dodson, V. N. 1970. Isozyme profiles and protein patterns in specific organ damage. *Toxicol. Appl. Pharmacol.* 16:411–423.
Cote, I. L., Rees, D. C., and J. R. Glowa. 1994. An introduction to the principles and methods of risk assessment, In *The vulnerable brain and environmental risks, vol. 3: Toxins in air and water*, eds. R. L. Isaacson and K. F. Jensen, pp. 185–206. New York: Plenum Press.
Cousins, R. J., and Leinart, A. S. 1988. Tissue-specific regulation of zinc metabolism and metallothionein genes by interleukin I. *FASEB J.* 2:2884–2890.
Coye, M. L., Lowe, I. A., and Maddy, K. J. 1986. Biological monitoring of agricultural workers exposed to pesticides: II. Monitoring of intact pesticides and their metabolites. *J. Occup. Med.* 28:28–36.
Crump, K. S. 1984. A new method for determining allowable daily intakes. *Fundam. Appl. Toxicol.* 4:854–871.
Davis, M. E., and Berndt, W. O. 1994. Renal methods for toxicology. In *Principles and methods of toxicology*, 3rd ed., ed. A. W. Hayes, pp. 871–894. New York: Raven Press.
Dean, J. H., Luster, M. I., Munson, A. E., and Amos, H. (eds.) 1985. *Immunotoxicology and immunopharmacology*, New York: Raven Press.
DeCaprio, A. P. 1997. Biomarkers: Coming of age for environmental and risk assessment. *Environ. Sci. Technol.* 31:1837–1848.
Depledge, M. H. 1994. The rational basis for the use of biomarkers as ecotoxicological tools, In *Nondestructive Biomarkers in vertebrates*, ed. M. C. Fossi and C. Leonzio, pp. 271–297. Boca Raton: CRC Press.
Dews, P. B. 1986. On the assessment of risk. In *Developmental and behavioral pharmacology*, eds. N. Krasnegor, J. Gray, and T. Thompson, pp. 53–65. Hillsdale, NJ: Lawrence Erlbaum.
Dourson, M. L., Knauf, L. A., and Swartout, J. C. 1992. On reference dose (RfD) and its underlying toxicity database. *Toxicol. Ind. Health.* 8:171–189.
Dourson, M. L., Felton, S. P., and Robinson, D. 1996. Evaluation of science-based uncertainty factors in noncancer risk assessment. *Reg. Toxicol. Pharmacol.* 24:108–120.
Duncan, R. C. and Griffith, J. 1985. Monitoring study of urinary metabolites and selected symptomatology among Florida citrus workers. *J. Toxicol. Environ. Health* 16:509–521.
Ehrenberg, L., Moustacchi, E., Osterman-Golkar, S., and Ekman, G. 1983. Dosimetry of genotoxic agents and dose-reponse relationships of their effects. *Mutation Res.* 123:121–182.
El-Masri, H., Reardon, K. F., and Yang, R. S. H. 1997. Integrated approaches for the analysis of toxicologic interactions of chemical mixtures. *Crit. Rev. Toxicol.* 27:175–197.

Engel, D. W., and Brouwer, M. 1989. Metallothionein and metallothionein-like proteins: Physiological importance. *Adv. Comp. Environ. Physiol.* 4:53-75.

Eto, M. 1974. *Organophosphorus pesticides: Organic and biological chemistry.* Cleveland, OH: CRC Press.

European Economic Community. 1994. *Technical guidance on risk assessment of existing substances in the context of commission regulation (EC) no. 1488194 in accordance with council regulation (EEC) no. 793193 on the evaluation and control of existing substances,* draft. EEC.

Farmer, P. B., and Bailey, E. 1989. Protein-carcinogen adducts in human dosimetry. *Arch. Toxicol. Suppl.* 13:83-90.

Fay, R. M., and Feron, V. J. 1996. Complex mixtures: Hazard identification and risk assessment. *Food Chem. Toxicol.* 34:1175-1176.

Feron, V. J., Groten, J. P., Jonker, D., Cassee, F. R., and van Bladeren, P. J. 1995. Toxicology of chemical mixtures: Challenges for today and the future. *Toxicology* 105:415-427.

Forkert, P. G., Mirehouse-Brown, P., Park, S. S., and Gelboin, H. V. 1988. Distribution and induction sites of phenobarbital- and 3-methylcholanthrene-inducible cytochromes P-450 in murine liver: Immunohistochemical localization with monoclonal antibodies. *Molec. Pharmacol.* 34:736-743.

Forkert, P. G., Vessey, M. L., Park, S. S., Gelboin, H. V., and Cole, S. P. C. 1989. Cytochromes P-450 in murine lung: An immunohistochemical study with monoclonal antibodies. *Drug Metab. Dispos.* 17:551-555.

Foran, J. A. 1998. Regulatory implications of hormesis. *BELLE Newsletter* 7 (1):11-13.

Fossi, M. C., and Leonzio, C. 1994. *Non-destructive biomarkers in vertebrates.* Boca Raton, FL: CRC Press.

Foster, R., Elcombe, C. R., Boobis, A. R., Davies, D. S., Sesardic, D., McQuade, J., Robson, R. T., Hayward, C., and Lock, E. A. 1986. Immunocytochemical localization of cytochrome P-450 in hepatic and extrahepatic tissues of the rat with a monoclonal antibody against cytochrome P-450c. *Biochem. Pharmacol.* 35:4543-4554.

Foulkes, E. C. 1993. Functional assessment of the kidney. In *Toxicology of the Kidney,* 2nd ed., eds. J. B. Hook and R. S. Goldstein, pp. 37-60. New York: Raven Press.

Fowle, J. R. III. 1989. Summary and perspectives: Panel discussion on toxicology and exposure assessment: state of the art. *J. Am. Coll. Toxicol.* 8:865.

Franklin, C. A., Fenske, R. A., and Grenhalgh, R. 1981. Correlation of urinary pesticide metabolite excretion with estimated dermal contact in the cause of occupational exposure to guthion. *J. Toxicol. Environ. Health* 7:715-731.

Franklin, C. A., Muir, H. I., and Moody, R. 1986. The use of biological monitoring in the estimation of exposure during application of pesticides. *Toxicol. Lett.* 33:127-136.

Friedman, R. L., and Stark, K. T. 1985. Alpha-interferon induced transcription of HLA and metallothionein genes containing homologous upstream sequences. *Nature (London)* 314:637-639.

Fritz-Niggli, H. 1995. 100 years of radiobiology: Implications for biomedicine and future perspectives. *Experientia* 51:652-664.

Fukuto, T. R. 1972. Metabolism of carbamate insecticides. *Drug Metabol. Rev.* 1:117-151.

Furst, A. 1987. Hormetic effects in pharmacology: Pharmacological inversions as prototypes for hormesis. *Health. Physics* 52:527-530.

Galen, R. S. 1975. Multiphasic screening and biochemical profiles: State of the art. In *Progress in clinical pathology,* Vol. 6, ed. M. Stefanini and H. D. Isenberg, pp. 83-110. New York: Grune and Stratton.

Garvey, J. 1984. Metallothionein: Structure/antigenicity and detection/quantitation in normal physiological fluids. *Environ. Health Perspect.* 54:117-127.

Gaylor, D. W. 1989. Quantitative risk analysis for quantal reproductive and developmental effects. *Environ. Health Perspect.* 79:243-246.

Gaylor, D. W., and Slikker, W., Jr. 1990. Risk assessment for neurotoxic effects. *Neurotoxicology* 11:211-218.

Gaylor, D. W., and Slikker, W., Jr. 1992. Risk assessment for neurotoxicants. In *Neurotoxicology: Principles of route-to-route extrapolation for risk assessment*, eds. H. Tilson and C. Mitchell. New York: Elsevier.
Gingerich, W. H. 1982. Hepatotoxicology of fishes. In *Aquatic toxicology*, vol. 1, ed. L. J. Weber, pp. 55–105. New York: Raven Press.
Gingerich, W. H., and Weber, L. J. 1979. *Assessment of clinical laboratory procedures to evaluate liver intoxication in fish*, EPA/600/3/79/088. Duluth, MN: Environmental Protection Agency.
Gooch, J. W., Elskus, A. A., Kloepper-Sams, P. J., Hahn, M. E., and Stegeman, J. J. 1989. Effects of ortho- and non-ortho substituted polychlorinated biphenyl congeners on the hepatic monoxygenase system in scup. *Toxicol. Appl. Pharmacol.* 98:422–433.
Groten, J. P., Schoen, E. D., van Bladeren, P. J., and Feron, V. J. 1994. Subacute toxicity of a combination of nine chemicals in rats: A two-level factorial design to predict interactive effects. *Toxciologist* (abstract No. 1153).
Grue, C. E., Fleming, W. J., Busby, D. G., and Hill, E. F. 1983. Assessing hazards of organophosphate pesticides to wildlife. *Trans. North Am. Wildl. Natl. Res. Conf.* 48:200–220.
Guengerich, F. 1982. Microsomal enzymes involved in toxicology-analysis and separation. In *Principles and methods of toxicology*, ed. A. Hayes, pp. 609–634. New York: Raven Press.
Guth, D. J., Jarabek, A. M., Wymer, L., and Hertzberg, R. C. 1991. *Evaluation of risk assessment methods for short-term inhalation exposure*, paper no. 91.173.2, Presented at the 84th Annual Meeting of the Air and Water Waste Management Association, Vancouver, BC, Canada.
Haasch, M. L., Wejksnora, P. J., Stegeman, J. J., and Lech, J. J. 1989. Cloned rainbow trout liver P_1450 complmentary DNA as a potential environmental monitor. *Toxicol. Appl. Pharmacol.* 98:362–368.
Hallenbeck, W. H. 1986. In *Quantitative risk assessment for environmental and occupational health*, eds. W. H. Hallenbeck and K. M. Cunningham, pp. 1–2. Chelsea, MI: Lewis Publishers.
Hamer, D. H. 1986. Metallothionein. *Ann. Rev. Biochem.* 55:913–951.
Hammock, B. D., Gee, S. J., Cheung, P. Y. K. 1987. Utility of trace analysis. In *Pesticide science and Biotechnology*, eds. P. Greenhaigh and T. R. Roberts, pp. 309–316. London: Oxford/Blackwell.
Hammock, B. D., and Mumma, R. A. 1980. Potential of immunochemical technology for pesticide analysis. In *Pesticide analytical methodology*, American Chemical Society Symposium Series 136, eds. J. Harvey and G. Zweig, pp. 321–351. Washington, DC: American Chemical Society.
Hammond, P. B., and Belile, R. P. 1980. Metals. In *Casarett and Doull's toxicology: The basic science of poisons*, J. Doull, C. D. Klassen, and M. O. Amdur, pp. 409–476. New York: MacMillan.
Hammond, G. L., Lai, Y. K., and Market, C. L. 1982. Diverse forms of stress lead to new patterns of gene expression through a common and essential metabolic pathway. *Proc. Natl. Acad. Sci. U. S. A.* 79:3485–3488.
Hedges, L. V., and Olkin, I. 1985. *Statistical methods for meta-analysis*. San Diego: Academic Press.
Hertzberg, R. C. 1989. Fitting a model to categorical response data with application to species extrapolation of toxicity. *Health Physics* 57:405–409.
Hertzberg, R. C., and Miller, M. 1985. A statistical model for species extrapolation using categorical response data. *Toxicol. Ind. Health.* 1:43–57.
Hinton, D. E., Baumann, P. C., Gardner, G. R., Hawkins, W. E., Hendricks, J. D., Murchelano, R. A., and Okihiro, M. S. 1992. Histopathologic biomarkers. In *Biomarkers: Biochemical, physiological, and histopathological markers of anthropogenic stress*, eds. R. J. Huggett, R. A. Kimerle, P. M. Mehrle, and H. L. Bergman, pp. 155–209. Chelsea, MI: Lewis Publishers.
Hodson, P. V., Blunt, B. R., Spry, O. J., and Austen, K. 1977. Evaluation of erythrocyte aminolevulinic acid dehydratase activity as a short-term indicator in fish of a harmful exposure to lead. *J. Fish. Res.* 34:501–508.
Holland, H. T., Coppage, D. L., and Butler, P. A. 1967. Use of fish brain acetylcholinesterase to monitor pollution by organophosphorus pesticides. *Bull. Environ. Contam. Toxicol.* 2:156–162.
Honeycutt, R. C. 1986. NACA overview on assessment of mixer-loader-applicator exposure to pesticides. *Toxicol. Lett.* 33:175–182.
Huggett, R. J., Kimerle, R. A., Mehrle, P. M., Bergman, H. L., Dickson, K. L., Fava, J. A., McCarthy, J. F., Parrish, R., Dorn, B. P., McFarland, V., and Lahvis, G. 1992. Introduction. In *Biomarkers*:

Biochemical, physiological, and histological markers of anthropogenic stress, ed. R. L. Huggett, R. A. Kimerle, P. M. Mehrie, Jr., and H. L. Bergman, pp. 1–4. Boca Raton, FL: Lewis Publishers.

Human Ecology and Risk Assessment. 1995. Special Issue: EPA uncertainty factor workshop. *Hum. Ecol. Risk. Assess.* 1:459–662.

Jarabek, A. M. 1994. Inhalation RfC methodology: Dosimetric adjustments, and dose-response estimation of noncancer toxicity in the upper respiratory tract. *Inhalation Toxicology.* 6 (Suppl.): 301–325.

Jarabek, A. M. 1995. The application of dosimetry models to identify key processes and parameters for default dose-response assessment approaches. *Toxicol. Lett.* 79:171–184

Jarabek, A. M., and Hasselblad, V. 1991. *Inhalation reference concentration methodology: Impact of dosimetric adjustments and future directions using the confidence profile method*, paper 91-173.3. Presented at the 84th Annual Meeting of the Air and Water Waste Management Association, Vancouver, BC.

Jarabek, A. M., and Hasselblad, V. 1992. Application of bayesian statistical approach to response analysis of non-cancer toxic effects. *Toxicologist* 12 (abstract No. 305).

Jonker, D., Woutersen, R. A., van Bladeren, P. J., Til, H. P., and Feron, V. J. 1990. 4-week oral toxicity study of a combination of eight chemicals in rats: Comparison with the toxicity of the individual compounds. *Food. Chem. Toxicol.* 28:623–631.

Jonker, D., Woutersen, R. A., van Bladeren, P. J., Til, H. P., and Feron, V. J. 1993. Subacute (4-week) oral toxicity of a combination of four nephrotoxins in rats: comparison with the toxicity of the individual compounds. *Food. Chem. Toxicol.* 31:125–136.

Kachmar, J. F., and Moss, D. W. 1976. Enzymes. In *Fundamentals of clinical chemistry*, ed. N. W. Tietz, pp. 652–660. Philadelphia: W. B. Saunders.

Kagi, J. H., and Kojima, Y. 1987. Chemistry and biochemistry of metallothionein. *Experientia (Suppl.)* 52:35–61.

Kagi, J. H., and Nordberg, M. (eds.) 1978. *Metallothionein.* Basel: Birkhauser.

Kapour, M., and Lewis, J. 1987. Alteration of the protein synthesis pattern in *Neurospora crassa* cells by hypothermal and oxidative stress. *Can. J. Microbiol.* 33:162–168.

Karin, M. 1985. Metallothionein: Proteins in search of function. *Cell* 4:9–10.

Keyse, S. M., and Tyrrell, R. M. 1989. Heme oxygenase is the major 32 kda stress protein induced in human skin fibroblast by uva radiation, hydrogen peroxide, and sodium arsenite. *Proc. Natl. Acad. Sci. U. S. A.* 86:99–103.

Kimmel, C. A. 1990. Quantitative approaches to human risk assessment for non-cancer health effects. *Neurotoxicology* 11:189–198.

Kimmel, C. A., and Gaylor, D. W. 1988. Issues in qualitative and quantitative risk analysis for developmental toxicology. *Risk Anal.* 8:15–20.

Kleinow, K., Melancon, M. J., and Lech, J. J. 1987. Biotransformation and induction: Implications for toxicity, bioaccumulation, and monitoring of environmental xenobiotics in fish. *Environ. Health. Perspect.* 71:105–119.

Kloepper-Sams, P. J., and Stegeman, J. J. 1989. The temporal relationshiops between P450E protein content, catalytic activity, and mRNA levels in the teleost *Fundulus heteroclitus* following treatment with β-naphthoflavone. *Arch. Biochem. Physics.* 268:525–535.

Klotz, A. V., Stegeman, J. J., and Walsh, C. 1984. An alternative 7-ethoxyresorufin-O-deethylase activity assay: A continuous visible spectrophotometric method for measurement of cytochrome P-450 monooxygenase activity. *Anal. Biochem.* 140:138–145.

Kraus, J. F., Mull, R., and Kurtz, P. 1981. Monitoring of grape harvesters for evidence of cholinesterase inhibition. *J. Toxicol. Environ. Health.* 7:19–31.

Krewski, D. C., Brown, C., and Murdock, D. 1984. Determining "safe" levels of exposure: safety factors or mathematical models. *Fundam. Appl. Toxicol.* 4:S383–S394.

Lave, L. B. 1982. In *Quantitative risk assessment in regulation*, ed. L. B. Lave, p. 6. Washington, DC: The Brookings Institution.

Lavy, T. L., and Mattice, J. D. 1986. Progress in pesticide exposure studies and future concerns. *Toxicol. Lett.* 33:61–71.

Lehman, A. J., and Fitzhugh, O. G. 1954. 100-fold margin of safety. *Assoc. Food Drug Officials U.S. Quart. Bull.* 18:33–35.

Lindquist, S. 1986. The heat shock response. *Ann. Rev. Biochem.* 55:1151–1191.
Lu, A. Y. H., and West, S. 1980. Multiplicity of mammalian microsomal cytochromes P-450. *Pharmacol. Rev.* 31:277–296.
Lu, F. C. 1988. Acceptable daily intake: Inception, evolution, and application. *Reg. Toxicol. Pharmacol.* 8:45–60.
Lu, F. C., and Sielken, R. L. 1991. Assessment of safety/risk of chemicals: inception and evolution of the ADI and dose-response modeling procedures. *Toxicol. Lett.* 59:5–40.
Luster, M. I., D. R., Blank, J. A., and Dean, J. H. 1987. Molecular and cellular basis of chemically-induced immunotoxicity. *Ann. Rev. Pharmacol. Toxicol.* 27:23–49.
Luster, M. I., Munson, A. E., Thomas, P. T.; Holsapple, M. P., Fenters, J. D., White, K. L., Lauer, L. D., Germolec, D. R., Rosenthal, G. J., and Dean, J. H. 1988. Development of a testing battery to assess chemical-induced immunotoxicity: National Toxicology Program's guidelines for immunotoxicity evaluation in mice. *Fundam. Appl. Toxicol.*10:2–19.
Mauderly, J. L. 1993. Toxicological approaches to complex mixtures. *Envrion. Health Perspect. Suppl.* 101 (4):155–164.
Mayer, F. L., Versteeg, D. J., McKee, M. J., Folmar, L. C., Graney, R. L., McCume, D. C., and Rattner, B. A. 1992. Physiological and nonspecific biomarkers. In *Biomarkers: Biochemical, physiological, and histological markers of anthropogenic stress*, eds. R. J. Huggett, R. A. Kimerle, P. M. Mehrle Jr., and H. L. Bergman, pp. 5–85. Chelsea, MI: Lewis Publishers.
McCarthy, J. F., Adams, S. M., Jimenez, B. D., and Shugart, L. R. 1989. Environmental monitoring of biological markers in animals and plants. In *Proceedings 2nd US-USSR Symposium on: Air Pollution Effects on Vegetation*, eds. R. D. Noble, J. L. Martin, and K. F. Jensen, pp. 187–196. Broomall, PA: Northeastern Forest Experiment Station.
Miller, D. S. 1981. Heavy metal inhibition of p-aminohippurate transport in flounder renal tissue: Sites of $HgCl_2$ action. *J. Pharmacol. Exp. Ther.* 219:428–434.
Miller, E. C., and Miller, J. A. 1981. Mechanism of chemical carcinogensis. *Cancer* 47:1055–1069.
Miller, E. C., and Miller, J. A. 1985. Some historical perspectives on the metabolism of xenobiotic chemicals to reactive electrophiles. In *Bioactivation of foreign compounds*, ed. M. W. Anders, pp. 3–28. Orlando, FL: Academic Press.
Moody, D. E., Taylor, L. A., Smuckler, E. A., Levin, W., and Thomas, P. E. 1983. Immunohistochemical localization of cytochrome P-450 in liver sections from untreated rats and rats treated with phenobarbital or 3- methylcholan-threne. *Drug. Metab. Dispos.* 11:339–343.
Moromoto, R., Tissieres, A. and Georgopoulos, C. (eds.) 1990. *The role of the stress response in biology and disease*. Cold Spring Harbor, NY: Cold Spring Harbor Laboratory.
Moseman, R., and Oswald, E. 1980. Development of analytical methodology for assessment of human exposure to pesticides. In *Pesticide analytical methodology*, American Chemical Society (ACS) Symposium Series 136, eds. R. Cannizaro, H. Dishburger, and J. Sherma, pp. 251–257. Washington, DC: ACS.
Mull, R., and McCarthy, J. F. 1986. Guidelines for conducting mixer/loader-applicator studies. *Vet. Hum. Toxicol.* 28:328–336.
Mumma, R. O., and Brady, J. F. 1987. Immunological assays for agrochemicals, In *Pesticide science and biotechnology*, ed. R. Greenhaigh and T. R. Roberts, pp. 341–348. London: Oxford/Blackwell.
Mumtaz, M. M., DeRosa, C. T., and Durkin, P. R. 1994. Approaches and challenges in risk assessment of chemical mixtures. In *Toxicology of chemical mixtures*, ed. R. S. H. Yang, pp. 565–596. New York: Academic Press.
Mumtaz, M. M., Sipes, I. G., Clewell, H. J., and Yang, R. S. H. 1993. Risk assessment of chemical mixtures: Biologic and toxicologic issues. *Fundam. Appl. Toxicol.* 21:258–269.
Munro, I. C. and Krewski, D. R. 1981. Risk assessment and regulatory decision making. *Food Cosmet. Toxicol.* 19:549–560.
Murthy, M. S., Calleman, C. J., Osterman-Golkar, S., Segergack, D., and Svensson, K. 1984. Relationships between ethylation of hemoglobin, ethylation of DNA and administered amount of ethyl methanesulfonate in the mouse. *Mutat. Res.* 127:1–8.

National Academy of Sciences/National Research Council 1983. *Risk assessment in the Federal government*: *Managing the process*. Washington, DC: National Academy Press.

National Academy of Sciences/National Research Council. 1987. Biological markers in environmental health research. *Environ. Health. Perspect.* 74:3–9.

National Academy of Sciences/National Research Council. 1988. *Complex mixtures*. Washington, DC: National Academy Press.

National Academy of Sciences. 1989. *Biologic markers of reproductive toxicology*, pp. 15–35. Washington, DC: National Academy Press.

National Academy of Sciences/National Research Council. 1994. *Science and judgment in risk assessment*. Washington, DC: National Academy Press.

National Toxicology Program. 1993. *Toxicity studies of a chemical mixture of 25 groundwater contaminants administered in drinking water to F344 / N rats and B6C3F$_1$ Mice*, NTP Technical Report Series No. 35, NTP Publication 93–3384.

Nebert, D. W. 1979. Multiple forms of inducible drug-metabolizing enzymes: A reasonable mechanism by which any organism can cope with adversity. *Mol. Cell. Biochem.* 27:27–46.

Nebert, D. W. and Gelboin, H. V. 1968. Substrate-inducible microsomal aryl hydrocarbon hydroxylase in mammalian cell culture. *J. Biol. Chem.* 243:6242–6249.

Nogawa, K. Yamada, Y., Kido, T., Honda, R., Ishizaki, M., Tswitsmi, I. and Kobayaski, E. 1986. Significance of elevated urinary N-acetyl-β-D-glucosaminidase activity in chronic cadmium poisoning. *Sci. Total Environ.* 53:173–178.

Ortiz de Montellano, P. R. 1986. *Cytochrome P-450: Structure, mechanism, and biochemistry*, New York: Plenum Press.

Osterman-Golkar, S., Ehrenberg, L., Segerback, D., and Hallstrom, I. 1976. Evaluation of genetic risks of alkylating agents: II. Haemoglobin as a dose monitor. *Mutation Res.* 34:1–10.

Paperiello, C. W. 1998. Risk management and risk management implications of hormesis. *BELLE Newsletter* 7(1):28–30.

Parke, D. V. 1990. Induction of cytochromes P-450: General principles and biological consequences. In *Frontiers in biotransformation*, vol. 2: *Principles, mechanisms and biological consequences of induction*, eds. K. Ruckpaul and H. Rein, pp. 1–34. London: Taylor and Francis.

Paustenbach, D. J. 1995. The practice of health risk assessment in the United States (1975–1995): How the U.S. and other countries can benefit from that experience. *Hum. Ecol. Risk Assess.* 1:29–79.

Patton, J. F. 1978. Indocyanine green: A test of hepatic function and a measure of plasma volume in the duck. *Comp. Biochem. Physiol.* 60A:21–24.

Payne, J. F., Fancey, L. L., Rahimtula, A. D., and Porter, E. L. 1987. Review and perspective on the use of mixed-function oxygenase enzymes in biological monitoring. *Comp. Biochem. Physiol.* 86C:233–245.

Peakall, D. B. 1994. Biomarkers: The way forward in environmental assessment. *Toxicol. Ecotox. News* 1(2):55–60.

Pereira, M. A., and Chang, L. W. 1981. Binding of chemical carcinogens and mutagens to rat hemoglobin. *Chem. Biol. Interact.* 33:301–306.

Pereira, M. A., Lin, L. H. C., and Chang, L. W. 1981. Dose dependency of 2-acetylaminofluorene binding to liver DNA and hemoglobin in mice and rats. *Toxicol. Appl. Pharmacol.* 60:472–478.

Perera, F. P. 1987. Molecular cancer epidemiology: A new tool in cancer prevention. *J. Natl. Cancer Inst.* 78:887–898.

Philip, D. H. and Sims, P. Polycyclic aromatic hydrocarbon metabolites: Their reactions with nucleic acids. In *Chemical carcinogens and DNA*, vol. 2, ed. P. L. Grover, pp. 29–57. Boca Raton, FL: CRC Press.

Plaa, G. L. and Charbonneau, M. 1994. Detection and evaluation of chemically induced liver injury. In *Principles and methods of toxicology*, 3rd ed., eds. A. W. Hayes, pp. 839–870. New York: Raven Press.

Preuss, P. W., and Ehrlich, A. M. 1987. The environmental protection agency's risk assessment guidelines. *J. Air. Pollut. Control. Assoc.* 37:784–791.

Recknagel, R. O., and Glende, E. A. Jr., 1973. Carbon tetrachloride hepatotoxicity: An example of lethal cleavage. *CRC Crit. Rev. Toxicol.* 2:263-297.
Ratanasavanh, D., Beaune, P., Baffet, G., Rissel, M., Kremers, P., Guengerich, F. P., and Guillouzo, A. 1986. Immunocytochemical evidence for the maintenance of cytochrome P-450 isozymes, NADPH cytochrome C reductase, and epoxide hydrolase in pure and mixed primary cultures of adult human hepatocyte. *J. Histochem. Cytochem.* 34:527-533.
Renn, O. 1998. Implications of the hormesis hypothesis for risk perception and communication. *BELLE Newsletter.* 7(1):2-9.
Ries, S. K. 1976. Subtoxic effects on plants in two herbicides. In *Herbicides*, pp. 313-344.
Rodgers, K. E., Devens, B. H., and Imamura, T. 1992. Immunotoxic effects of anticholinesterases. In *Clinical and experimental toxicology of organophosphates and carbamates*, eds. B. Ballantyne and T.C. Marrs, pp. 211-222. London: Butterworth-Heinemann.
Rodricks, J. V., Brett, S. M., and Wrenn, G. C. 1987. Significant risk decisions in federal regulatory agencies. *Reg. Toxicol. Pharmacol.* 7:307-320.
Sagen, L. 1989. On radiation, paradigms, and hormesis. *Science* 245:574.
Sanders, B. 1990. Stress proteins: Potential as multitiered biomarkers. In *Biomarkers of environmental contamination*, ed. J. F. McCarthy and L. R. Shugart, p. 165. Boca Raton, FL: Lewis Publishers.
Saunderman, F. W., and Horak, E. 1981. Biochemical indices of nephrotoxicity exemplified by studies of nickel nephropathy. In *Organ-directed toxicity, chemical indices and mechanisms*, eds. S. S. Brown and D. S. Davis, pp. 55-67. New York: Pergamon Press.
Schenkman, J. B., Robie, K. M., and Jansson, I. 1977. Aryl hydrocarbon hydroxylase: Induction, In *Biological reactive intermediates/formation: Toxicity and inactivation*, ed. D. S. Follow, J. Kocsis, J. J. Snyder, and R. Vainio. New York: Plenum Press.
Scheuhammer, A. M. 1987. Erythrocyte α-aminolevulinic acid dehydratase in birds: The effects of lead and other metals. *Toxicology.* 45:155-163.
Schlesinger, M. J., Ashburner, M., and Tissieres, A. 1982. *Heat shock from bacteria to man*, pp. 1-440. Cold Spring Harbor, NY: Cold Spring Harbor Laboratory.
Segerback, D., Calleman, C. J., Ehrenberg, L., Loforth, G., and Osterman-Golkar, S. 1978. Evaluation of genetic risks of alkylating agents: IV. Quantitative determination of alkylated amino acids in hemoglobin as a measure of the dose after treatment of mice with methylmethanesulfonate. *Mutat. Res.* 49:71-82.
Shafik, T. M. 1980. Analytical approaches for determining human exposure to pesticides. *J. Environ. Sci. Health.* B15:1023-1058.
Shafik, T. M., and Bradway, D. E. 1976. Worker re-entry safety VIII: The determination of urinary metabolites—an index of human and animal exposure to non-persistent pesticides. *Res. Rev.* 62:59-77.
Sharma, R. P. 1981. *Immunologic considerations in toxicology*, vols. 1 and 2. Boca Raton, FL: CRC Press.
Sharma, R. P. and Tomar, R. S. 1992. Immunotoxicology of anticholinesterase agents. In *Clinical and experimental toxicology of organophosphates and carbamates*, ed. B. Ballantyne and T. C. Marrs. pp. 203-210. London: Butterworth-Heinemann.
Shoaf, C. R. 1991 Current assessment practices for non-cancer endpoints. *Environ. Health Perspect.* 95:111-119.
Sielken, R. L. Jr., and Stevenson, D. E. 1998. Some implications for quantitative risk assessment if hormesis exists. *Hum. Exp. Toxicol.* 17:259-262.
Simonsen, L., Lund, S. P., and Hass, U. 1996. An approach to risk assessment. *Neurotoxicology* 17:815-824.
Skipper, P. L., and Tannenbaum, S. R. 1990. Protein adducts in the molecular dosimetry of chemical carcinogens. *Carcinogenesis* 11:507-518.
Smith-Sonneborn, J. 1992. The role of the stress protein response in hormesis. In *Biological effects of low level exposure to chemicals and radiation*, ed. E. J. Calabrese, pp. 41-52. Chelsea, MI: Lewis Publishers.
Smolowitz, R. M., Hahn, M. E., and Stegeman, J. J. 1991. Immunohistochemical localization of cytochrome P-450lA1 induced by 3,3' 4,4'-tetrachlorobiphenyl and by 2,3,7,8-

tetrachlorodibenzofuran in liver and extrahepatic tissues of the teleost *Stenotomus chrysops* (SCUP). *Drug Metab. Dispos.* 19:113–123.

Stebbing, A. R. D. 1982. Hormesis: The stimulation of growth by low levels of inhibitors. *Sci. Total Environ.* 22:213–234.

Stebbing, A. R. D. 1985. Organotins and water quality: Some lessons learned. *Marine Pollut. Bull.* 16:383–390.

Stegeman, J. J., Brouwer, M., DiGiulio, R. T., Forlin, L. Fowler, B. A., Sanders, B. M., and VanVeld, P. A. 1992. Molecular responses to environmental contamination: Enzyme and protein systems as indicators of chemical exposure and effect. In *Biomarkers: Biochemical, physiological, and histological markers of anthropogenic stress*, ed. R. J. Huggett, R. A. Kimerle, P. M. Mehrle, and H. L. Bergman, pp. 235–335. Boca Raton: Lewis Publishers.

Stevens, D. K., Bull, R. J., Nauman, C. H., and Blancato, J. N. 1991. Decision model for biomarkers of exposure. *Reg. Toxicol. Pharmacol.* 14:286–296.

St. Omer, V. E. V., and Rottinghaus, G. E. 1992. Biochemical determination of cholinesterase activity in biological fluids and tissues. In *Clinical and experimental toxicology of organophosphates and carbamates*, ed. B. Ballantyne, T. C. Marrs, and W. N. Aldridge, pp. 15–46. Oxford: Butterworth and Heinemann.

Stonard, M. D., and Evans, G. O. 1994. Clinical chemistry. In *General and applied toxicology*, eds. B. Ballantyne, T. Marrs, and P. Turner, pp. 303–332. New York: M. Stockton Press.

Stroo, W. E., and Hook, J. B. 1977. Enzymes of renal origin in urine as indicators of nephrotoxicity. *Toxicol. Appl. Pharmacol.* 39:423–434.

Subjeck, J. R., and Shyy T. 1986. Stress protein systems of mammalian cells. *Cell Physiol.* 19:C1–C17.

Tannenbaum, S. R., Skipper, P. L., Greeen, L. C., Obiedzinski, M. W., and Kadlubar, F. 1983. Blood protein adducts as monitors of exposure to 4-aminobiphenyl. *Proc. Am. Assoc. Cancer Res.* 24:69.

Tarloff, J. B. and Goldstein, R. S. 1994. In vitro assessment of nephrotoxicity, In *In vitro toxicology*, ed. S.C. Gad, pp. 149–193. New York: Raven Press.

Thakker, D. R., Yagi, H., Levin, W., Wood, A. W., Conney, A. H., and Jerina, D. M. 1985. In *Bioactivation of foreign compounds*, ed. M. W. Anders, pp. 177–242. Orlando, FL: Academic Press.

The Presidential/Congressional Commission on Risk Assessment and Risk Management. 1997. *Risk assessment and risk management in regulatory decision-making*, final report (volume 2). Washington, DC: Author.

Thomas, P. T., and House, R. V. 1995. Preclinical immunotoxicity assessment. In *CRC Handbook of Toxicology*, eds. M. J. Derelanko and M. A. Hollinger, pp. 294–316. Boca Raton, FL: CRC Press.

Thorgeirsson, S., Glowinski, I. B., and Mc Manus, M. E. 1983. Metabolism, mutagenicity and carcinogenicity of aromatic amines. *Rev. Biochem. Toxicol.* 5:349–386.

Toxicology Excellence for Risk Assessment. 1996. *Evaluation of science-based uncertainty factors in non-cancer risk assessment*, Full Report Prepared for Heatlh and Environmental Sciences Institute, Cincinnati, OH.

Truhaut, R. 1991. The concept of the acceptable daily intake: An historical review. *Food Add. Contam.* 8:151–162.

Trump, B. F., McDowell, E. M., and Arstilia, A. U. 1980. Cellular reaction to injury. In *Principles of pathobiology*, 3rd ed., eds. R. B. Hill and M. F. LaVia, pp. 20–111. New York: Oxford University Press.

Tucker, S. M. Rrice, R. J., and Price, G. R. 1980. Characteristics of human N-acetyl-D-glucosaminidase isoenzymes as an indicator of tissue damage in disease. *Clin. Chim. Acta.* 102:29–40.

U.S. Environmental Protection Agency. 1984. Proposed guidelines for carcinogenicity, mutagenicity, and developmental toxicant risk assessment. *Fed. Reg.* 49:46294–46331.

U.S. Environmental Protection Agency. 1986a. Guidelines for carcinogenic risk assessment, *Fed. Reg.* 51:33992–34003, Washington, D.C.

U.S. Environmental Protection Agency, 1986b Guidelines for mutagenicity risk assessment, Fed. Reg. 51:34006-34012.
U.S. Environmental Protection Agency. 1986c Guidelines for Exposure Assessment. Federal Register, 51:34042-34050.
U.S. Environmental Protection Agency. 1986d. Guidelines for the health risk assessment of chemical mixtures. Fed. Reg. 51:34014-34025.
U.S. Environmental Protection Agency. 1987. Applicator exposure monitoring: Pesticide Assessment Guidelines, NTIS PB87-133286. Springfield, VA. National Technical Information Service, U.S. Dept. of Commerce.
U.S. Environmental Protection Agency. 1988a. Proposed guidelines for assessing female reproductive risk. Fed. Reg. 53:24834-24847.
U.S. Environmental Protection Agency. 1988b. Proposed guidelines for assessing male reproductive hazard. Fed. Reg. 53:24850-24869.
U.S. Environmental Protection Agency. 1989. Decision model for the development of biomarkers of exposure, EPA/600/x-89/163. Washington, DC: Author.
U.S. Environmental Protection Agency. 1990. Technical support document on health risk assessment of chemical mixtures, EPA/600/8-90/064. Cincinnati, OH: EPA Environmental Assessment and Criteria Office.
U.S. Environmental Protection Agency. 1992. Guidelines for exposure assessment. Fed. Reg. 57:22888-22938.
U.S. Environmental Protection Agency. 1994a. Principles of neurotoxicity risk assessment: Notice. Fed. Reg. 59:42360-42404.
U.S. Environmental Protection Agency. 1994b. Guidelines for reproductive risk assessment, EPA/600/AP-94/001. Washington, DC: Author.
U.S. Environmental Protection Agency. 1996. Proposed guidelines for carcinogen risk assessment. Fed. Reg. 6l:17960-18011.
Utley, W. S., and Mehendale, H. M. 1989a. Pentobarbital-induced cytosolic cytoprotective mechanisms that offset increases in NADPH cytochrome P-450 reductase activity in menadione-mediated cytotoxicity. Toxicol. Appl. Pharmacol. 99:323-333.
Utley, W. S., and Mehendale, H. M. 1990a. Phenobarbital-induced cytoprotective mechanisms in menadione metabolism: The role of glutathione reductase and DT-diaphorase. Int. J. Biochem. 22:957-967.
Utley, W. S., and Mehendale, H. M. 1990b. Cytoprotective mechanisms that offset phenobarbital-induced increment in O2 generated from quinone recycling. In Proceedings of the International Conference on Biological Oxidation Systems, vol.1, eds. C. C. Redddy, G. Hamilton, and K. M. Madhyastha, pp. 183-200. San Diego, CA: Academic Press.
Vanderlaan, M., Watkins, B. E., and Stanker, L. 1988. Envrionmental monitoring by immunoassay. Envrion. Sci. Technol. 22:247-254.
Vasilic, Z., Drevenkar, V., Frobe, Z. 1987. The metabolites of organophosphate pesticides in urine as an indicator of occupational exposure. Toxicol. Environ. Chem. 14:111-127.
Vogt, R. F. 1991. Use of laboratory tests for immune biomarkers in environmental health studies concerned with exposure to indoor air pollutants. Envrion. Health Perspectives 95:85-91.
Vos, J. G. 1977. Immune suppression as related to toxicology. CRC Crit. Rev. Toxicol. 5:67-101.
Vos, J. G. 1980. Immunotoxicity assessment: Screening and function studies. Arch. Appl. Toxicol. Suppl. 4:95-108.
Voss, G., and Sachsse, K. 1970. Red cell and plasma cholinesterase activities in microsamples of human and animal blood determined simultaneously by a modified acethythiocholine/DNTB procedure. Toxicol. Appl. Pharmacol. 16:764-772.
Weeks, B. A., Anderson, D. P., DuFour, A. P., Fairbrother, A., Goven, A. J., Lahvis, G. P., and Peters, G. 1992. Immunological biomarkers to assess environmental stress. In Biomarkers: Biochemical, physiological, and histological markers of anthropogenic stress, eds. R. J Huggett, R. A. Kimerle, P. M. Mehrie, and H. L. Bergman, pp. 211-234. Chelsea, MI: Lewis Publishers.
Weil, C. S. 1972. Statisticx versus safety factors and scientific judgement in the evaluation of safety for man. Toxicol. Appl. Pharmacol. 21:454-463.

Weiss, C. M. 1965. Use of fish to detect organic insecticides in water. *J. Water Pollut. Control Fed.* 37:647–658.

Welch, W. J. 1990. The mammalian stress response: Cell physiology and biochemistry of stress proteins. In *The role of the stress response in biology and disease*, eds. R. Moromoto, A. Tissieres, and C. Georgopoulos. Cold Spring Harbor, NY: Cold Springs Harbor Laboratory.

Welch, W. J., Mizzen, L. A., and Arrigo, A. P. 1989. Structure and function of mammalian stress proteins. In *Proteins*, cds. M. L. Pardue, J. R. Feramusco, and S. Lindquist, pp. 187–206. New York: Alan R. Liss.

Wilkinson, J. H. 1970. Clinical application of isoenzymes. Clin. Chem. 16:733–739.

World Health Organization (WHO) 1982. *Field surveys of exposure to pesticides, standard protocol VBC/82.1*. Geneva: Author.

Wroblewski, F., and LaDue, J. S. 1956. Glutamic pyruvic transaminase in cardiac and hepatic disease. P.S.E.B.M. 91:569–571.

Yang, R. S. H. 1994. Introduction to the toxicology of chemical mixtures, In *Toxicology of chemical mixtures: Case studies, mechanisms, and novel approaches*, ed. R. S. H. Yang, p. 1. San Diego, CA: Academic Press.

INDEX

Acid gases, 167
Air pollutants, 1, 163, 167, 267
Allowable daily intake (ADI), 65
American Conference of Governmental Industrial Hygienists (ACGIH), 4, 235
Animal studies, 96, 97, 99, 100, 101, 102, 194
Antagonism, 5
Arsenic, 211
Arsenobetaine, 211

Behavioral performance, 66, 79
Benchmark dose, 108
Benchmark dose approach, 138
Beta curve, 95
Bioavailability, 20
Biomarkers, 274
Body surface area, 115
Bosnia, 169
Bright lines, 266
Bromodeoxyuridine, 102

Cadmium, 97
Cancer risk, 9, 169,187
Carcinogenicity, 12, 19, 21, 47, 199, 200, 212, 227, 229, 251
Chemical mixtures, 266, 297
Chloracne, 12
Cholinergic supersensitivity, 85
Citrus thrips, 101
Clean Air Act, 1, 261, 267
Confused flour beetle, 101
Copper, 97
Cost-benefit analysis, 148
Cotton stainer, 99
Covariates, 66
Cross-species extrapolation, 112
Cytochrome P450, 281

Daphnids, 96
Data analysis, 148
DDT, 100
Decision support software (DDS), 50, 147, 149

Delaney Amendment, viii, 2, 223
Dermal absorption, 165
Di-(2-ethyl-hexyl) phthalate, 109
Dicofol, 101, 102
Dieldrin, 101
Diisopropylfluorophosphate (DFP), 78
Dimethylarsenic, 211
Dinocap, 102
Dioxins, 187
Diphenylhydantoin, 102
Dose response, 2, 19, 203, 205, 217, 274, 294
Drinking water advisory, 206
Drinking water standard, 216

Economic analysis, 267
Egyptian cotton leafworm, 100
Environmental exposure, 164
Environmental justice, 220
Environmental Protection Agency (EPA), 1, 9, 20, 23, 27, 51, 53, 175, 188, 193, 214, 218, 227, 267, 270
Epigenetic, 14
Esfenvalerate, 101
Ethanol, 67
Exposure assessment, 8, 175, 185, 217, 266, 273, 288

Fate and transport, 184, 187
Fathead minnow, 96
Food and Drug Administration, 4, 252, 267, 270
Food Drug and Cosmetic Act, viii, 223
Formaldehyde, 192, 201, 202
Formetanate, 101
Fraction-of-diet, 115
Furans, 187

GA, 187
Gasoline, 191
GB, 187
GD, 187
Geographic Information Systems (GIS), 168

Genotoxic, 14, 47
Green peach aphid, 99
Gulf War Syndrome, 47, 71, 72, 78

Harmonization, 21, 271
Hazard characterization, 203
Hazard evaluation, 3
Hazard identification, 8, 217, 273
Hazard index, 9, 185
HD (mustard), 187
Health risk assessment, 183, 223, 274
Health risk management, 262
Heavy metals, 96, 167
Hormesis, 95, 98, 284, 298
Human equivalent dose, 193, 199
Human studies, 194
Hydra, 97
Hydrochloric acid, 186
Hypothermia, 80

Immune system disorders, 72, 293
Immunotoxins, 47
Ingestion, 165
Inhalation, 165, 186, 1998
Initiators, 14
Intelligence quotient (IQ), 66, 67, 68, 69

Kidney toxicity, 195, 199, 200
K-hit model, 127

Lead, 67, 97
Lewisite, 187
Logit, 131
Log-probit model, 132
Low dose, 95, 230
Lowest-observed-adverse-effect-level (LOAEL), 195, 196

Malathion, 101
Mantel-Bryan, 123
Margin of exposure, 197
Maximum contaminant level (MCL), 213, 227
Maximum contaminant level goal (MCLG), 213
Mercury, 188
Metallothioneins, 281
Methylene chloride, 235
Methyl tertiary butyl ether (MtBE), 191

Mice, 97
Mites, 100
Mosquito, 101
Multihit model, 127
Multiple chemical sensitivity (MCS), 47, 58, 71, 75, 80, 82, 84
Multistage model, 125
Mustard (HD), 187

National Academy of Sciences/National Research Council, 1, 16, 51, 187, 216, 219, 272
Neurotoxicant, 47, 57
Neurotoxicity, 61, 197
Noncancer effect/risk, 9, 165, 169
Nonlinear dose response, 132
No-observed-adverse-effect-level (NOAEL), 4, 48, 65, 138, 195, 196

Occupational Safety and Health Administration (OSHA), 235, 267
Oil fires, 166
One hit model, 108
Organoleptic effect, 202
Oxygenate, 191

Paint strippers, 235, 240, 244, 248, 255
Particulates, 167
PBPK, 118
Peer review, 267
Peroxisome proliferators, 226
Pesticides, 57, 75, 99
PCBs (polychlorinated biphenyls), 67
Performance, 66, 69, 70, 79
Persian Gulf War, 47, 71, 167
Pharmacokinetic model, 128
Pollutants, 167
Polychaete worms, 97
Polycyclic aromatic hydrocarbons (PAHs), 167
Post-traumatic stress disorder, 72
Potentiation, 48, 59, 60
Probit model, 122
Promoters, 14
Proposed Guidelines (carcinogenic risk assessment), 229
Pyridostigmine, 75, 76, 85

INDEX 313

QSAR (Quantitative Structure Activity Relationship), 20
Quantitation of exposure, 109

Red Book, 7, 225
Reference dose (RfD), 48, 65, 165, 294
Regulatory, 52
Relative exposure levels (RELs), 186
Remedial action analysis, 148
Reproductive toxicity, 95, 196
Risk analysis, 10, 39
Risk assessment 1, 2, 8, 24, 51, 57, 62, 66, 163, 177, 183, 212, 223, 253, 261, 271
Risk characterization, 8, 52, 165, 168, 217, 220, 274
Risk communication, 12, 16, 33, 242, 266
Risk (dose) analysis, 148
Risk management, 1, 12, 52, 261, 263, 271
Risk reduction, 51

Safe Drinking Water Act Amendment, 214, 219
Sampling, 175
Scaling, 114
Science policy, 53
Sea urchins, 97
Sensitivity, 47
Selenium, 97
Slope factor, 9, 19, 165, 187
Smoking, 67
Sodium fluoride, 101
Space Maximal Acceptable Concentration (SMAC), 70

Stress proteins, 281
Susceptibility factors, 116
Superfund, 7, 166, 187, 267
Surveillance, 175
Synergism, 5

Taiwan, 213
Target endpoint, 10
Tertiary butyl alcohol (TBA), 192, 201
Threshold Limit Value (TLV), 4, 69, 166, 185, 186
Threshholds, 108
Time-weighted average (TWA), 237
Tobacco, 67
Toluene, 69
Toxicity assessment, 8, 165
Trichlorethylene (TCE), 224

Uncertainty factors (UF), 9, 48, 65, 215, 274, 294
U-shaped curve, 95

Veterans Administration Health Registries, 175
Virtual safe dose (VSD), 110
Volatile organic compounds (VOCs), 167

Weibull, 130
Western corn rootworm, 101

Zinc, 97